# Conditioning Factors for Cardiac Necroses

EÖRS BAJUSZ

Institut de Médecine et de Chirurgie Expérimentales, Université de Montréal

With a foreword by Professor HANS SELYE, Montreal

30 figures and 35 tables

19 63

BASEL (Switzerland) S. KARGER NEW YORK

**Distributed in North America simultaneously by**
**Intercontinental Medical Book Corporation, New York, N.Y.**

Verlag S. Karger AG, Arnold-Böcklin-Strasse 25, Basel (Switzerland)

---


Printed in Switzerland by Buchdruckerei Stäfa AG, Stäfa ZH
Clichés: Steiner & Co., Basel

# Index of Contents

**Foreword by Professor Hans Selye** . . . . . . . . . . . . . . . . . . . VII

**General Introduction** . . . . . . . . . . . . . . . . . . . . . . . . . 1

PART I. REVIEW OF RELATED LITERATURE

**Conditioning governing interactions in the pathogenesis and prevention of diseases**

I. **Definitions and terminology, with a historical survey of the modern literature** . . . . . . . . . . . . . . . . . . . . . . . . 12
General-Adaptation-Syndrome. Stressor. Systemic stress. Irritation syndrome. Historical development of both concepts. Conditioning. Permissive or supportive actions. Pavlovian use of conditioning. Biologic meaning of adaptation. Necrotizing cardiopathies.

II. **The theory of conditioning and pluricausal diseases** . . . . . . . . . 22
Types of pathogens. Conditioning agent. Heterotypic conditioning. Positive and negative conditioning. Unilateral conditioning. Selective conditioning. Interrelation between pharmacologic property and conditioning action. Metacorticoid conditioning. Concept of pluricausal diseases.

III. **Experimental examples of conditioning** . . . . . . . . . . . . . . . . 31
Topical irritation arthritis. Chronic polyarthritis. Hormonal polyarthritis. Anaphylactoid inflammation. Circulatory changes. Muscular atrophy. Muscular fatigue. Muscular contractions. Focal skeletal muscle necrosis. Examples of neurohumoral conditioning.

IV. **Stress as conditioning agent: how do nonspecific adaptive reactions alter susceptibility to disease?** . . . . . . . . . . . . . . . . . . . . . 42
Stress concept. Systemic damage. Systemic defense. Resistance. Conditioning actions of stress: Walker carcinoma; tissue injuries; congenital abnormalities; anaphylactic shock; bacterial infections; scleroderma; gastric erosions; actions of hormones and drugs.

a) *Neuroendocrine relationships in adaptive reactions* . . . . . . . . . . . . . 51
Hypothalamo-hypophyseal-system: neurosecretion and neurohormones. Neurohypophysis. Adenohypophysis: corticotrophin; pituitary-adrenal-

activation; aldosterone; regulation of trophic, adaptive hormones other than ACTH.

b) *Actions of stress and corticoids at the cellular level* . . . . . . . . . . . . . 80
Distinction between corticotypic and non-corticotypic actions of stress. Actions of stress at the cellular level. Actions of corticoids at the cellular level: cell permeability; electrolyte metabolism. How stress and corticoids act at cellular level: a hypothesis.

V. **Conditioning as applied to cardiovascular pathology: stimuli influencing the resistance of the heart muscle** . . . . . . . . . . . . . . . . 92
Primary cardiotoxic agents and conditions: plasmocid; papain; cardiac glycosides; potassium deficiency. Secondary (indirectly acting) cardiotoxic agents: sulfonamides; agents influencing the onset of arteriosclerosis. Potential cardiotoxic agents: corticoids, electrolytes and stress—direct effects of corticoids upon the heart, neural pathways of stress reactions—; nicotine. Miscellaneous agents and conditions: factors that provoke cardiac changes characteristic of rheumatic fever; relationship between pancreas and cardiovascular disease.

VI. **Conclusions and outline of problems** . . . . . . . . . . . . . . . . 112

PART II. PERSONAL INVESTIGATIONS

**Conditioning factors for cardiac necroses**

I. **General methodology and glossary** . . . . . . . . . . . . . . . . 118

II. **Sensitization of the heart muscle: positive conditioning actions** . . . 125

*A. Stress, corticoids and steroids of the vitamin-D group:*
a) Sensitization with Me-Cl-COL for the induction of cardiac lesions by diverse stressor agents . . . . . . . . . . . . . . . . . . . . . . . 125
b) Interaction between steroid hormones in the production of the ESCN 135
c) Conditioning by corticoids for the production of cardiac lesions with noradrenaline . . . . . . . . . . . . . . . . . . . . . . . 141
d) Sensitization by DHT for induction of cardiac lesions by various agents 146

*B. Electrolytes and electrolyte-steroid interactions:*
a) The role of sodium in stress-induced cardiac necrosis . . . . . . . 149
b) Sensitization by DHT and calcium acetate for the induction of cardiac lesions by various agents . . . . . . . . . . . . . . . . . . . 155
c) Interactions between electrolytes, corticoids and DHT in the production of cardiovascular disease and nephrocalcinosis . . . . . . . . . . . 160

*C. Dietary deficiencies and other sensitizing factors:*
a) Sensitization by K-deficiency for the production of myocardial necrosis by various stressor agents . . . . . . . . . . . . . . . . . . 167

b) Sensitization by K- or Mg-deficiency for the production of myocardial necroses by papain . . . . . . . . . . 171
c) Influence of variations in dietary intake of chlorides upon diverse necrotizing cardiopathies . . . . . . . . . . 175
d) Sensitization by chloride deficiency to corticoid-induced cardiac necroses 187
e) The age factor in the production of various experimental cardiopathies 190

III. **Desensitization of the heart muscle: negative conditioning actions** . 197

*A. Stress, hemodynamic changes and stimuli influencing stress-induced cross-resistance:*
a) Adaptation to the cardiac necrosis-eliciting effect of stress . . . . . . 197
b) Induction of cross-resistance to cardiotoxic agents . . . . . . . . . . 204
c) Influence of blood pressure upon the production of myocardial necroses by various agents . . . . . . . . . . 210
d) Prevention of cross-resistance to cardiotoxic agents by low chloride intake . . . . . . . . . . 216

*B. Electrolytes:*
a) Prevention of stress-induced cardiac necrosis by oral administration of electrolytes . . . . . . . . . . 224
b) Prevention by $MgCl_2$ and KCl of the myocardial necroses normally produced by proteolytic enzymes . . . . . . . . . . 228
c) Effect of various chlorides upon the development of $NaClO_4$-induced cardiac lesions . . . . . . . . . . 232

*C. Dietary deficiencies and other desensitizing factors:*
a) Provocation and prevention of K-deficiency by various ions . . . . . 234
b) Effect of Na-deficiency upon necrotizing cardiopathies produced by various agents . . . . . . . . . . 239
c) Effect of pregnancy upon myocardial lesions produced by various agents 245

IV. **Development of new techniques for the induction of experimental cardiovascular disease** . . . . . . . . . . 250
a) Simple techniques for the surgical occlusion of coronary vessels in the rat and the ECG alterations so induced . . . . . . . . . . 250
b) Production of dissecting aneurysms by chronic isoproterenol treatment 271

V. **General summary and conclusions** . . . . . . . . . . 274

VI. **References** . . . . . . . . . . 292

# Acknowledgments

It is with great pleasure that I record my gratitude to Professor Dr. Hans Selye, Director of the Institut de Médecine et de Chirurgie expérimentales, Université de Montréal, for his constant advice, guidance, criticism and support given to me throughout the period of present study and investigation.

Some experiments were done in co-authorship with Doctors S. Grasso, Y. Lemire, P. Mendell, M. Nadasdi and S. Renaud, whose valuable cooperation is gratefully acknowledged.

I wish to thank the personnel of the Institut de Médecine et de Chirurgie expérimentales, Université de Montréal, for their general helpfulness during my stay in the Institute for the present work.

The investigations carried out by me and described in this thesis were made possible through Fellowships received from the Muscular Dystrophy Association of Canada (1957/58) and from the Gustavus and Louise Pfeiffer Research Foundation (1959/61) as well as through grants from The National Medical Research Council of Canada (Consol. Gr. No. 11), The Canadian Arthritis and Rheumatism Society and the National Institutes of Health, U.S. Public Health Service (Grants Nos. A-1641-C2, B-2037-C2 and H-3688-C3).

I am greatly indebted also to the following firms for their generous supplies of the compounds as indicated:

The Upjohn Company for 6α-methyl-11β-hydroxyprogesterone, 6α-methyl-11-keto-progesterone, 6α-methyl-21-fluoro-11β,17α-dihydroxy-$\Delta^{1,4}$-pregnadiene-3,20-dione, 6α-methyl-9α, 21-difluoro-11β, 17α-dihydroxy-$\Delta^{1,4}$pregnadiene-3,20-dione, 6α-methyl--21-desoxy-cortisol, 6α-methyl-9α,21-desoxy-cortisol, 6α-methyl-cortisol, 'Medrol', 9α-fluoro-cortisol, 2α-methyl-9α-chloro-cortisol;

Lederle Laboratories for $\Delta^{1}$-fluoro-16-hydroxy-cortisol, 'Triamcinolone';

The Squibb Institute for 9α-fluoro-16α-hydroxy-16α,17α-acetonide-cortisol;

Schering Corporation for estradiol, 'Progynon', methyl-testosterone, 'Oreton-M' and desoxycorticosterone acetate, 'Cortate';

The Sterling-Winthrop Research Institute for noradrenaline;

Dr. A. Wander, A.G. for dihydrotachysterol, 'Calcamin';

Parke, Davis and Company for vasopressin, 'Pitressin';

Lilly Research Laboratories for plasmocid.

Finally, I would like to thank the Editors and Publishers of the following periodicals: Acta endocrinologica, American Heart Journal, American Journal of Cardiology, American Journal of Pathology, American Journal of Physiology, Angiology, and Zeitschrift für Vitamin-, Hormon- und Fermentforschung, for granting permission to reproduce some illustrations from my original publications.

## Foreword

The concept of conditioning factors for cardiac necroses has received a great impetus through the systematic investigations of Doctor EÖRS BAJUSZ. He has explored this field for many years with considerable assiduity and originality, not only contributing numerous new observations, but also novel and stimulating interpretations of the observed facts.

The view that certain diseases are dependent upon the simultaneous presence of various factors is not a new one. Many instances of it came to light before we began to speak of "pluricausal diseases". However, the experimental investigations described in this monograph have contributed a great deal to illustrate the manifold mechanisms through which pluricausal diseases can develop and opened the way to further research, not only on experimental animals, but also in clinical medicine.

The bulk of the work before us was performed in this Institute and formed the basis of the author's Ph. D. thesis. However, many interesting additional experiments on related subjects were carried out by the author in his new position at the Department of Pathology of our University. These most recent findings are described in the form of an addendum, which brings the reader right up to date regarding the status of our knowledge concerning the role of conditioning factors upon the development of cardiac necroses.

In view of the ever increasing interest both among basic-research men and clinicians in the biochemical mechanism responsible for cardiac necroses, I believe that many readers will welcome the appearance of this carefully documented and stimulating monograph.

HANS SELYE

Université de Montréal, 1963

# General Introduction

One of the most striking memories I have of my early days at medical school is that of my bewilderment when our professor of bacteriology, A. IVANOVICS, told us that it was impossible to culture leprosy in animals and in contrast that certain bacteria that found themselves quite at home with animals could not, if inoculated into the human organism, produce the symptoms that were observable in animals. Although I did not realize it at that time, this pointed to the very potent idea that it is only rarely the case that 'disease has a single cause', but in most instances some internal and/or external factors determine the disease susceptibility of the organism. It was only ten years later that I learned of Professor SELYE's concept of *conditioning* agents as well as his experiments which in fact gave the explanation to this question which had so deeply troubled me in medical school.

As known, human type of tuberculosis bacilli do not cause tuberculosis in the rat. Administration of cortisone, of course, likewise fails to cause tuberculosis in itself; however, if both agents act simultaneously, the rat will develop fatal tuberculosis. On the other hand, it was also shown that the animal can be protected against the disease otherwise produced under these conditions, if it receives simultaneous treatment with somatotrophic hormone (STH). Thus, these experiments clearly revealed that the pathogenic factor is not only the presence of tuberculosis bacilli in the animal organism, but a pathogenic situation that includes, among other factors, a certain balance between glucocorticoids and hypophyseal hormones, such as cortisone and STH (599).

In fact, it has long been observed that variations in disease susceptibility are dependent on climate, diet, social conditions, or pregnancy and aging, that is, on environmental factors and internal conditions, which produce—as we would say it today—nonspecific effects in the organism. It was also early established that a variety of diseases react more or less favorably to such diverse means as fever therapy, balneotherapy, bloodletting, electroshock and physical exercise. Epidemiological observations, furthermore, indicated different patterns of disease not only in different societies but also in different groups within the same society. Certain ailments were observed to be more prevalent in one ethnic group or in one social class; other diseases, such as cancer, may be endemic within a society but may affect different body sites among different segments of a heterogeneous population. What are the factors underlying such differences; how do non-specific agents, e.g., muscular work, fasting and overeating, heat and cold, influence the disease susceptibility of the organism; what are the methods for studying their actions and interrelationships?

During more recent years, three concepts of SELYE helped to open this complex field for scientific enquiry; that of stress (597), that of the pluricausal diseases (628) and that of conditioning (605). Each of them will be discussed on the following pages, but here it would be appropriate simply to point out that the concept of stress and that of the pluricausal diseases holds that '*many diseases have no single cause,* no specific pathogen, but are largely due to non-specific stress and to pathogenic situations that result from inappropriate responses to such nonspecific stress'. The concept of conditioning, furthermore, tells us that 'the pathogenic actions of many agents and especially those of the hormones depend upon a variety of conditioning factors. Thus the effect of hormones as well as of other agents is always being modified by conditioning factors (the 'constitution' or 'terrain'), which are different in every individual, and indeed, in every part of the individual'. The importance of such conditioning influences is particularly striking in the regulation of stress reactions, because, in the final analysis, they are the factors that usually determine whether exposure to noxious agents will be met by a physiologic adaptation syndrome or by a 'disease of adaptation'.

With the evolution of modern medicine, effective means have been developed to control and prevent the spread of various epidemic diseases; increased medical knowledge and improved public health measures have sharply decreased infant mortality and extended the human life span. These advances in medical technology have developed and spread more rapidly than advances in our understanding of man's interrelationship with his natural and social environment. Gradually, however, it has come to be recognized that health and disease are due to multidimensional processes involving a complex of interactions between external and internal conditioning factors.

Disease is, in a sense, that alteration of living cells or tissues that jeopardizes their survival due to a changed environment. This definition introduces the idea of environmental conditioning in any concept of disease. Conditioning influences of environmental as well as internal factors are, indeed, extremely important since a phenomenon that may appear to be pathologic under one condition is not in another. When we find eight or nine million red cells per cubic millimeter in the people living on the highest plateaus of the Andes, we do not consider this pathologic because it helps them to survive in that particular environment. If we make the same observation at sea level, we certainly worry over the health of the individual. This definition of disease stresses, furthermore, as its criterion, survival, which is, of course, the basic dynamic force of any living thing. It seems to be better to define disease in terms of survival than to characterize it in terms of health, since health is also a very relative concept. Finally, this definition is a reminder that there is no function without structure; functional changes may often reveal themselves in structural abnormalities of degeneration and necrosis. We have heard so much in the past of so-called purely functional diseases, and much time has been spent in discussing this without referring to the indispensable basis for any function, which is structure.

We may say, that disease can never occur without the combination of two orders of factors converging in time and space, that is, there must be stimuli from the environment, and response from the organism. The stimuli from the environment can be classified into physical, biological, and emotional stimuli. These three classes interact with each other, and the use of the inclusive term, 'stressors', gives an inclusive, conceptual way of presenting the subject. The response of the organism is an attempt to adapt or defend itself, and as such, involves the pathways of the General-Adaptation-Syndrome. We are now becoming more aware of physical and emotional stresses that foster anxieties that are manifested in disease. Experimental observations also increasingly lend support to the hypothesis that multicausal factors are operative in the pattern of many diseases.

For example, it is evident that the final outcome of an infection depends upon the ability of the organism to mobilize its defense reactions immediately after being challenged by a bacterial invasion. Whatever direction we may progress in depth with our analysis from the onset of infection, we always meet observations showing that the success of the defense reactions of the organism depends on a number of conditioning interactions. Undoubtedly, mobilization of polymorphonuclear neutrophilic leukocytes, invested with phagocytic power, forms an important component of these defenses; increasing evidence points to the conditioning participation of the adrenals in this regard (221, 222, 239). On the other hand, it was also shown that the effect of antibiotics is also under the influence of external and internal conditioning agents (517).

Such conditioning factors underlying the disease susceptibility of the myocardium are analyzed in the present monograph and methods are described for studying their interrelationships. These investigations will show that in many instances a multiplicity of causes are needed to produce that alteration of cardiac tissue which creates its maladaptation, structural abnormalities, and even death.

For many years there has been considerable speculation and investigation concerning the possible role of stressful life situations as well as that of an altered production or metabolism of corticoid hormones in the pathogenesis of cardiac necrosis and related cardiovascular disease. The opinion of many present-day investigators is reflected in the following editorial comment of OLIVER AND BOYD (480) published in 1957 in the British Heart Journal: 'The remarkable social and economic changes of the century are undoubtedly stressful to some people. Increasing stress might favor the development of clinical coronary disease by disturbing normal endocrine balance and thus influencing both cholesterol metabolism and the coagulation and fibrinolytic systems. Similarly, long continued environmental stress might disturb the autonomic control of the coronary arteries'. One may put forward the working hypothesis that cardiac necroses and some related cardiovascular disease, in a broad aspect, may be end-products of altered reactivity of body processes in their response to changes in intrinsic and extrinsic environmental influences. Final evidence to support such notions is still lacking, but, as it will be seen during the discussions on the following pages, several clinical observations and experimental findings tend to support this view.

Stress, for the purpose of this monograph, is considered to be present when the adaptive mechanisms of the living organism are activated or strained. The results are by no means specific, and a simple analysis of pathways, through which stressor stimuli can influence the normal functions of organs or organ-systems, itself presents a complex problem. Our present knowledge on neuroendocrine relationships, on adrenocorticosteroid biogenesis and metabolism, as well as on the metabolic actions of hormones, although by no means complete, is extensive enough to make it apparent that there are numerous possible defects of physiologic processes that may result from inappropriate responses to stress.

For example, no longer may one think in the simple terms of overproduction or underproduction of corticoids, as was customary a few years ago. It is now well established that there are many corticoids, that these are formed by an orderly series of reactions whose rates are influenced by specific enzymes, that they vary considerably and even may be antagonistic in their metabolic effects, that each is metabolized in a characteristic way, that there may be simultaneous overproduction of one and underproduction of another, and that one may be metabolized at a normal rate while simultaneously another can be metabolized at an abnormal manner. All of these factors have to be considered in order to understand a given disease state and to find effective measures for prevention.

The problem is only further complicated by the fact that the variability of response to stress of the human being may be immense, varying from invention or artistic creation, on the one hand, to surrender or death on the other. Among this great variety of possible reactions to stressful circumstances are a host of alterations in visceral function, including the elements of the heart or more precisely those of the cardiovascular system as a whole. Let me illustrate, by an example, the complexity of conditioning interactions that may occur in the development of cardiopathies.

As it is known, cardiac disease is perhaps the most common immediate cause of death among diabetics. Arteriosclerosis of the cardiac vessels has been considered as an important factor which would explain the frequent occurrence of angina pectoris and myocardial infarcts, among diabetics.

Statistical studies indicate that diseases of the coronary arteries are found in about 60% of all diabetics over 50 years of age, in contrast to less than 15% in non-diabetic patients (168, 464). Numerous experimental findings and clinical observations suggest that a number of factors (diet, stressful life experiences, etc.) can condition to the onset of coronary artery disease (pp. 95–97). On the other hand, there is evidence that myocardial lesions—quite similar to those seen in potassium-deficient animals—can occur in patients with diabetic acidosis (531). In this instance, the focal necroses with round-cell infiltration may be due to hypokalemia (which often occurs in diabetic acidosis as a consequence of dehydration), or may be conditioned by an insufficient exogenous supply of potassium, by the diuretic and dilution effects of intravenous glucose and saline therapy, or by the potassium-fixing effect of insulin (613). It has been shown in animal experiments that the development of this type of cardiac lesion is greatly aggravated by the presence of Mönckeberg-sclerosis (651) as well as by exposure to various stressful conditions (639).

It is known, furthermore, that poor diabetic control decreases myocardial reserve in the heart damaged by coronary artery disease or hypertension. Such hearts may not be able to meet ordinary demands, and angina, congestive failure, or myocardial necrosis results. Insulin overdosage also can induce not only angina, but sometimes tachycardia, elevation of systolic arterial and venous pressure, increase in stroke volume as well as in cardiac output and cardiac work, arrhythmias, ST-T changes in the ECG, congestive heart failure, and myocardial infarction (143). From all these abnormalities, how many are due to a direct action of insulin, and which are nonspecific, secondary changes owing to the obvious disturbance of the hormonal balance, is not known at present. The active participation of the pituitary-adrenal axis in carbohydrate metabolism strongly suggests the second possibility. At any rate, as already mentioned, necrotizing cardiopathies are more often observed in diabetic acidosis than in hyperinsulinism. Thus, in analysing the alterations of the diabetic organism that may lead to cardiac disease, we have to look for conditioning factors that influence the onset of diabetic acidosis and ketosis.

Let me recall in this connection that, just as in the pancreatectomized animal, acidosis and ketosis develop in spontaneous diabetes mellitus, when the disturbance in carbohydrate metabolism becomes severe. Ketosis occurs mostly because of an increased fat and protein utilization; the formation of ketone bodies from fatty acids and amino acids is increased. Consequently, excessive amounts of ketone bodies appear in the blood and urine. The degree to which this occurs is determined not only by the severity of the defect in carbohydrate utilization and by the metabolic load, but also by a number of conditioning factors (e.g., adrenocortical and gonadal steroids), as shown in the following diagram:

Mechanisms of Ketogenesis

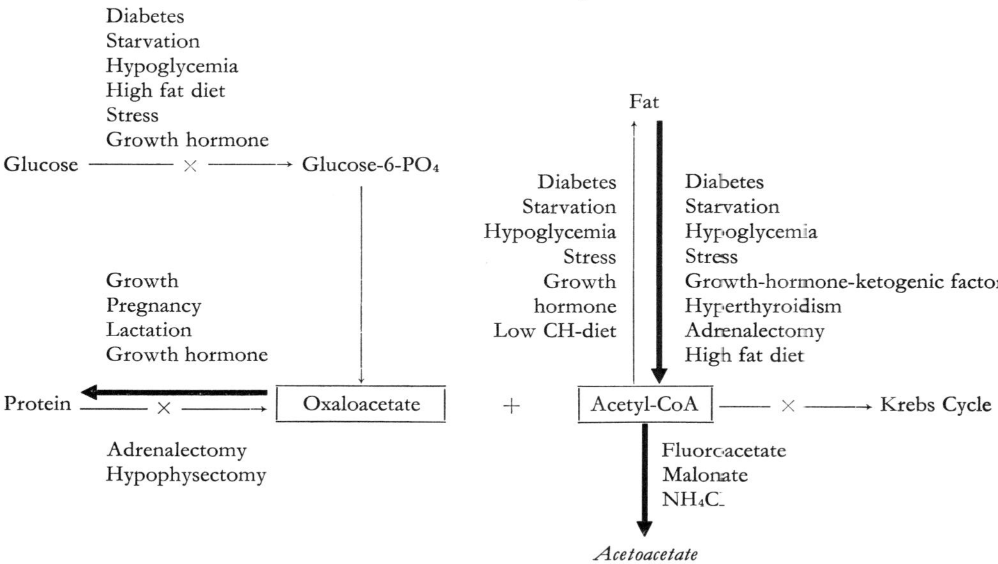


Mechanisms of Antiketogenesis

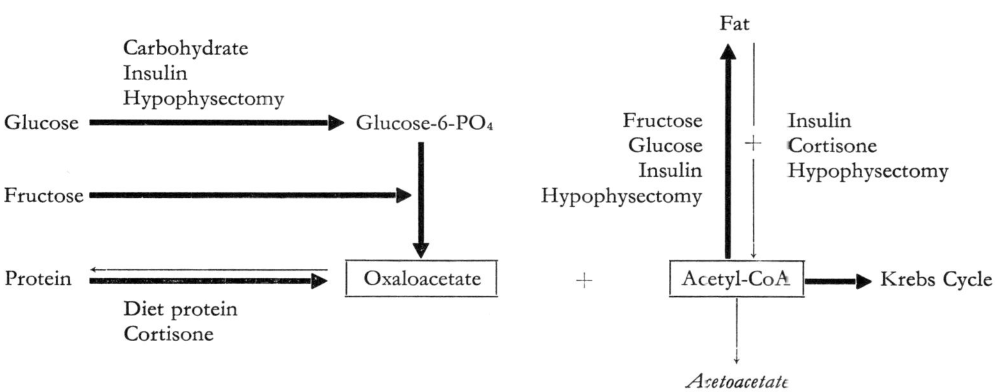


Schema of ketogenesis and prevention of ketosis, as influenced by conditioning factors

This diagram reduces the phenomenon of acidosis to its simplest term, i.e., the balance between production and utilization of acetyl-CoA by diverse pathways. Ketogenesis is presented by the situation in which there is an excess of acetyl-CoA which 'drains off' as acetoacetate. Conversely antiketogenesis follows when the metabolic pattern favors utilization of acetyl-CoA by fat synthesis and oxidation in the Krebs cycle. As indicated, a number of conditioning (nutritional and hormonal) factors can influence different steps in these biochemical processes, directly or indirectly and in diverse ways. (For the literature, upon which this diagram is based, see the references: 143, 394, 717, 726.)

On the following pages additional examples of conditioning interactions will be reviewed and described along with original observations made concerning the reactivity of the myocardium. The many new facts and problems which recently came to light during these studies on necrotizing cardiopathies clearly reveal the difficulties of such correlative research. Numerous, earlier, isolated observations, as well as in the investigations on homogeneous animal material showed that cardiac necroses can be produced by a variety of drugs, physical agents, allergens and infections. A part of this work will be discussed in the present thesis while many related data have already been summarized in two earlier monographs (613, 628).

The realization that so many, essentially dissimilar factors can produce myocardial necrosis in experimental animals, as well as the variability of the results produced by the same potentially cardiotoxic agent under different experimental conditions, made the evaluation of the findings rather difficult. However, an evaluation of the results based on the concept of 'conditioning' appears to supply at least some explanation: differences in the diet, the stressor effect of the pathogens and the stress-susceptibility of the animal may be important factors that alter the reactivity of the myocardium.

One of the most interesting results of the present investigations is the demonstration that the production of necrotizing cardiopathies by basically different means is uniformly aggravated by certain agents (i.e., corticoids, sodium salts, dietary deficiencies in potassium, magnesium and chloride, sudden stress situations, age and coronary sclerosis) and prevented by others (i.e., chlorides, dietary sodium deficiency, adaptation to stressor agents and the condition produced by pregnancy). Thus, the production of experimental cardiopathies may largely depend upon conditioning factors, that sensitize or desensitize the heart muscle to potentially cardiotoxic agents or environmental influences.

As a practical conclusion, I may say that the old art of reading symptoms and treating them by what appear to depress them best is fast disappearing in medical science. It becomes more and more clear that disease is, at least to a certain extent, a biological expression of inadequate adaptation resulting from conditioning influences. This is perhaps what should be taught to the students in medical schools, and this phenomenon against which they are going to fight all their lives cannot be understood without correlative studies in depth that should give equal importance to both the internal, as well as external conditioning stimuli, and the response of the organism. The real sense of the words that SELYE wrote as early as 1952 now becomes increasingly clear:

'In due course, a somewhat more unified concept of pathology has been established, in which the most varied manifestations of disease are considered to have a tripartite pathogenesis consisting of: 1. the direct actions of exogenous agents, 2. endogenous factors that inhibit this action, and 3. endogenous factors that facilitate this action' (601).

# PART I

## Review of related literature

## Conditioning Governing Interactions in the Pathogenesis and Prevention of Diseases

## I. Definitions and Terminology, with a Historical Survey of the Modern Literature

No physiologist ever formulated a more pregnant concept than CLAUDE BERNARD (81) when he wrote: 'All the vital processes have but one aim: to maintain the constancy of conditions required for life in our internal environment which is an essential element of our free and independent existence'. Thus, as CLAUDE BERNARD so ably put it, the organism is an entity, a whole, from which no single part can be isolated. It became then gradually clear that in this complex organism, there are systems of correlation among the different cells which influence each of them when another is the victim of an aggression. As the eminent French physiologist, LABORIT, admitted in his recent book on 'Stress and Cellular Function' (379): 'It was the success, the wide circulation and the intellectual appeal of HANS SELYE's papers that compelled us to seek a relationship between the autonomic and endocrine phenomena participating in adaptive reactions of the organism'.

The story of HANS SELYE's 'Adaptation Syndrome' started in 1936, when he discovered a new syndrome induced by the administration of certain crude ovarian extracts. This syndrome consisted of three phenomena: adrenal enlargement, thymicolymphatic involution and gastrointestinal ulcers. Initially he thought that this syndrome was due to a new hormonal factor, which consequently now was to be purified. However, it turned out that not only were purer preparations less active, but also crude extracts of other organs produced the same syndrome. Reasoning that the mere toxicity of all these impure extracts might account for this effect, he injected damaging agents like formalin which also appeared to elicit the triad of manifestations even more clearly than before.

Nevertheless, it seems that a scientific worker should always keep his mind extremely supple when considering his experimental results, especially when they are negative. It suddenly occurred to SELYE that this syndrome of response to 'damage as such' might be a general unspecific reaction to all noxious stimuli, and that any agent which acts acts upon the body may produce this unspecific syndrome (601).

From these observations developed the theory of the *General-Adaptation-Syndrome* (G-A-S). The first detailed review of this concept has been published in a book form in 1950 (597). Each following year an 'Annual Report on Stress' (677) appeared, containing new facts and amendments. A review of this concept is given on p. 43. Here we simply note that the G-A-S is the sum of all non-specific systemic defense reactions of the body which ensue upon continued exposure to stress. The term *'stressor'* or *'alarming stimulus'* denotes agents which can cause *systemic stress*. The latter may be defined as 'a state manifested by a specific syndrome which consists of all non-specifically induced changes in a biologic system' (625). Any change affecting a living organism is a stressor since it elicits some efforts to resist this change and therefore at least mild manifestations of the G-A-S. In fact, a survey of the modern literature now clearly shows that actually any stimulus can serve as a stressor, depending on the manner of its application.

The extensive work on experimental cardiopathies alone has revealed that a large number of stimuli (e.g., cold, heat, restraint, muscular exercise, drugs, trauma) all aggravate the development of cardiac necrosis in animals (613, 628). GAGNON AND FORSHAM (228), in a recent review, cite 19 stressors that invariably activated the pituitary-adrenocortical system. This list includes varieties of drug and hormone treatments, use of intense or novel stimuli, 'psychic' stressors and infectious materials. Significant is the fact that not only direct intervention (surgical, pharmacological or physical) but indirect (neurogenic and psychogenic) stimulation can induce G-A-S. MASON (420), for example, has shown that such factors as the presence or absence of persons in a room, the changes from one room to another, or the application of previously shock-associated stimuli could produce measurable stress-response. CHRISTIAN (118) has reported both laboratory and field studies in which what he calls socio-psychological stimulation of size of animal colony has affected internal hormonal events associated with the stress syndrome. The studies of PORTER *et al.* (495) suggest, furthermore, that gastric ulcer can be produced in monkeys placed under psychic stress. BASOWITZ *et al.* (64) using paratroopers, COOK AND WHERRY (129) studying submarine crews, MASON (420) with pilots, DAVIS *et al.* (147) with combat infantry-men, amongst others, have demonstrated that lifethreat and social-status-threat situations could serve as stressors. Thus, it appears from the modern literature that systemic insults (e.g., injury, injection of foreign substances, heat, cold, neuromuscular strain) and neuro- and psychogenic stimulation (e.g., anticipation of pain, uncertainty, anxiety-provoking situations or situations made noxious only as a result of prior conditioning) may both invoke patterns of stress. Depending on the length, severity and time of exposure, both may lead to adaptation or maladaptation.

Sorting out the conditions which give rise to protective effects from those which lead to disease is an extremely important current area of active research. One clear clue is the factor of timing. In this Institute as elsewhere, studies show that 'critical periods' exist for the production of stress effects as well as for the 'readiness' of the organism to adapt itself. Slow adaptation, through systematically-increased exposure to stressor agents, appears able to modify thresholds of reactivity; stimuli earlier intolerable may be experienced without inducing maladaptation.

Even before Selye made his early discoveries leading to the stress theory, another concept was born in France, which is known as the *'irritation syndrome'*. It was shown by Reilly and co-workers (516) that the typhoid endotoxin produces its well-known intestinal lesions by means of the vegetative nerve fibers. When a very small amount of typhoid endotoxin, which normally does not exert any harmful effect, was placed in contact with the splanchnic nerves, a rapid development of intestinal hemorrhages and necrotic ulcers was observed. They demonstrated, furthermore, that it is not necessary for an irritating stimulus to be in close contact with sympathetic fibers; if the stimulus is strong enough, these fibers are indirectly affected and lesions will occur unless the tissues are denervated. However, the intimate mechanism of the irritation syndrome is not yet definitely established. It is also true that this syndrome reveals only one aspect of the stress reactions.

The general impression of the *historical development of both concepts,* the stress theory and the irritation syndrome, is that they started from different random observations on either endocrine or autonomic nervous phenomena and consequently have developed to generalized theories. It is interesting to see how the research in both fundamentally different lines converged in another field, namely the central nervous system. It has become evident that the brain stem mechanisms, particularly the hypothalamic area, are the major site of stress control, while at the same time the school of REILLY was forced to consider the same structures as governing the entire stress mechanism. It should be recalled at this point that the stress concept was widely criticized saying that SELYE assigned no important role to the nervous system. This is, however, not the case and in fact he early recognized the importance of nervous pathways. He wrote in 1952 (601): 'the important investigations of RICKER, REILLY and SPERANSKI focused our attention upon the nervous system as an important link in the pathogenesis of disease in general. Our work on the adaptation syndrome re-emphasized this point showing that nervous irritation is an extraordinarily powerful stressor. Transection of the spinal cord, psychic stress, hypothalamic lesions, all tend to produce G-A-S manifestations qualitatively similar to those elicited by other agents, but of unusual intensity.... Certainly, much could be gained by a further elucidation of the manifold interrelations which exist during stress, between the two great co-ordinating systems of the body: the nervous and the humoral systems'. Most probably, the observations that adrenalectomy and hypophysectomy do not abolish the G-A-S turned interest towards higher brain structures while searching for factors regulating ACTH secretion (625).

It is often said that only facts build science. This may be true insofar that they represent the necessary building material, but it is also known that the architecture determines the usefulness of the building. It is the concept which fertilizes the scientific mind and gives the impetus to further fruitful research. SELYE is certainly right in stating that to his mind 'the most important contribution of research on stress is that it has furnished an objective, scientific basis for the development of a new approach to the treatment of disease. This is neither specific causal nor specific symptomatic therapy, but a treatment based upon the initiation and perfection of Nature's own auto-pharmacological responses' (601).

The mechanism of interaction in metabolism between corticoids and response to stress has been the subject of extensive investigations during the past 25 years. These studies have finally led to the conclusion that it is immaterial whether we say that the hormone influences (conditions) the effect of the non-hormonal stimulus, or vice versa since synergism between both factors is necessary to obtain an optimal response. This interpretation actually contains the very concept of *'conditioning'* and *'conditioning agents'*, for which the following definitions may be found in the relevant literature:

'Conditioning is a generic designation to include synergism, antagonism, potentiation, induction of reactivity where such would otherwise not exist and qualitative changes in reactivity.'

'Conditioning factors are substances or circumstances which influence response to an agent, for instance, a hormone. In other words, conditioning factors have little or no pathologic activity but can significantly alter the response to a stimulus.'

It has long been known that biologic reactions depend not only upon the nature of the evocative stimulus, but also upon other factors (e.g., age, diet, pregnancy or disease) that condition reactivity. Such interactions may take many forms, variously described in pharmacology as sensitization, desensitization, summation, potentiation, synergism, antagonism, blockade or reversal of effect, etc. As a generic term for all these types of interactions, the designation 'biochemical conditioning' has been suggested.

In 1936, Selye and Collip (671) performed certain experiments that called their attention to the importance of conditioning effects exerted by internal secretions: hormones proved to enable various stimuli to produce reactions that would not occur unconditionally, that is, without the aid of a hormonal sensitization. More precisely it was observed that large doses of oestrone cause hypertrophy of the adrenal cortex and of the corpora lutea, and full development of the mammary gland in normal rats, while none of these effects were obtained after the pituitary had been removed. In hypophysectomized rats treated with anterior pituitary extracts (in order to prevent the endocrine glands from atrophying), such oestrone treatment remained without effect on the adrenal cortex or the mammary gland, but did cause ovarian enlargment. It was shown, furthermore, that stressors such as formaldehyde, which caused marked adrenal hypertrophy in the normal, but not in the hypophysectomized animal, remained without effect, even if the adrenal cortex was prevented from undergoing atrophy by the administration of pituitary extract. From these findings a general law, regulating hormone actions, was deduced in the following terms: 'the fact that a certain stimulus is active in the presence, but inactive in the absence of the pituitary does not necessarily prove that it acts by way of stimulating the output of a certain pituitary principle. It is equally possible that stimuli, usually influencing a pituitary-controlled tissue, are inactive after hypophysectomy only because of the atrophy of the tissue on which they should act. Thus, for instance, it is theoretically possible that estrin may be unable to act on the atrophic gonad and adrenal cortex of a hypophysectomized animal, simply because the atrophic tissue is no longer able to respond. Similar considerations may be extended to the action of any stimulus affecting an endocrine-controlled tissue. Such stimuli may induce the endocrine to produce more hormones, or they may act directly upon the tissue, but only if this tissue is maintained in a responsive condition by the simultaneous hormonal stimulus, received from the endocrine in question' (671). It was possible to establish with the experimental arrangements outlined above whether the stimuli, the effects of which depend upon the integrity of the pituitary, act through one or other of the possible pathways. Thus, it has become clear that: 1. the effect of stressors (e.g., formaldehyde) on the adrenal appears to be an indirect one due to pituitary stimulation, and 2. estrin, besides its pituitary stimulating action, has a direct effect on the ovary, while it has no direct action upon the adrenal or the mammary gland.

As will be shown later in this monograph, these considerations apply to any physiologic response, and are by no means limited to hormone actions.

Experimental observations showed that the interaction between potentially pathogenic stimuli (e.g., stressors) and adaptive hormones may become the chief mediators in many pathologic conditions. For example, traumatic shock produces hyperglycemia in the intact, but hypoglycemia in the adrenalectomized rat (672). If an adrenalectomized rat is maintained on threshold doses of adrenocortical extracts (which in themselves cause no hyperglycemia), it can again respond to surgical shock normally, that is by marked rise in blood sugar. Apparently the stress of traumatic injury does not merely raise the blood sugar through excessive production of glucocorticoids, nor do the glucocorticoids exert their maximal hyperglycemic action by themselves. We may conclude that the metabolic changes incident to stress produce favorable conditions for the manifestation of the hyperglycemic effect of the glucocorticoids. Thus, neither the glucocorticoids nor the trauma can be considered as the cause of the response, but the interaction between these agents make conditions suitable to altered or normal response.

A rather similar concept has been developed by INGLE (320, 321) who refers to this type of effect as a *'permissive' or 'supportive' action.* According to this concept, the hormones play only a supporting role in the reactions to stress (e.g., trauma). In these terms the corticoids make conditions suitable for a normal response to trauma and as such presumably are tending to subserve homeostasis. The role of hormones in the etiology of diseases would then be considered as secondary (permissive) to other factors (179). There are certain differences in the basic ideas of these two concepts; this latter serves also as a useful working hypothesis for the elucidation of the role of hormonal-nonhormonal interactions in various pathologic processes such as peptic ulcer, hypertension, inflammation, etc. INGLE (320) admits the great value of the theory of conditioning saying: 'My views are not incompatible with the concepts of SELYE, who also assumes that adjustments in adrenal cortical functions normally support homeostasis. It cannot be denied that homeostatic mechanism can break down and that aging, disease, and death can be defined in these terms'. It is perhaps most important that it was demonstrated by both groups of workers that during severe stress, the adrenals can secrete damaging amounts of hormones. For example, when diabetes is produced by pancreatectomy, exposure to stress will suddenly kill such animals with signs of hypoglycemic shock. When the diabetic animal is adrenalectomized, the diabetes disappears. The primary cause of pancreatic diabetes is, of course, lack of insulin, but the conditioning action of corticoids is essential for its manifestation. It is peculiar, yet true, that corticoid hormones must be present to manifest certain diseases.

It should be recalled that according to the concept of conditioning this term refers to the sensitizing and desensitizing effect of pre-exposure or simultaneous exposure to stress or to adaptive hormones on a particular organ or system. Thus, the term 'conditioning' as used in this monograph should not be confused with its *Pavlovian use*. However, some recent neuroendocrine studies clearly revealed that even specific, neural reflex-mechanisms may be conditioned by humoral factors, and vice versa, endocrine functions may be basically altered by purely nervous mechanisms.

As is well known, PAVLOV (487) introduced the term 'conditioning' to describe the effects of pairing a neutral stimulus with one capable of eliciting a given response. Under appropriate conditions, a series of such pairings would lead to eliciting the response by the previously neutral stimulus alone. 'Conditional' reflexes (often mistranslated into English as 'conditioned' reflexes), or conditional responses are developed always through the repetitive pairing of two classes of stimuli: 1. unconditional stimuli which evoke innate or firmly established reflexes which are relatively stable and permanent; and 2. conditional stimuli which are ineffective prior to reinforcement in evoking the effects of unconditional stimuli. The response produced by the unconditional stimulus is termed an unconditional response, and the response acquired as a result of pairing a conditional stimulus with an unconditional stimulus and ultimately produced in full or in part by the conditional stimulus alone is designated a conditional response. PAVLOV (487) showed, for example, that the nature of the sensory stimulus, viz. whether auditory, visual, tactile or olfactory, determines the amplitude of the salivary conditional reflex.

Extensive research has revealed, furthermore, that conditioning is possible not only of motor and exocrine reactions, but for endocrine and visceral responses as well. BYKOV (99) summarized a vast Russian literature showing the conditionability of a variety of visceral processes through the use of both exteroceptive and interoceptive stimuli. Thus conditioned diuresis was established to a particular room, to a distinct stimulus (e.g., horn), to injection of water into the stomach; inhibition of this response was likewise able to be controlled as a result of the systemic pairing of stimuli. Heart and vascular conditioning, splenic conditioning, respiratory conditioning and conditioning of HCl-secretion by the stomach have all been demonstrated in response not only to stimulation via the exteroceptive sensory pathways, but in response to physiologically neutral solutions after pairing with hormones, such as thyroxine. Further, it has been shown that both chemical and neural stimulation of internal organs can serve as conditional as well as conditioned-stimuli to overt responses which are induced through separate means. Finally, a complex system of interrelations has been demonstrated between chemical (i.e., hormonal and metabolic) and neural receptor and response systems—interrelationships which may be modified by experimental conditioning.

It is reasonable to assume from the observations just outlined that neuroendocrine reflex mechanisms actively participate in physiologic reactions governing the adaptive processes of the organism in its constantly changing environment. Consequently, we have arrived at the point where a survey of the modern literature will be useful concerning the *biologic meaning of adaptation.*

If one goes back to the classical writings of some of the great authors, such as DARWIN, one will often find information shadowed and outlined, general truths that hold up later and which are very useful to the experimenter. In DARWIN's work on the emotional expressions, one now sees many instances of sudden changes which were discovered by general observational methods, but which would certainly fall into the category of defense or adaptation mechanisms. Later, as experimental medicine developed, several early investigators have attempted to elucidate the mechanisms of adaptive phenomena. RICKER, SPERANSKY, REILLY, HOFF and many others have gathered important data concerning the role of the nervous system in such non-specific defense reactions as fever, polymorphonuclear leukocytosis, inflammation, etc. (516, 719). In the domain of what is called 'physiologic stress' W. CANNON's studies helped us to understand the part played by the sympathetic nervous system and its humoral effector substances (104, 105). CLAUDE BERNARD focused our attention on the importance of balanced states within the 'milieu interior' of the organism (81) and HANS SELYE offered a powerful unifying theory in his concept of systemic stress and the processes of adaptation (597).

I started my discussion with DARWIN because the term adaptation now is also being employed widely among proponents of evolution, especially in relationship to cultural change and cultural evolution. For example, according to STEWARD (729) 'the concept of environmental adaptation underlies all cultural ecology'. According to SIMPSON (703), 'adaptation is intimately involved in almost all evolutionary processes'. For MURDOCK (461), 'the net effect of the various processes of cultural change is to adapt the collective habits of human societies progressively over time to the changing conditions of existence'. BEALS AND HOIJER (67) lean heavily on the proposition that 'life itself is an adaptive mechanism', while HONIGMANN (310) wrote 'adaptation, adjustment and stress are emergency functions of the living organism' and 'the stress theory is broad enough to include all other concepts'. GOLDSCHMIDT (235) has recently given great prominence to such terms as 'fitness' and 'adjustment', which he seems to equate with 'adaptive changes' and 'adaptive patterns'.

In general, while the anthropologists usually supply a definition of adaptation, no definitions are commonly attempted by biologists, apparently because it is felt that the prominence of the concept in biology makes its meaning self-evident. The authors of a recent and representative biology textbook, however, analyze the problems of adaptation and, after stressing the difficulties biologists experience with this concept, they supply the following definition: 'An adaptation is an aspect of the organism that promotes its general welfare and survival, or the welfare and survival of the species to which it belongs in the environment it usually inhabits' (704).

It is clear that, as defined above and as used in biologic science, the concept of adaptation must be distinguished from the concept of stress: the latter was advanced for studying the regulation of the body's adaptive or defense mechanisms that are suddenly mobilized by environmental influences. The most significant aspect of the stress concept is, furthermore, the fact that initially adaptive reactions may themselves become harmful. Analyzing this dual capacity of stress reactions continues to be one of the most fascinating characteristics of modern stress research.

Recent investigations of the physiopathology of stress resulted in a better insight into the complex relationship between electrolytes, steroids and stress, which plays a fundamental role in the pathogenesis of certain *necrotizing cardiopathies*. The term cardiac necrosis, or necrotizing cardiopathy will be used in general to denote focal necroses of cardiac muscle that, unlike the true cardiac infarcts, are not due to acute vascular obstruction, but presumably to biochemical changes in the myocardium.

It has been well known for half a century that focal myocardial necroses, followed by inflammation, can occur in man, either as an apparently separate disease (FIEDLER's myocarditis) or as a part of systemic infections (192, 724). A review of the literature has shown, furthermore, that cardiac glycosides (396), vitamin-D derivatives (578) adrenaline (182, 194), forced muscular exercise (97), potassium and magnesium deficiencies (566), electrolyte-corticoid interactions (615)—i.e., a number of apparently quite unrelated agents—can elicit essentially similar lesions in the myocardium of experimental animals. The first effort at presenting a synoptic view of this field was made by SELYE a few years ago in a monograph on 'The Chemical Prevention of Cardiac Necroses' (613). As the work along these lines progressed it has been pointed out that necrotizing cardiopathies are usually caused by complex pathogenic situations and not by any one specific pathogen. Subsequently, by applying the concept of pluricausal disease, the name 'pluricausal cardiopathies' has been suggested (628). It has become obvious during these investigations that, in animals, a great variety of cardiac lesions (e.g., hyalinization, necrosis, calcification, acute inflammation or fibrosis, and various types of coronary sclerosis) can be produced, if two or more agents are applied in the proper amounts and sequence.

The recognition of the pluricausality of certain necrotizing cardiopathies makes it tempting to apply the concept of stress and that of conditioning, in order to see whether there are conditioning factors capable of selectively sensitizing or desensitizing the heart to the effect of various agents known to be potentially cardiotoxic. The main task of the present monograph is to clarify some of the problems which have so arisen.

## II. The Theory of Conditioning and Pluricausal Diseases

In order to understand the part played by conditioning interactions in the pathogenesis of pluricausal disease we must learn to distinguish between three *types of pathogens:*

1. directly acting stimuli, primary pathogens;
2. indirectly acting stimuli, secondary pathogens;
3. conditionally acting stimuli, potentially pathogenic agents.

The first type invariably produces disease under any circumstances. Thus, these are stimuli that act upon their targets directly and their effects do not depend upon the given condition of the organism. For example, a complete occlusion of all renal vessels results in necrosis of the kidney, or long-acting, intensive cold produces permanent alterations in the affected area. In general, such stimuli affect the receptive cells, even in vitro, since the immediate response they elicit is independent of the rest of the body.

Indirectly acting stimuli are those that exert some actions on a certain organ or organ-system, but the pathologic manifestations observed are only secondary consequences of a primarily altered function. Agents exhibiting specific blocking or activating properties on some basically important physiologic mechanism (e.g., gastric secretion, hypothalamic regulating centers) may belong in this category. Thus, these secondary pathogens in themselves do not affect the target organ at all. They act upon another organ or pathway and induce it to produce pathologic alterations in the target-organ. The hypophyseal trophic hormones may also be cited as examples of such indirectly acting stimuli whose mediated pathogenic effects depend, in some instances, entirely upon the reactivity of endocrine end-organs (e.g., gonads, thyroid, adrenal cortex).

Conditionally acting stimuli produce disease only under special circumstances. They may be directly or indirectly acting agents, yet depending upon the circumstances, the receptive cells may or may not respond. But while the former are obligatory, the conditionally acting stimuli are potential, pathogens. For example, desoxycorticosterone (DOC) causes nephrosclerosis, but only if the diet of the experimental animals contains sufficient amounts of sodium chloride. To some extent of course, the action of all stimuli depend upon the condition of the target-cells. In some instances, however, the target is almost always optimally sensitive to the potentially pathogenic agents, while, in others, the response is greatly influenced by activating or inactivating agents. These modifying agents may themselves be directly, indirectly or conditionally acting stimuli. Thus, there are many possible gradations between these three classes of stimuli and their interactions may result in diverse pathologic conditions.

Humoral and nervous mechanisms help to adjust the activity of different organ systems to changing conditions in the organism or its surroundings. In the humoral mechanism, hormones play a particularly important role. During the last 25 years, subsequent to the formulation of the stress concept, it has been amply demonstrated, that, in response to a variety of stressors (trauma, infections, intoxications, nervous stimuli, etc.), the body reacts in a rather stereotyped manner by secreting certain hormones, such as ACTH, and corticoids. The resulting excess in these 'adaptive hormones' furnishes essentially useful defense reactions. On the other hand, in certain circumstances a similar excess of the 'adaptive hormones' can become the cause of disease, or, at least, can condition the body to the production of morbid changes. For example, the excessive secretion of ACTH and of anti-inflammatory corticoids is useful because it helps the organism to survive during an emergency and because it suppresses excessive inflammatory reactions; but at the same time, it can also be harmful, in that it may enhance the spread of infections, or condition to the production of peptic ulcer (for lit. see: 597). Interestingly, hormones (especially the corticoids) actively participate in the pathogenesis of several maladies, but they do not actually elicit them.

Consequently, one may think that the *conditioning agent* could be defined as one that is inert in itself but prepares the target organ for the actions of another agent, which later would be the primary pathogen. Experience has shown that this definition is not always applicable (605). The following examples may serve to illustrate this.

Experiments dealing with the pathogenesis of cardiac necroses showed that combined treatment with corticoids (e.g., fluorocortisol) and a number of Na-salts (e. g., $NaHCO_3$, NaCl, Na-citrate, -glutamate,

-succinate) predisposes the cardiac muscle for necrotizing changes elicited by stressor agents (42, 638). Here, neither the Na-salts nor the corticoids, alone or in combination produce, in themselves, any histologically detectable cardiac damage. Undoubtedly, the subsequent exposure to stress is responsible for the induction of cardiac necrosis. Thus, both the corticoid and the Na-salts are conditioning agents in the sense of the original definition, while stress can be considered as the pathogen. Still, sometimes a sharp distinction between the conditioning and conditioned agent (i.e., primary pathogen) is not possible. For example, the concurrent administration of the same corticoid (fluoro-cortisol) with a number of other Na-salts (especially, phosphates, sulfates, sulfites and perchlorate), without subsequent exposure to stressor agents has been found to produce the ESCN (Electrolyte-Steroid-Cardiopathy with Necrosis). But, here again, neither the steroid hormone nor the Na-salt produces similar changes when given alone (613). In this case, we cannot actually indentify the conditioned factor; hence, only the combination is active in the production of the cardiac disease. In such instances of sensitization it is immaterial whether we say that agent A (e.g., corticoid) conditions for the actions of agent B (e.g., Na-salt) or vice versa. Thus, a singular type of conditioning is encountered when concurrent treatment with a hormone and a non-hormonal stimulus produces an effect that cannot be duplicated by either agent alone, irrespective of dosage. This type of interaction is usually designated (625) as *heterotypic conditioning,* because its result is the synthesis of a new biologic reaction type. However, as it was demonstrated above, conditioning is sometimes truly unilateral in that agent A or the condition produced by A + B (e.g., corticoid + Na-salt) decisively influences the production of a certain reaction with agent C, a primary pathogen (e.g., stress). It is interesting to note here that, in both examples enumerated, the appearance of the histologically detectable changes of the myocardium are identical: 1. the accumulation of a strongly fuchsinophilic material, which eventually displaces all other elements within the cardiac muscle fibers and results in 2. infarctoid foci consisting of massive, necrotic patches in which the fibers are gradually absorbed and replaced, first by histiocytes, later by connective tissue. This consideration actually indicates that apparently different conditioning interactions can result in the development of essentially the same disease.

Experimental observations suggested, furthermore, that it is useful to distinguish between *positive and negative conditioning* actions, on the basis of successful production, aggravation, or prevention of pathologic manifestations.

The effect of glucocorticoids upon thymus involution is a positive conditioning action. In adrenalectomized rats, neither a stressor (e.g., trauma) nor a subthreshold amount of a glucocorticoid (e.g., cortisol) causes thymus involution, but if the trauma is applied subsequent to treatment with doses in themselves ineffective of cortisol, pronounced thymolysis occurs (557a). In other words, the corticoid can create conditions favorable for the induction of thymolysis by a stressor.

The antiphlogistic effect of glucocorticoids furnishes an example of negative conditioning. Here, the hormone does not support or permit the effect of the phlogogenic irritant; on the contrary, it actually prevents it. In rats, the injection of croton oil into a subcutaneous air-sac ('granuloma-pouch', technique), or of formalin into the paw ('topical arthritis' test), induces marked inflammation under ordinary conditions, but this effect can be supressed by doses of ACTH or of antiphlogistic corticoids (e.g., cortisol), which under similar circumstances produce no striking effect upon non-irritated connective tissue (594, 595).

However, when agent A (e.g., cortisol) itself does not exhibit a certain action (e.g., inflammation) but merely influences this effect of another agent B (e.g., formalin), we may speak of *unilateral conditioning*. Positive conditioning (or sensitization) of this sort has already been discussed, e.g., the decrease of heart's resistance to stress following corticoid + electrolyte pretreatment. Thus, here agents A — B prepare the target organ to the necrotizing action of agent C (e.g., stress), although A + B themselves are completely devoid of the ability to produce such a reaction. Unilateral negative conditioning (or deconditioning) is, to a certain extent, the inhibition of inflammation by antiphlogistic corticoids as well as the prevention of osteolathyrism by cortisol or thyroxin, which will be discussed in detail later (611). It should be noted, however, that in order to appraise such interactions completely, all the characteristic effects of both agents have to be analyzed.

In such analysis we must ask ourselves, for example, not only to what extent an anti-inflammatory hormone influences the effect of inflammatory irritants, but also to what extent agents that cause inflammation affect the action of the corticoid. If we do this, we shall find that, here again, the actions of both agents are often mutually affected as a result of their concurrent application to the same organism.

However, it is true that in some instances the type of the resulting response is predominantly that of the one or the other agent. For example, the production of a minute cutaneous inflammatory focus by a topical irritant can be totally prevented (negatively conditioned) by systemic treatment with cortisol, but such an inflammation exerts no detectable effect on the systemic actions (catabolism, thymolysis, etc.) of the corticoid. On the other hand, a severe inflammation, such as generalized peritonitis, is not only conditioned by, but in its turn conditions for, such systemic corticoid actions. Still, in such cases it may be argued that the distinction is based merely on quantitative differences (597).

Another interesting example of unilateral conditioning by a hormone was discovered in the course of the studies of Selye *et al.* (612, 669, 670, 695), on osteolathyrism. The skeletal lesions of osteolathyrism induced in rats by lathyrogens (e.g., Lathyrus odoratus seeds or aminoacetonitrile, AAN) can be prevented by certain hormones (cortisol and thyroxin) and greatly aggravated by others (STH and prolactin). Thus, in rats receiving subthreshold amounts of AAN, severe, crippling skeletal deformities are induced by concurrent treatment with minute amounts of STH. This effect of STH is truly unilateral, because, in themselves, even the highest tolerable doses of growth hormone fail to induce any changes resembling lathyrism. Here, it is particularly evident that the hormone conditions for the action of the non-hormonal agent and not vice versa, since concurrent treatment with AAN not only fails to enhance the typical growth effects of STH but actually abolishes them, presumably owing to the destructive lesions in the growth cartilage plates and to the general antianabolic effect of severe lathyrism.

The term *selective conditioning* was introduced earlier (625) on the basis of observations showing that in many cases the conditioning agent affects one particular action of another stimulus with great selectivity. As an example, let me quote the finding that desoxycorticosterone (DOC) predisposes the rat for the production of nephrocalcinosis by $Na_2HPO_4$, but does not significantly alter other effects of this salt (e.g., its ability to produce phosphate tetany). Similarly DOC sensitizes the animals for the production of aortal aneurysms by lathyrogenic compounds (such as AAN), but it does not inhibit the characteristic effect of these drugs upon the skeleton. By combined treatment with cortisol and DOC, it has even been possible to reverse the normal morphologic syndrome of experimental osteolathyrism; this corticoid combination caused lathyrogens to produce aortal aneurysms in the virtual absence of bone lesions, and that, under conditions in which bone lesions would normally have occurred in the absence of aortal aneurysms. Furthermore, it has been possible to induce a predisposition for giant callus formation at the site of bone fractures, by pretreatment with lathyrogens in the rat (611).

At this point it is important to note that any knowledge concerning *interrelation between pharmacologic properties and conditioning actions* of agents (e.g., corticoids) is of great practical value, since it is sometimes possible to selectively increase or abolish specific actions and consequently modify or depress conditioning influences. However, pharmacologic interactions and conditioning interactions are two basically different problems.

By pharmacologic interaction we understand that two independent actions can have the property of influencing each other. When two compounds are given together and the combined effect is stronger than could be predicted from the effect of each separate compound, the pharmacologists speak of a potentiation of the effect. It is generally accepted that a simple synergism of the effects of two compounds is an indication that the two compounds have the same site of action in the organism. An antagonism between the effects might also suggest that the two compounds have the same site of action and that, for example, a depressing action of one component in suitable doses counteracts a stimulating effect of the other.

If the conditions were as simple as that, the study of the synergistic, potentiating, and antagonistic effects of stimuli (for example, that of potentially cardiotoxic agents) would give many important clues to the understanding of the pathogenesis of disease. However, in the extremely complicated organ-systems, such as the endocrine, nervous and circulatory systems, it is not even possible to conclude that two agents have the same or different site of action when they potentiate each other's pathogenic effects. If, for example, two compounds given in combination exert inhibitory effect on the normal cardiac functions, they are 'cardioactive' compounds, but beyond that no conclusions can be drawn. It is not possible to conclude that, because two compounds or stimuli applied in combination exert a depressive effect, they are both depressant. One might have a depressing effect of one nerve center, and the other a stimulating effect of another nerve center, the normal function of which it is to inhibit the first nerve center; or they might be both depressants, one depressing an inhibiting center, but they might be both stimulants, one of them stimulating an inhibiting center. Although such considerations are obvious, they must be kept in mind when attempting to explain some of the apparent paradoxes in the mutual effects of conditioning interactions.

This short theoretical discussion clearly reveals that an analysis of compounds from a purely pharmacological point of view is a different problem than the study of conditioning actions in a given pathogenic situation. People are not all exposed to the same conditioning factors; also, the reactions caused by the latter may vary with the individual. In experiments on animals, more objective tests can be applied in order to study a possible negative or positive conditioning interaction. Yet, even here it may be difficult enough to evaluate the effect. Furthermore, it is necessary to use large doses of various compounds as well as strong acting stimuli in animals in order to get constant and measurable effect. With such doses or agents, the effects may be somewhat qualitatively altered and certain fundamental mechanisms be completely hidden from observation. Therefore, any theoretical conclusion drawn from such experiments must be treated with reservation.

Another important point is that diseases resulting from conditioning interactions do not necessarily become manifest during the action of sensitizing agents (e.g., during exposure to stress). This is clearly demonstrated by the observation that temporary overdosage with DOC can initiate a self-sustaining hypertension that eventually leads to death, long after hormone administration has been discontinued (220, 248, 546). This type of interaction has been called *metacorticoid conditioning,* thereby emphasizing that it continues beyond the period of hormone administration. These experiments provided additional evidence that absolute or relative hypercorticoidism represents a common pathway through which various agents can produce pathologic change (e.g., hypertensive disease). In fact, recently GREEN (247) and STURTEVANT (732)—reviewing the similarities and differences between human and experimental hypertension—concluded that essential hypertension is simulated most closely, in both its physiologic and anatomic characteristics, by the post-DOC, or metacorticoid syndrome. It seems reasonable to view all forms of experimental hypertension (the neurogenic, renal, renoprival and hormonal) as the result of interventions at different segments of a common, highly integrated, homeostatic mechanism which, as a unit, is fundamentally involved in resistance to stress (658).

The recognition that many agents or stimuli produce pathologic manifestations only under certain circumstances resulted in the *concept of pluricausal diseases* (628). Examples of pluricausal diseases may be seen as follows: Chronic polyarthritis caused by administration of DOC in rats sensitized with high NaCl intake; muscular atrophy which results from cortisol administration in an area conditioned by circulatory deficiency; muscular cramps due to $NaClO_4$ administration in the methylchlorocortisol pretreated animals,; and the electrolyte-steroid cardiopathies that develop as a consequence of combined corticoid-electrolyte treatment. In this last mentioned case the effect of the potentially pathogenic corticoids (e.g., cortisol, fluorocortisol) is nonspecific. They produce no cardiac lesion by themselves but, by appropriate conditioning with certain electrolytes, they can produce essentially different types of cardiopathies depending primarily on the chemical characteristic of the salt administered. In other words, the same steroid can predispose the rat for the production of qualitatively dissimilar lesions, but different electrolytes are necessary to elicit one or another type of change. Thus, in such instances it is immaterial whether we say that corticoids condition for the actions of electrolytes or vice versa. The corticoids and electrolytes are both conditioning factors that when given in a combination become pathogenic and cause a typical 'pluricausal cardiopathy'.

The observations discussed here clearly show that, the manifold, interacting mechanisms governing the development of pluricausal diseases are very complex. Hence, conditioning interactions between factors that affect tissue responses cannot be predicted with any degree of reliability on theoretical grounds and must be subjected to experimental verification in each instance. Yet, great progress is being made concerning the understanding of the development of pluricausal diseases despite the intrinsic difficulties of working in these areas, where so much must be learned by inference about systems and interactions which are not directly observable in the functioning organism. In addition to this major handicap to rapid progress, there are limitations inherent in the circumstances of the different particular laboratories with regard to available means, methods and species of subjects. Thus, one laboratory studies rats exclusively, another rabbits, dogs, a third monkeys or men. One laboratory relies on electrolyte determinations in blood and tissues primarily, a second uses histologic techniques, a third purely pharmacologic tests, or clinical evaluation of subjective states. One laboratory places its animals for days in cold, a second applies electrical stimulation for minutes, a third uses naturally diseased patients in hospitals, or artificially induces 'psychic' stress in, sometimes already damaged, subjects. Generalizations from each of these situations must be carefully checked against comparable studies. Contradictory findings must be evaluated as to species used, experimental conditions applied, etc.

However, through frequent review and evaluation from different points of view, considerable progress can be made toward clarifying the multitude of problems in this field. It is not enough to obtain or collect new data from the living organism; we need to correlate them in order to understand the development of disease. Therefore, unifying concepts that are based on integration leading from analysis to synthesis seem to be extremely helpful for the experimenter.

In *summary* we may say that the concept of conditioning and of pluricausal diseases teaches us that the regulation of tissue reactivity, for instance, through corticoids, often determines whether the body succumbs to disease or resists a potential pathogen by means of adaptation. Thus, the general consequence of stress (e.g., of trauma or emotional disturbance), and particularly the effect of the adaptive hormones, largely depends upon conditioning factors, some of which are external (diet, temperature, light) others internal (heredity, constitution, previous exposure to stress, etc.). A state of stress is produced in the body through multiple pathways, its effect always being modified by the variable specific actions of the eliciting agents and by the conditioning factors that differ in every individual and, indeed, in every part of the individual. These factors can affect the various targets and pathways selectively and, thereby, vary the manifestations of what in essence is but a single stress response (601).

If we use this concept as a guide in analyzing the pathogenesis of pluricausal diseases, we must always consider both the conditioning interactions and the response of the organism. It is now evident that nonspecific adaptive reactions can act as defensive and disease-producing factors, depending upon conditioning circumstances. The pathogenicity of stimuli may depend upon nutritional factors, previous stressful experiences, age, etc. That is why it is often very difficult to decide which among the many factors is necessary for the production of disease; which is the primary pathogen, which are the conditioning factors, and which factors are useful in the prevention of disease. Usually the full pathogenic situation must be analyzed in order to understand the pluricausality of a morbid change.

It is, of course, true that the regulation of body's defense mechanism can be considered from different standpoints. Since defense is a general effort of the organism as a whole, every organ system participates in this reaction, e.g., the nervous system, endocrine system, heart and blood circulation, respiratory system, gastrointestinal system, muscular system, etc. It is possible to examine in detail one site of the pathways, or the changes in one specific organ. The conclusions so obtained are, however, very limited, since it is impossible to designate one site, one organ or one system which would be responsible for the regulation and integration of the adaptive reactions. This indicates a need for correlative approaches and suggests a growing demand for integrative research. Consequently, the individual scientist finds himself in the predicament of requiring greater and greater knowledge of the development of the whole medicine, even if his research area is only a small portion of the total spectrum of the adaptation mechanisms of the organism.

## III. Experimental Examples of Conditioning

It is important to note that although only very intense overdosage with corticoids produces manifestation of disease, even small amounts of these hormones can decisively influence the effect of certain nonhormonal pathogens. For example, the *'topical irritation arthritis'* produced by the injection of formalin or other irritants into the paw of a rat can be prevented by relatively small doses of glucocorticoids and aggravated by mineralocorticoids. Both the antiphlogistic effects of glucocorticoids and the prophlogistic actions of mineralocorticoids are more evident in the adrenalectomized than in the intact animals, presumably because, in the latter, endogenous corticoids of the opposite type can interfere with the actions of the hormones that are injected (595). Here, the specific pathogen primarily responsible for the arthritis is undoubtedly the formalin (or other irritant). Whether a given dose can actually exhibit its potential inflammatory action largely depends, though, upon the balance between mineralocorticoids and glucocorticoids, that is, upon the balance between positive and negative conditioning influences. Interestingly, according to the type of irritant utilized and the stage of development attained, the histologic picture of the topical irritation arthritis can quite closely resemble rheumatic lesions (678). In the acute stage, this is particularly evidenced by edema of the synovial membrane, hyalinization of connective tissue and exudation into the metatarsal-joint cavities, while the chronic lesions are more comparable to the rheumatoid type of arthritis, with the formation of a chondroid pannus and erosion of the articular cartilage.

As is known, one of the major distinctions between the arthritis of rheumatic fever, rheumatoid arthritis and osteoarthritis is that the first mentioned is the most acute, and the last the most chronically developing lesions. Accordingly, the arthritis of rheumatic fever is most common among the youngest age group, while osteoarthritis is most frequent in the oldest. Some experimental studies (597), however, pointed out that irritants usually cause increasingly less acute inflammatory reactions with advancing age. Even the topical irritation arthritis (as caused by the injection of formalin) more closely resembles rheumatic, rheumatoid or osteoarthritic, in young, middle-aged and senile rats respectively. Consequently the hypothesis was advanced that the underlying mechanism in all these arthritides may be essentially similar, the differences being mainly due to incidental conditioning factors. The production of the polymorph or pulmonary, osseous, cutaneous and miliary types of tuberculosis by the same agent, would be a somewhat comparable case.

When implanted into 'granuloma-pouches' (606), Murphy Rat Lymphosarcoma (MRLS) tissues cause the formation of a large amount of viscous exudate. Upon intravenous or intraperitoneal injection, this exudate tends to produce a *chronic polyarthritis* in the rat. The joint lesions are particularly severe in adrenalectomized animals maintained on DOC and can be prevented by cortisone. The polyarthritis-producing factor in the tumor exudate has not yet been identified. It is evident, however, that the adrenal cortex plays a decisive role in the development of these lesions (679). Among the pituitary hormones, STH aggravates while ACTH prevents this polyarthritis. Interestingly enough, prolonged treatment with a crude pituitary extract rich in STH itself also produces polyarthritis, especially in hypophysectomized animals (608). These joint lesions may serve as experimental models in the study of clinical problems pertaining to the action of systemic inflammatory agents on certain specific tissue area. They demonstrate once again the important conditioning role of hormonal factors in the development of non-endocrine diseases.

The *hormonal polyarthritis,* produced by overdosage of DOC in the rat, usually develops in the metatarsal or metacarpal joints. 'Aschoffnodule-like' granulomas in the heart and vascular lesions, resembling rheumatic myocarditis, were also observed in the same DOC-treated animals (674, 675, 685, 693). Unlike many other manifestations of DOC overdosage, arthritis is not definitely more pronounced or frequent in unilaterally nephrectomized than in intact rats. Furthermore, involvement of the joints is much less constant than are other lesions (e.g., cardiovascular and renal changes). Studies concerning the role of the adrenal cortex in the production of joint lesions showed that under the influence of DOC, adrenalectomized animals developed arthritis much more easily than did intact controls. Thus, it seems that some adrenal principle normally antagonizes the arthritis-producing effect of DOC. It appeared that microscopic signs—such as inflammatory infiltrations in the synovial membranes and the periarticular connective tissues—are quite regularly present in the adrenalectomized, but not in the intact, DOC-treated rats. Here, the increased DOC sensitivity was ascribed to the absence of the adrenal glucocorticoids. In experiments in which the effect of DOC and cortisone—singly or in combination—was examined in rats with arthritis, it was found that cortisone not only inhibits the development of joint lesions, but even overcomes the aggravation normally induced by DOC. It was also observed that a high glucocorticoid-mineralocorticoid quotient favors the absorption of edema and granulation tissue from the periarticular structures (693). Apparently, in the production of experimental arthritis the ratio between mineralocorticoids and glucocorticoids plays an important role.

The so-called *'anaphylactoid inflammation'* that ensues in rats, following the intraperitoneal or intravenous administration of egg-white, dextran and other macromolecular substances, is similarly influenced by corticoids as is the development of experimental arthritis (676). It was also revealed that stress does not act upon inflammatory responses to topical irritation only through an increase in corticoid production. Even in the absence of the adrenals, stress can sensitize (condition) the tissues to the antiphlogistic effect of a given amount of corticoid. Thus, even moderate amounts of endogenous corticoids can become highly effective during stress (606) Supression by these hormones of the most diverse clinical inflammatory diseases (e.g., in rheumatology, ophthalmology, and dermatology) furnished ample evidence in support of the thesis that stress can suppress inflammation through both, increased production and enhanced activity of adaptive hormones (for lit. see: 597, 677). Since inflammation is a basic mechanism of many diseases, this type of conditioning may have fundamental importance.

It is interesting to note that *circulatory changes* are extremely effective in conditioning hormonal actions. For instance, experimental interference with the circulation in a circumscribed tissue area can strikingly alter topical reactivity to irritants and to the antiphlogistic effect of cortisol. Thus, certain vascular territories can be selectively conditioned to the anti-inflammatory actions of corticoids. Conversely, when tissue damage is severe, such selective conditioning may induce a seemingly paradoxical reversal of the cortisol effect with the hormone enhancing inflammation. However, here—as was repeatedly shown (607)—cortisol and impairment of circulation facilitate the necrotic rather than the inflammatory response to irritants. Similarly, it was possible to dissociate the individual actions of DOC overdosage by this type of selective conditioning. It was observed that partial constriction of certain mesenteric vessels can selectively desensitize the part of the vascular tree in which the pulse pressure is diminished, so that, here (unlike in the rest of the mesenteric arterial system), periarteritis will not develop (656). Consequently it may be concluded that a decrease in pulse pressure acts as a negative conditioning agent, for mineralo-corticoid hormones.

Another observation suggested that the increase of the adreno-cortical hormone secretion, which is produced by various stressors, can play an important role in the development of *muscle atrophy* in a region selectively conditioned by a latent vascular deficiency (23, 24). Experiments on the rat revealed that ligature of one common iliac artery causes a latent circulatory disturbance in the corresponding limb, but does not produce any marked involution in the triceps surae muscle. If, after this operation, the animals are exposed to the chronic effects of various stressor agents, the triceps surae muscle of the vasoligated side undergoes atrophy. This selective muscular involution is intensified by administration of cortisol. On the other hand, a mild muscular exercise which predisposes for the development of compensatory vascular changes, even when combined with cortisol administration, results in less muscle atrophy. It was concluded that in the presence of a latent circulatory deficiency, the actual blood glucocorticoid level may be a pathogenic factor of primary importance in the development of muscular atrophy. Thus, these investigations indicated that an interference with the circulation, too slight to produce any manifest disturbance in itself, can selectively condition muscular tissue for the production of local atrophy by exogenous or endogenous corticoids.

In view of the wide, and manifold, therapeutic uses of glucocorticoids, the mechanism through which they influence or cause disease is of considerable interest to the experimenter. It is noteworthy that, in the experimental arrangement just described, the cortisol (whether subcutaneously administered or produced in excessive amounts in the body by stress) must have been carried to the muscles of the limbs, by the blood-stream. Therefore, it is somewhat difficult to explain that a reduction of the circulation increases the catabolic effect of the hormone selectively in the muscle area with the diminished arterial blood supply. Yet, an earlier experiment also showed that the atrophy of a muscle (triceps surae), that follows severance of its motor nerves can be further enhanced by certain hormones which produce intense catabolism (e.g., cortisol, estradiol, thyroxin) and delayed by anabolic hormones (e.g., STH and testosterone) (28, 634). The disuse atrophy of a limb, that follows immobilization in a plaster cast, is also significantly aggravated by cortisol or chronic exposure to stressor agents (25). More precisely, slight atrophy of the triceps surae muscle of the rat was produced by immobilization of one hind limb in a plaster of Paris cast. The development of disuse atrophy was significantly aggravated when the immobilized animal was exposed to stressors and/or treated with cortisol. These results indicated that immobilization of one limb, which did not produce any visible local damage through compression, can act as a conditioning factor which selectively sensitizes the muscular tissue to the catabolic effect of endogenous and exogenous corticoids. It is most probable that this type of conditioning is due to a circulatory disturbance caused by the immobilization; thus, experimentally produced vascular deficiency and application of plaster cast may act through the same pathways in this regard. It is true, however, that, when measured by direct methods, an increased blood flow can be demonstrated as a result of immobilization in a plaster cast. This finding does not contradict the above assumption, because an increased rate of blood flow does not necessarily indicate a greater blood volume, i.e., an increased arterial blood supply to the disused muscular tissue.

Another instance of conditioning by corticoids for a noninflammatory process was discovered in the course of studies on *muscular fatigue* (43, 637). Oral administration of $NaClO_4$ greatly increases the fatigability of skeletal muscle, so that rats normally able to run for about three hours in a standard running mill collapse with fatigue within 10 minutes when pretreated with this salt. Glucocorticoids (e.g., cortisol or triamcinolone) restore working ability to essentially normal levels, under similar conditions.

Overdosage with $NaClO_4$ also produces *muscular contractions* to which the rat can be greatly sensitized by thyroparathyroidectomy, parathyroidectomy and certain mineralocorticoids, such as $2\alpha$-methyl-$9\alpha$-chlorocortisol (Me-Cl-COL) or DOC. Conversely, glucocorticoids, such as cortisol and triamcinolone, exert a potent protective effect against this type of muscular dysfunction (43). The prophylactic effect of cortisol against $NaClO_4$ intoxication is fairly specific: this hormone offers no protection against the muscular contractions induced by an excess of $Na_2HPO_4$ in similar circumstances. It is especially noteworthy that, owing to its catabolic effect, cortisol greatly reduced the body weight of these experimental animals and yet offered protection against a dose of $NaClO_4$ inducing pronounced muscular contractions in the much larger, unpretreated controls.

It will be noted here, as in so many instances, the corticoids do not produce a morbid derangement, but merely condition for or against it. The specific pathogen primarily responsible for the muscular cramps is undoubtedly the perchlorate, but whether a given dose of $NaClO_4$ can actually exhibit its potential convulsive action largely depends upon the balance between positive and negative conditioning influences. The effect of glucocorticoids upon $NaClO_4$-induced muscular contractions is a striking example of what is called 'negative conditioning'.

Subsequent experiments in the rat indicated that the motor disturbances elicited by sudden overdosage with $NaH_2PO_4$ and $NaClO_4$ are qualitatively different. $NaH_2PO_4$ produces a tetany-like condition, with generalized continuous tremor and occasional fits of generalized clonic convulsions. $NaClO_4$, on the other hand, induces no tremor, but rather persistent, tonic extensor cramps, predominantly in the hind legs. Among a great variety of stressors, only those associated with increased muscular work (exercise in a revolving cage, forced restraint, electric shocks) enhanced the susceptibility to acute phosphate intoxication, while all the stressor agents that were examined elicited marked muscular contractions following treatment with threshold doses of $NaClO_4$. Thus, the muscular action of $NaClO_4$ (unlike that of $NaH_2PO_4$) is greatly enhanced even by stressors which do not act primarily upon muscle (637).

In view of the previously mentioned observation that glucocorticoids impart a resistance against the muscular actions of $NaClO_4$ intoxication, it is unexpected that all stressors should have an inverse effect. The stressors which were used in these experiments have previously been shown to augment glucocorticoid production. Hence, it must be concluded that they augment sensitivity to $NaClO_4$ more markedly than they inhibit it by the enhancement of glucocorticoid secretion. The analysis of such specific conditioning by non-specific stress reactions furnishes a promising, but not yet clarified, field for future research.

Electrolyte-steroid conditioning interactions also play an important role on the development of *focal skeletal muscle necrosis*. It will be recalled that in 1863 ZENKER described focal necrosis of voluntary muscle fibers in patients dying from typhoid fever. Since that time similar changes in the skeletal muscles have been reported in humans dying from a variety of acute infectious diseases, myasthenia gravis, muscular dystrophy, dermatomyositis and lupus erythematosus. Experimentally, such muscular lesions occur when there is a deficiency of vitamin E, thiamine, ascorbic acid, vitamin A or potassium; they are also seen in rats given an excess of vitamin D, as well as in rabbits and certain strains of mice after overdosage with cortisone or cortisol (Lit.: ELLIS [173]). In spite of our increased knowledge of the histologic characteristics of this so-called Zenker-degeneration, nothing is known as yet of the etiology and pathogenesis of focal muscular necroses. Therefore, it will be especially interesting to review some recent experiments showing the occurrence of a morphologically similar type of necrosis of individual muscle fiber segments in the rat after combined treatment with certain electrolytes plus steroids.

It is interesting to note that after sudden overdosage with $NaClO_4$, even when the animals die in extensive muscular cramps, there is no histologically detectable alteration in the voluntary muscle. On the other hand the rats become highly resistant to the convulsive effect of this electrolyte when the daily dose is gradually raised. However, when the rats are sensitized with Me-Cl-COL, chronic treatment with perchlorate produces severe degenerative changes of skeletal muscles; initial partial myolysis followed by interstitial edema, while in a later stage inflammatory, phagocytic processes occur around isolated necrotic fibers (40).

Subsequent investigation revealed that rats fed a potassium- or magnesium-deficient diet for a short period became very sensitive to the myotoxic effect of $NaClO_4$. Thus, dietary deficiencies in either potassium or magnesium can substitute for the sensitizing (conditioning) action of Me-Cl-COL. In such animals, the perchlorate elicits particularly severe motor disturbances and marked degenerative changes in the skeletal muscles. The occurrence of all these pathologic manifestations can be inhibited (negatively conditioned) by the concurrent administration of various chlorides (e.g., KCl, $MgCl_2$, NaCl, $NH_4Cl$, $CaCl_2$) alone or in combination. In this respect, KCl and $MgCl_2$ were equally effective in both potassium- and magnesium-deficient animals (657). However, not only the conditioning effect of potassium- or magnesium deficiencies can be abolished or at least markedly diminished with the administration of various chlorides, but these 'desensitizing' electrolytes also prevent the muscular necrosis that normally ensues after combined corticoid plus $NaClO_4$ treatment.

Dietary chloride excess or deficiency also actively conditions for the induction of neuromuscular disorders. An otherwise ineffective oral dose of $Na_2HPO_4$ produces intensive muscular cramps in the rat when the chloride content of the diet is either increased to 1.62% or decreased to 0.035%, from a basic 0.935%. In rats kept on high chloride diet for 14 days, injection of fluorocortisol produces muscular dysfunction, with only a slight tremor but rather persistent, tonic extensor cramps, predominantly in the hind legs. On the other hand, sensitization with low chloride diet not only significantly aggravates the calcium deposition in the muscular tissue due to combined dihydrotachysterol plus Ca-acetate administration, but in rats so treated also induces the development of acute paralysis (49, 50).

It is interesting that in the experiments just summarized the skeletal-muscle lesions were modified by electrolytes in the same manner as the cardiac lesions that also developed under these experimental conditions and will be discussed later. With respect to the pathogenesis of both types of lesion, it would be difficult to decide which among the various factors (dietary deficiencies, corticoids, electrolytes, etc.) is actually the fundamental 'primary pathogen' and which is the modifying, or conditioning factor, responsible for aggravation. Dietary deficiency of potassium or magnesium can, in itself, result in similar muscle lesions if the rats are fed the diet for a much longer period than in the experiment in question (202, 204, 566). On the other hand, long-term administration of $NaClO_4$ also produces muscular necrosis, at least in the suitable sensitized animals (42, 626). Furthermore—as it was already stressed—, both in man and in experimental animals, similar necroses can occur under diverse conditions. Presumably, this type of lesion is not characteristic of any one specific pathogen but represents, rather, a basic reaction of muscle to injury. Virtually nothing is known of the factors that determine whether necrosis will affect skeletal and/or cardiac muscles in any given set of pathogenic circumstances. It is noteworthy, however, that, in the experiments shortly outlined, both the cardiac and the skeletal muscle necroses were prevented by the administration of various chlorides.

As we have seen from the model experiments just summarized, the toxic effect of various adaptive hormones depends largely upon a variety of conditioning factors. Both the production of these hormones and their effect upon individual target organs are decisively influenced by heredity, age, nutritional state, and similar conditioning factors. There are many additional observations to support this view. For instance, the hyalinosis resulting from treatment with crude lyophilized anterior pituitary (LAP) is enhanced by a high protein diet, while restriction of food intake can completely abolish the renal and vascular lesions that normally follow prolonged treatment with DOC. Also, STH fails to stimulate growth, inflammation, and lymphatic-tissue development in adrenalectomized rats unless the animals are maintained with salt supplements or a threshold dose of DOC. Furthermore, as it will be shown later, stress itself can become a conditioning factor in altering tissue reactivity. This may explain why the same stress-producing agent can cause diverse pathologic manifestations in different individuals. It has been observed that a brief overdosage with DOC, especially in combination with LAP and STH, may cause permanent renal and cardiovascular damage in NaCl-sensitized animals. Upon cessation of the administration of both hormone and NaCl, the rats appear to be in perfect health and yet, during the following months, they develop progressively increasing and eventually fatal nephrosclerosis, hypertension, periarteritis nodosa, and cardiac-nodule formation. Exposure to stressors can facilitate the development of all these lesions (Lit.: SELYE AND BAJUSZ [656]).

These observations indicated that not only an increase or decrease in hormone production, but also a change in hormone activity, may sensitize or desensitize the tissues to potentially pathogenic agents. This type of interaction is due to faulty conditioning and, hence, need not be reflected by any absolute change in hormonal levels. As was illustrated in various experimental examples, in themselves well tolerated amounts of hormones (e.g., DOC, Me-Cl-COL, STH) can acquire severe pathogenic potencies, owing to changes in the metabolic conditions that determine susceptibility to their potentially toxic effects. Therefore, an increase in corticoid activity must not be equated with an increase in hormone secretion. In most instances examined, glucocorticoids afforded a positive, while mineralocorticoids a negative conditioning effect. However, this is not always the case. For example, ASHWIN (15) observed that reserpine given to adrenalectomized rats produces diarrhea and gastrointestinal hemorrhage with high mortality. Administration of mineralocorticoids (e.g., DOC) protected (negatively conditioned) the animals from this action of reserpine.

Finally let me cite a few *examples of neurohumoral conditioning* of many recent studies, to indicate the consistent nature of findings of neurohumoral interrelations and the usefulness of conditioned responses as measures of experimentally introduced changes.

In one study, COOK *et al.* (130) demonstrated that adrenaline, noradrenaline and acetylcholine should serve as conditioned stimuli to a shock avoidance response. Control injections of saline were ineffective as conditioned stimuli. In a second study, GUTMANN AND JAKOUBEK (260) were able to show a significant rise in blood-sugar levels during repeated 10-minute waiting periods in a special cage prior to administration of electric shock to rats. Bilateral lesions of the mid-line thalamic nuclei—a part of the brainstem-reticular formation—abolished this 'metabolic preparatory response'. The authors concluded that the thalamic mid-line nuclei are of great importance in the elaboration of the conditioned hyperglycemic preparatory reaction to nociceptive stimulation. Afferent signals apparently activate these thalamic nuclei, and it is probable that impulses from the diencephalic reticular ascending system induce, via hypothalamic centers, neurohumoral mechanisms participating in stress situations (see also pp. 65–70). Similar neuroendocrine conditioning interaction was established by APPLEZWEIG AND MOELLER (11) in rats. These authors found consistently greater difficulty in establishing avoidance responses in hypophysectomized animals as compared with controls, whereas escape responses were learned with equal rapidity. Such distinction was observed also by SOLOMON AND WYNNE (715) in sympathectomized dogs. These findings on anticipatory behavior would further affirm a close neurohumoral relation in conditioning interactions. The fact that varied types of interruptions of neurohumoral circuits produce the same interference with avoidant behavior may be only further evidence that the organism is supplied with alternate adaptive routes, permitting shifts from one to another means of self-regulation.

Another interesting example of neurohumoral conditioning is the influence of the hypothalamo-hypophyseal-adrenal system upon the stomach and the gastric responses to stress. In order to understand the neuroendocrine relationships integrating the gastric and peptic glands into the general endocrine system it should be pointed out that there are two possible pathways by which stress may be relayed from the hypothalamus to the stomach. The neurogenic transmission is by way of the anterior hypothalamus to the vagal centers and the vagus nerve. Direct electrical stimulation of the anterior hypothalamus produces a prompt increase in gastric secretion of hydrochloric acid, which is abolished by vagotomy (494). This vagal phase of secretion is activated by smell, ingestion of food, and psychic stressor stimuli. The second, hormonal phase of gastric secretion is mediated through the adrenal cortex to the stomach by way of the hypothalamus and pituitary. This pathway was postulated by the observations in man of an increase in gastric HCl and pepsin secretion during ACTH administration unaffected by vagotomy but requiring an intact adrenal gland (720). Consequently, it was suggested that chronic emotional and physical stress might be transmitted to the stomach by a neurohumoral pathway through the hypothalamic-pituitary-adrenal mechanism independent of the vagus nerve and gastric antrum, and that acute or chronic peptic ulcer might be induced in man through this neuroendocrine mechanism (244, 245).

Evidence for such conditioning actions in the development of gastric ulcers was recently presented by Gray and Ramsey (243). These authors showed that under normal circumstances the stomach enjoys a semi-autonomous role relative to the adrenal cortex, requiring the presence of normal adrenocortical function for acid-peptic activity. During conditions of stress, however, the stomach is more directly under adrenocortical control: the adrenal gland exerting a conditioning action upon the stomach potentiating its response to other secretory mechanisms. Stress (even moderate emotional stimuli, such as fear, rage, anxiety, hostility) produces an increase in gastric acid, pepsin, and urinary uropepsin to levels usually seen in peptic ulcer disease. In fact, the ulcer due to exposure to stress in experimental animals is closely simulated by the ulcer produced by the prolonged administration of ACTH or corticoids (see also p. 48). Increased corticoid activity seems to interfere with the normal function of the mucous protective barrier and tissue repair. It is probable, however, that the neurogenic pathways, through which stress is mediated to the stomach via the anterior hypothalamus and the vagus nerve, also participate in the pathogenesis of gastric ulcers. In this route, stress may result in alteration in gastric motility, vascular reactivity and secretory activities. The conditioning interactions which may participate here are multiple, since, although ACTH can enhance the response of the organism to stress and thus predispose it to ulceration, ACTH itself, or the glucocorticoids, are capable of producing gastric lesions, as had been documented in man and in experimental animals. The importance of the hypothalamic-gastric pathway was especially emphasized by the demonstration of focal hemorrhages and ulcerations in the stomach following experimental lesions in the hypothalamus and brain stem (344).

All these observations show that interference with the normal function of neurohumoral regulatory mechanism, just as dietary factors, previous stress situations, or altered metabolic activities of organs, all can selectively increase or decrease the responsiveness of target cells to the potentially pathogenic actions of various agents. The recognition of such interactions between the specific primary pathogen and the nonspecific conditioning factors that alter the response to it is of fundamental importance in both clinical and experimental medicine.

## IV. Stress as Conditioning Agent: How do Nonspecific Adaptive Reactions Alter Susceptibility to Disease?

Notoriously, stress itself is one of the most active conditioning factors. Consequently the analysis of the specific conditioning by nonspecific stress furnishes a promising field for stress research. It may be stated, furthermore, that in experimental medicine, the polymorphism of the stress response is no longer a hypothesis, but an established fact. It is important to keep this in mind, because perhaps the most frequently disputed question is that, depending upon conditions, stress can produce or prevent a number of essentially different physiologic and pathologic phenomena. It will be shown later in this chapter that in certain cases the same stress reaction can selectively produce or suppress the same pathologic manifestations (e.g., cardiac necroses), depending upon conditions that the experimenter can control at will. Stress is by no means the only factor that can affect the disease-producing ability of pathogens (e.g., the necrotizing action of potentially cardiotoxic agents), but it is a factor common to so many pathogens and, therefore, extremely important in this sense. It selectively alters the responsiveness of numerous individual targets in the organism. At this point, in order to understand how stress conditions for disease, it may be useful to summarize briefly the basic aspects of *stress concept*. Of course, it would be impossible to touch upon all aspects of this topic in a few pages and for more details one should refer to earlier monographs (597, 601, 609, 625, 677) as well as recent reviews of the author (21, 27, 33, 36, 37, 635, 636, 652, 656), upon which the following outline is largely based.

Experiments of SELYE in animals showed that the most characteristic manifestations of the stress-response are: adrenocortical enlargement with histologic signs of hyperactivity, thymicolymphatic involution with certain concomitant changes in the blood count (eosinopenia, lymphopenia, polynucleosis), and gastrointestinal ulcers, all frequently accompanied by other manifestations of damage or shock (580, 583).

Notably, while during this reaction all the organs of the body showed involution or degenerative changes, the adrenal cortex actually flourished on stress. It was suspected, therefore, that this adrenal response plays a useful part in the systemic, nonspecific adaptive reaction, which was initially termed a 'call to arms' of the body's forces and named the 'alarm reaction' (582, 585).

Subsequent studies showed that the alarm reaction is only the first stage of a much more prolonged General-Adaptation-Syndrome (G-A-S). The latter comprises three distinct stages, namely:

1. the alarm reaction (A-R), in which adaptation has not yet been acquired;
2. the stage of resistance (S-R), in which adaptation is optimal;
3. the stage of exhaustion (S-E), in which the acquired adaptation is lost.

During continuous treatment with a stressor, 'after an initial enlargment the adrenal decreases in size and returns to normal, even though injection of the drug (such as adrenaline, histamine or morphine) that produced the initial enlargement is continued. In such cases, the lipoid content of the cortex also returns to normal and the thymus resumes its normal size. It seems, therefore, that the changes in these glands are not due simply to the presence of the toxic substance in the organism (as had previously been thought), but are the morphologic expression of an A-R, which enables the organism to meet critical situations efficiently'. This change in reactivity might have been due to specific adaptive reactions, but the results were the same when a state of stress was initiated with one agent and maintained with another. Hence, it was thought 'possible that nonspecific fever therapy and protein therapy act by eliciting such an A-R, which would help the organism to defend itself even against stimuli other than those that elicited the reaction' (581).

In order to elucidate the kinetics of this syndrome rats were adrenalectomized and then exposed to stressor agents. This experimental arrangement showed that in the absence of the adrenals stress can no longer cause thymicolymphatic involution or characteristic blood-count changes. When adrenalectomized rats were treated with the impure cortical extracts available at that time, it became evident that thymicolymphatic involution and the typical blood-count changes could be produced by adrenal hormones, even in the absence of the adrenals. Therefore, these changes were considered to be indirect results of stress mediated by corticoids (593). Conversely, the gastrointestinal ulcers and other manifestations of pure damage or shock were actually more severe in adrenalectomized than in intact animals and could be lessened by treatment with cortical extracts. It was concluded that these lesions are not mediated through the adrenals; in fact, they are actually combated by an adequate adrenocortical response to stressor agents.

But what stimulates adrenocortical function during stress? It was found that among many surgical interventions tried, only hypophysectomy prevents the adrenal response during A-R. Hence, it was concluded that stress stimulates the adrenal cortex through an adrenocorticotrophic hormone, now known as ACTH (585, 671).

When pure cortical steroids became available it was observed that the administration of mineralocorticoids (such as DOC) produces experimental replicas of the so-called hypertensive and inflammatory 'rheumatic' diseases; notably, nephrosclerosis, hypertension, vascular lesions (especially periarteritis nodosa and hyalin necrosis of arterioles) as well as arthritic changes resembling, in acute experiments, those of rheumatic fever and, after chronic treatment, those of rheumatoid arthritis (592, 693). Administration of glucocorticoids (such as cortisone or cortisol), on the other hand, were highly potent in causing thymicolymphatic involution and in eliciting the characteristic blood-count changes of the alarm reaction. They also tended to inhibit the inflammatory 'rheumatic-like' changes that can be elicited in animals by mineralocorticoids. Thus, in many respects, the two types of corticoid hormones antagonize each other (596).

The stressor always influences some tissue directly. In certain instances (e.g., hemorrhage, anoxia, total-body x-irradiation) many, if not all cells of the organism are injured owing to a direct action of the damaging agent; frequently (e.g., with trauma, or burns) however, the tissues directly affected by the stressor represent only a limited part of the body as a whole. Yet, even such circumscribed lesions can elicit systemic reactions; hence, it was assumed that the stimulus responsible for the latter must be carried to distant parts of the organism through one of the two great integrating mechanisms, the blood-circulation or the nervous system. Available data suggest that, depending upon the circumstances, either or both of these two integrators may carry such impulses from a directly injured area to other parts of the body.

Whether the eliciting stressor affects only a small part of the organism directly or whether it exerts an immediate action upon all cells, more or less generalized manifestations of *systemic damage* can ensue. Among these, we might mention increased capillary and cell-membrane permeability (with the resulting alterations in the chemical composition of inter- and intra-cellular fluid), hemoconcentration, tissue-catabolism, hypotension, hypothermia, clinical manifestations of 'shock', gastrointestinal erosions, etc.

No matter how such systemic damage is produced, it is always accompanied or followed by manifestations of *systemic defense,* or 'counter-shock'. Here again the mediation, from a limited area of tissue directly affected by the stressor, must occur through nervous and/or humoral pathways. It is probable that such systemic reactions in many instances do not depend upon the liberation of any specific mediator but are activated by a variety of derangements in the chemical composition of the blood and tissues as well as by nervous stimuli.

Thus, in the final analysis, resistance (i.e., disease susceptibility) of the organism is influenced on the one hand by systemic damage and on the other hand by the terminal effector stimuli of the hormonal and nervous defense systems. Interestingly, exposure to a systemic stressor causes characteristic changes in resistance not only to the particular agent to which the organism is exposed (specific resistance) but also to other stimuli (nonspecific or crossed resistance). Such nonspecific resistance induced by systemic stress can express itself either by an increased survival rate, following exposure to normally lethal pathogens, or by the prevention of local and systemic disease manifestations (e.g., inflammation, hypersensitivity reactions, cardiac and renal lesions) that otherwise result from either the topical or the systemic application of pathogens (for lit. see: 629). Under appropriate experimental conditions, it was possible to demonstrate, furthermore, that specific and nonspecific resistance can vary independently of each other, the former rising, while the latter diminishes, as a consequence of intense pretreatment (590).

Several examples on the *conditioning actions of stress* reactions were already discussed (pp. 23–27) and, here, we only enumerate some additional data in more detail.

Starvation and dehydration produce a disturbance in metabolism which might be considered a form of metabolic stress. Anabolism is replaced by catabolism and there is a mobilization of body's reserves. Griffiths and Hope (252) observed that acute starvation and dehydration reduce resistance of the rat to inoculated *Walker carcinoma* cells. Interestingly, chronic malnutrition, which probably allows some metabolic adaptation, was not effective in this respect. It is also known that the growth rate—but not the number of takes—of Walker tumors is significantly reduced by repeated exposure to stressor agents (e.g., forced immobilization). Thus, it seems that the degree of growth of this tumor depends on the degree of adrenocortical hyperactivity (311). Of course, a large tumoral mass itself elicits intense stress. Such tumor-induced stress situation have been observed to sensitize to the cardio- and nephrotoxic actions of antibiotics (527).

Leonard *et al.* (393) observed that cats treated with toxic doses of reserpine have more and greater *tissue injuries,* including perforation, than do untreated controls after esophageal perfusion with human gastric juice. Possible causes of the decreased tissue resistance may be:

1. increased ACTH release through hypothalamic stimulation with resultant corticoid secretion, 2. serotonin release, and 3. local factors such as vascular spasm or decreased blood flow because of hypotension. Selye (602, 603) found that if dilute croton oil is injected into the lumen of the granuloma pouch (for technic see ref. 603, 604) the wall becomes so resistant that, 10 days later, a hundred times the original concentration of the irritant can be withstood. Not only are the adjacent tissues (connective tissue, skin) protected from necrosis, but even the granulomatous membrane, though in direct contact with the strong irritant, remains virtually unaffected. If, under the experimental conditions just mentioned, pretreatment with dilute croton

oil is followed a few days later by the injection of other caustic or irritating solutions into the granuloma pouch, the wall proves to have become resistant, not only to croton oil, but also to normally necrotizing amounts of formic acid, hypertonic NaCl-solution, mustard oil, NaOH, HCl, trypsin, ox-bile, or even hot water (602). We are certainly dealing here with a nonspecific phenomenon that may be considered as a classical example of local crossed resistance.

Cortisone acetate produces *congenital abnormalities* (cleft palate) in offspring of treated pregnant mice, but usually only in small incidence. However, KALTER (335) observed that this pathogenic effect of cortisone is greatly enhanced by restriction of food intake, given during the middle third of pregnancy.

Experiments on guinea pigs showed that, during the so-called 'artificial hibernation', resistance to a normally fatal *anaphylactic shock* is greatly augmented. Even individual organs can be similarly protected by agents which cause a topical 'hibernation', in that they selectively diminish the vital activities of individual organs. For instance: thiourea-derivatives can protect the thyroid against the pathogenic actions of radioiodine; a ureteral calculus, which stops urine production, can protect renal tissue against nephrotoxic agents (327). The relationship between hibernation and the stress-induced cross-resistance would deserve further study. It is likely that in some instance stress also protects by virtue of interfering with the vitality of tissues. Notably, resistance to whole-body radiation is similarly enhanced by previous exposure to cold (62) as is resistance to toxic compounds (38).

Resistance to *bacterial infections* is either increased or decreased following exposure to X- and gamma-radiation. While large daily doses seem to decrease resistance in this respect, prolonged exposure to very small doses may actually increase resistance to bacterial infections of animals (265, 266, 401). Pretreatment with benzol, total-body X-ray irradiation, and toxic doses of nitrogen mustard almost completely suppressed the Shwartzman reaction normally induced by repeated injections of meningococcal toxin, in the experiments of BECKER (71). However, the acute toxicity of a single, massive dose of various bacterial toxins is usually potentiated by stress. PELLOJA (490), for example, observed that in the guinea pig the toxic effect of tetanus toxin is markedly increased by the administration of muscular extracts, the increased mortality being proportional to the crudeness of the extract. In experiments with rabbits to which a standard procedure of hemorrhage was applied, it was shown that the animals so treated could not safely withstand more than 1/400,000 the dose of a purified endotoxin that non-stressed rabbits can survive (574). Similar observations were described also by others (9,800), and it was even concluded that in toxin treated animals acute stress is at least as potent in inducing lesions and high mortality as is a preliminary sensitization by the toxin itself (748). On the other hand, DARE AND MONGEY (144) found that restraint decreases the response of rabbits to bacterial pyrogens. Severe restraint was more effective in this respect than moderate exposure to this stressor.

In rats pretreated with dihydrotachysterol, local trauma to the skin (e.g., that of epilation) produces calcinosis reminiscent of the so-called calcifying *scleroderma* ('sclérodermie calcaire'). However, if the animals are restrained just prior to the dihydrotachysterol-treatment, they become resistant to the production of such skin lesions by cutaneous trauma. Here again, we are dealing with a phenomenon of nonspecific resistance induced by stress (681).

The acute *gastric erosions* characteristic of the A-R can be elicited by most diverse stressors (trauma, burns, cold, etc.). Rather similar acute gastric ulcers are produced by histamine liberators, such as 48/80. These gastric lesions produced by 48/80 (as well as the accompanying anaphylactoid inflammation and shock) can actually be prevented by stressors, although under similar conditions of dosage and timing, stressors may also produce erosions of the A-R type (682). Here, the stressors applied induce increased resistance to a histamine liberator, and the gastrointestinal tract is the target organ.

The response of animals and man to the *actions of hormones and drugs* is also greatly altered by stress. For example, a few years after discovery of insulin, it was rapidly recognized that, in man, infections, shock and surgical interventions increase the need for this hormone and sometimes completely inhibit its hypoglycemic action (388). It was demonstrated that this condition could be reproduced in rabbits by injecting various infective and toxic agents, and only after the formulation of the stress concept was it evident that this inhibition of the hypoglycemic action of insulin is not due to any specific effect of the agents applied, but is a nonspecific consequence of the A-R (421). More recently, these original observations were confirmed by studies in man and in animals. In man, delay in the insulin response has been described after endocrine, hepatic or infectious diseases (297), neoplastic diseases (84, 415) and accidental injuries (575), the most severely injured group showing the least sensitivity to insulin. In animals, several authors were able to demonstrate a remarkable delay in the hypoglycemic action of this hormone in hypothermia (1, 446, 791), after moderate exercise (751) or anesthesia (445). Even such stressor agents as intensive sunshine, cold water, noise and moderate pain seem to have a definite action on the sensitivity of mice to insulin (773). Emotional and psychological factors may alter similarly the responsiveness of patients to oral antidiabetic compounds (157). However, certain reports seem to contradict the above findings, and state that, for example, physical exertion can induce a fatal hypoglycemia, following insulin administration (378, 751). It is probably the case that this opposite reaction occurs only in the S-E when the organism is no longer able to mobilize its glycogen reserves because of lack of adaptive hormones (597).

Depending on the doses used and on the chronology of the experiments, stress can protect animals against the toxicity of adrenaline, or increase their susceptibility to it. A-R produced by pretreatment with formalin, exposure to cold, forced muscular exercise, or surgical trauma increases the resistance of the rat to the subsequent intravenous injection of a lethal dose of adrenaline (587). SELYE (588) showed that this form of stress-induced nonspecific resistance is not only effective against the lung edema normally produced by adrenaline overdosage, but also against the fatal pulmonary changes caused by the intravenous injection of large amounts of physiologic NaCl solution in bilaterally nephrectomized rats. On the other hand, if prior to trauma adrenaline or noradrenaline is administered to rats at a dose that in itself has no lethal effect, a high mortality occurs even from moderate stressor stimuli (395). The stress of confinement, produced by crowding the animals together, induces a very high mortality in mice treated with small doses of amphetamine that were not lethal in themselves (112, 113, 295, 304); similar phenomenon was observed by WEISS AND LATIES (771) after electric stimulation in rats.

It is well known that in the presence of an injury in patients, anesthesia can aggravate an already active shock condition, or if shock is impending, anesthesia precipitates it. Studies on dogs subjected to hemorrhage showed well-defined differences in the circulatory reaction between normal and anesthetized animals (77). This finding was confirmed by ZWEIFACH *et al.* (800) in rabbits anesthetized with ether, nitrous oxide or cyclopropane. BEECHER (73) reported that thiopental sodium anesthesia is poorly tolerated in patients with large wounds and severe burns. According to another report of BEECHER (74) the depressant action of morphine is potentiated by trauma (particularly by hemorrhage and pneumothorax) and is dangerous in hypothyroidism, and in any kind of impaired liver function. An increase of morphine toxicity under adverse conditions has also been seen in rats and mice placed at different room temperatures (288). PRIORESCHI (498) described that forced immobilization or electrical stimulation causes a marked increase in the anesthetic activity of sodium bromide in rats. Certainly, it may be concluded from these observations that when the same change in the pharmacologic action of a drug is seen after such diverse conditions, it is no longer due to a specific effect of any one particular stimulus. The various agents and conditions enumerated above induce a similar pattern of changes in the organism, changes that are the result of the body's response to injury, and have been called the 'stress response'.

In *summary* we might say that all agents that act upon the body or any of its parts exert dual effects: 1. specific actions (which may modify the effects of other agents to a certain extent), and 2. nonspecific or stressor actions (through which they all activate stress-defense). The stressors act upon the target (the body or some part of it) directly and indirectly through the hypothalamo-hypophyseal-adrenal system or in other instances through the pituitary-adrenal axis (601). Through some as yet unknown pathways the 'first mediator' travels from the directly injured target area to the hypothalamus or in some instances directly to the anterior pituitary. It notifies the latter that a condition of stress exists and thus induces it to discharge ACTH. In connection with the hormonal defense reactions this activation of the anterior hypophysis is of special importance. During stress the increased ACTH output stimulates the adrenal-cortex to produce excessive amounts of corticoids. In other cases of stress, systemic nervous defense reactions operate through neuro-hormonal pathways. The hypothalamus is generally considered to be the center of the neuroendocrine adaptive mechanism. However, purely nervous defense reactions are also regulated by the hypothalamus. From here, autonomic fibers carry impulses throughout the body to the vascular tree and to the organs involved in metabolism. Such nervous stimuli play an extremely important role in gearing the organism for adaptation to environmental influences.

It was illustrated, furthermore, with a number of clinical and experimental findings that exposure to stressors can induce marked changes in tissue resistance as well as in the response of the organism in general. Under some conditions the potentially pathogenic actions of the most diverse agents are aggravated by stress; under other circumstances, the mortality, or disease normally produced by various pathogens can be prevented by pretreatment with stressors. This latter phenomenon may be ascribed to a kind of nonspecific adaptation. Interestingly, even adrenalectomy without corticoid substitution therapy does not completely prevent this type of induced resistance (or adaptation); thus at least certain forms of this systemic, nonspecific resistance must result from reactions other than mere stress-induced increase in corticoid secretion (586). It was also shown, that, under certain experimental conditions, true cross-resistance to the pathogenic effect of one stressor develops, if the animal is adapted to another fundamentally different, stressor agent. Thus, depending upon the time, duration and intensity of pretreatment, a variety of nonspecific stimuli can prevent or elicit disease manifestations in the suitably conditioned animals.

In the following pages an attempt will be made to examine the pathways through which a stressor elicits the systemic reactions characteristic of G-A-S as well as influences fundamental biochemical activities of organs. The hypothalamo-hypophyseal-adrenal interrelationships on the one hand, the actions of corticoids at cellular level, on the other hand, seem to be the most important in this complex problem. However, it is necessary to state, here, that in spite of the enormous increase in our knowledge concerning the neurosecretory function of the hypothalamus and as regards the multidimensional biochemical actions of steroid hormones, the principle of the stress-concept remains unchanged. It is now certain that the ACTH discharge is a nonspecific character of the pituitary response and that the primary physiologic function of ACTH is to stimulate the adrenal cortex. It is also clear that at least some reactions of the G-A-S do possess a defensive value, i.e., they facilitate adaptation to biologic stressors.

### *a) Neuroendocrine Relationships in Adaptive Reactions*

An increasing amount of clinical and experimental evidence supports the validity of the thesis that the central nervous system exerts some regulatory function over the pituitary. In the following pages, therefore, we shall discuss some problems of the hypothalamo-hypophyseal system and of the main pathways through which, it is thought, the central nervous system regulates the activity of endocrine end-organs. Of course, this is an artificial way of handling neuro-endocrine relationships of adaptive reactions, since not only does the nervous system play an important role in governing the secretory activities of endocrine glands, but the reverse is also true: the hormonal substances of endocrine organs may basically alter the function of purely nervous mechanisms. For example, clinical evidence has shown that lesions of the adrenal cortex can be considered the determining cause of neurologic disease (225).

Developments of the last decade, furthermore, have made it clear that the nervous system itself is, in a sense, a complex endocrine system producing humoral substances for the control of endocrine functions and, probably, also, of a number of other bodily functions. Thus, chains of alternating neural, neurohumoral, and hormonal links, which play a governing role in physiologic and pathologic conditioning processes, are so numerous that it would be impossible to correlate them on the pages of the present monograph. The anatomy of the neuroendocrine structure (249, 781), its phylogenetic aspects (561) and maturation (774), the neuroendocrine reflex (184, 467) and adaptation (118, 226, 300) mechanisms, the neurosecretion (227, 562) and the neuroendocrine substances (775) are all well defined complex problems; and even when summarized only briefly they fill the pages of a vast volume (237). Papers on clinical aspects of neuroendocrine correlations (8, 90, 98, 150, 197, 373, 476, 570, 571, 752, 761) as well as those on experimental findings showing hypothalamic or nervous influence on tumorigenesis (262, 342, 397, 754) well illustrate the wide variety of basically important problems involved in the simple designation 'neuroendocrinology'. Thus, one has to look for borderlines to be able to fulfil the task, since otherwise, we would have to go so far as to illustrate, for example, that the growth of mammalian populations is controlled by a sociopsychologic-physiologic feedback system that responds to changes in population density, and that the central nervous system (especially the sympathetic pathways), the hypothalamus and the pituitary are all involved in the mechanisms through which behavioral factors activate adrenocortical function and depress gonadal activities (118, 119).

*Hypothalamo-Hypophyseal System*

At the present time, research is governed by the assumption that hypothalamic regulation of the adenohypophysis is mediated by humoral agents transmitted from the median eminence to the anterior lobe by the portal vessels. However, a number of questions still remain unexplained in the problem as a whole. While it is certain that the hypothalamus exerts a degree of control that is necessary for hypophyseal functions, there is not sufficient evidence for considering this neutral region to be the main coordinating control system for endocrine adjustment reactions. Diencephalic areas seem to be critical for the emergence of normal internal secretory adjustment patterns; but whether these brain regions directly and autonomously control the endocrine pattern or merely influence background tonus—probably even this by stimuli originating in higher centers—cannot be determined definitely at this time.

The hypothalamus is a part of many complex neural circuits involving certain cortical and brain stem areas. It has connections with the prefrontal lobes, the gyrus cinguli, the rhinencephalon (limbic system) and the higher brain stem systems, such as the ascending reticular formation, etc. Thus, a great number of tracts leading into the diencephalon from higher and lower centers of the nervous system can and do mediate various categories of stimuli. In fact, the connections enumerated are both afferent and efferent. The hypothalamus in turn activates the neocortex, thus showing that the former is involved in an interplay of pathways: controls a complex pattern of autonomic and somatic functions, but also is regulated by cortical impulses. Furthermore, the interrelation of the two autonomic systems, the ergotropic and the trophotropic mechanisms, does not show a fixed and invariable pattern, but depends on the actual reactivity of the areas concerned, and in a matter of balancing interplay influenced by lower and higher structures (34). Most of these are too poorly understood as yet to allow any definite conclusion as regards neuroendocrine correlations forming the subject of the present discussion.

The origin, course, and terminal distribution of the central nervous efferent pathways concerned with the regulation of the anterior lobe function are not as well known as those concerned with the activities of the posterior lobe. Experiments conducted under grossly unphysiologic laboratory conditions show mechanisms of function and control of that specific model, but do not establish the applicability of the observed phenomena to spontaneous activity by intact animals or man. Hypothalamic lesion experiments, presently very popular, are of limited value, because the fine structural patterns of the hypothalamus–while probably very complex—are at the moment poorly understood. Consequently, we have no precise information concerning the functions of neurons destroyed or interrupted by an 'effective' lesion. Concepts of control mechanisms derived from such studies could be generally accepted only if the experimental model proved to be a realistic substitute for corresponding reactions of physiologic processes. However, we simply know that lesions in various parts of the hypothalamus may affect the secretion of trophic hormones differently, and there is already lack of agreement even on so fundamental a point as precise localization of such 'effective' lesions. Of course, many other problems are involved here, one of which was well emphasized by Kovács, Lissák and Endröczi (370) when they wrote: 'it cannot be stated with certainty whether the changes observed in the endocrine organs after destruction of the paraventricular nucleus are consequences of a disturbed regulation of the pituitary secretion of trophic hormones or whether the altered function of one single organ had initiated functional changes in the others'. New approaches are, therefore, urgently needed to attack the problems of the hypothalamo-pituitary relationships from new points of view.

Let me recall that, according to the well-known hypothesis of Harris and Green (Lit.: Harris (270])—which, in fact, basically helped the development of neuroendocrine thinking—the final hypothalamic path to the adenohypophysis, whatever its origin, consists of two parts: one, neural, terminating in the median eminence, and the other, vascular, via the hypophyseal portal vessels. However, there are observations to indicate that yet another, purely neural, part is involved in the hypothalamic final common path to the anterior lobe (439, 440). This last seems to be constructed solely of neurons that do not terminate in the external layer of the eminencia but extend further into the adenohypophysis and terminate among its glandular cells. If further confirmed, this finding may result in our seriously reconsidering the current ideas, since the fibers in question are probably always damaged by lesions of the median eminence that affect the function of the anterior lobe. It is now evident, furthermore, that the neurosecretory system of the diencephalon cannot be discussed solely in relation to the posterior lobe of the pituitary. However, it would be equally incorrect to interpret the functions of the hypothalamo-hypophyseal-adrenal axis in terms of 'neurosecretion' alone.

During the past years, a number of papers have dealt with additional morphologic (68, 69, 152, 153, 176, 253, 322, 352, 530), and functional (156, 201, 238, 449, 457, 510, 511, 518, 548, 789, 792) studies of diencephalic structure as well as of the hypothalamo-hypophyseal system; see also reviews of BARD (60), NAUTA (468) and of BAJUSZ (34, 35), KELLER (345) as well as SMITH *et al.* (710). A number of other reviews and symposia on various aspects of the subject of the hypothalamo-hypophyseal system have also appeared; such as written by K. BAUER (66), CODACCIONI (122), FIRKET (193), GRAUX (242), HUANT AND DUSSERT (317), KOVÁCS (369), KRIEGER (362), LEGAIT (390), NOBLE (474), RODECK (528, 529), SAFFRAN (543, 544) and SAYERS (552). H. C. BAUER (65) has written an excellent summary of endocrine and metabolic conditions related to pathology in the hypothalamus; other papers show the increased clinical interest in and the attempts to diagnose neuroendocrine disorders (5, 190, 241, 333, 413, 417, 442, 512, 539, 577, 762). Several recent observations are interpreted in terms of the classical 'feedback-theory' of HOSKINS (312), on the assumption that the circulating target organ hormones inhibit the activity of appropriate hypothalamic centers, and, thus, induce secondary suppression of pituitary trophic hormones (142, 303, 793).

*Neurosecretion and neurohormones.*—According to WELSCH's classification (775), we may distinguish between two types of substances produced by the neurons: 1. neurohumors (e.g., acetylcholine, noradrenaline, 5-hydroxytryptamine), which are short-range, brief-acting products, and 2. neurosecretory materials or substances (e.g., oxytocin, vasopressin, corticotrophin-releasing-factor), which serve mostly as long-range, long-acting coordinating agents. But since the neurohumors (products of ordinary neurons) and the neurosecretory materials (originating from neurosecretory cells) are all internal secretions with regulatory functions, the inclusive terms 'neurohormones' or 'neuroendocrine substances' have been suggested. The neurohormones are usually released into the circulation from storage centers and may act at many loci of the organism to regulate physiologic processes. The mechanisms of their storage and release have been studied in more detail in the simplest model-system, the adrenal medulla, but even here, they are, as yet, poorly understood (294). The hypothalamus and the neurohypophysis themselves contain a family of chemically related polypeptides with varying and sometimes overlapping, biological properties. Vasopressin (or antidiuretic hormone, ADH) and oxytocin, the so-called neurohypophyseal hormones, originate in the hypothalamus.

The neurosecretory material(s) (NSM) is assumed to originate from cells of the supraoptic and paraventricular nuclei and transported along their axon to the neural, and possibly the intermediate, lobe of the pituitary. It may be concluded from experimental observations that both the paraventricular and supraoptic nucleus contain vasopressin- and oxytocin-producing neurons that vary in relative abundance from species to species and that in some species the oxytocin-producing units predominate in the paraventricular area.

It was, moreover, established that the fibers of the supraoptico-hypophyseal tract laden with NSM enter into close association with loops of capillaries in the wall of the infundibulum, which convey blood to the adenohypophysis and, especially, to the pars tuberalis. Thus, possible neurohormones of the diencephalon may influence the adenohypophysis. Whether the NSM is identical or closely related to such neurohormones or whether it really enters into the capillaries of the median eminence has not been definitely established. It is true, however, as shown by histologic studies, that the neurosecretory droplets usually become progressively smaller with increasing proximity to blood vessels and beyond this point they cannot be identified. This would suggest that the NSM is carried to the anterior lobe by the portal venous system of the pituitary. As it is known, the anterior pituitary does not receive direct arterial blood. The afferent blood channels are the thin-walled portal vessels that arise from a rich network of capillaries formed by branches of the superior hypophyseal arteries that come off the internal carotids. The venous drainage is into the cavernous sinus. The special anatomical arrangement of the portal system which breaks up to form sinusoids provides intimate contact between the circulating blood and the hormone-secreting cells of the adenohypophysis.

As another possibility, the NSM may enter the vessels at the third ventricle, reaching the adenohypophysis via the systemic circulation. This would serve to explain discrepancies showing that while complete division of the pituitary stalk is regularly associated with the derangement of physiologic functions dependent upon the neurohypophysis, there is considerable doubt about the extent of the disturbances this operation provokes in processes governed by the adenohypophysis. Conclusions varying from complete hypopituitarism to 'no effect' are to be found in the literature and more recent experiments also indicate that sectioning of the pituitary stalk (i.e., separation of the portal venous system) does not inhibit the menstrual cycle in the monkey (307) or the normal stress-response in the dog (366). In accordance with these experimental observations the group of OLIVECRONA (316) claims that after section of the pituitary stalk in man, an adequate production of both cortisol and aldosterone takes place. Hypophysectomy, however, is followed by an immediate diminution or even cessation of cortisol production, whereas aldosterone continues to be secreted not only in normal quantities, but sometimes in markedly increased amounts.

The NSM is believed to be a glyco-lipo-protein complex rich in polysaccharide as well as in -SH and -SS- groups containing polypeptides; its chemical structure remains unknown. It probably represents neurosecretion with a number of different physiologic potencies. For example, MAETZ *et al.* (407a) extracted a new, presumably hormonal, principle from the neurohypophysis, which exhibited an effect on active sodium transport through the cell membranes. In general, however, during the last years, investigators have done little more than test staining combinations (100, 267, 319, 443) or observe the microscopically visible amounts of NSM under various experimental conditions (10, 12, 19, 206, 217, 315, 355, 356, 471, 522). Indeed, cytologic observations showed at least a partial distinction in the functions of the paraventricular and the supraoptic nuclei, by the variations in their response to diverse light conditions (195). In the region ventral to the supraoptic nuclei, the amount of NSM was most abundant in the rats exposed to continuous illumination as compared with animals kept under usual laboratory light-conditions (controls); it was least in those maintained in permanent darkness. In the posterior lobe, the NSM was plentiful in the controls, but reduced in both groups subjected to extensive light or darkness. Added light increases the secretion and release of NSM, since large amounts of the material appeared along the neurosecretory axons, while the pars nervosa was relatively depleted. The central nervous system obviously plays a role in these phenomena: an intact retina and optic nerve are essential in the transmission of light stimulus. It is interesting to note here that, in birds, visible radiations induce gonadostimulation. Evidence presented by BENOIT AND ASSENMACHER (78) indicates that a neurosecretory link between the hypothalamus and adenohypophysis is involved in this photosexual reflex.

Recent studies on the hypothalamic neurosecretory system as well as on the structure and blood supply of the pituitary are in favor of functional interrelationships between the neurohypophysis and adenohypophysis (71, 91, 137, 152, 306, 551, 756). This view is further substantiated by the observations of Nikitovitch-Winer and Everett (472, 473) on cytologic and functional restitution of pituitary grafts re-transplanted from the kidney to median eminence. The authors believe that the degenerative phenomena and the functional deficiencies observed when the pars distalis is removed from its original site are caused by the loss of hypothalamic influences, stimuli probably mediated by the hypophyseal portal vessels. This most likely concerns the secretion of corticotrophin, thyrotrophin, follicle stimulating and luteinizing hormones.

*Neurohypophysis*

Scharrer's conception that the ADH and oxytocin are produced in the hypothalamus itself has at long last been accepted. The neurohypophysis is concerned with the storage and release of these two hormones. The stored ADH (and probably oxytocin also) is released into the blood stream by nervous impulses arising in the supraoptic and paraventricular nuclei and conducted by the supraoptico-hypophyseal tract to the neurohypophysis.

Three factors appear to act as trigger mechanisms in the release of ADH: 1. the osmolar pressure of extracellular fluid, 2. the volumetric changes in extracellular fluid and, 3. the central nervous system response to direct stimulation. An increase of 1–2% in the extracellular osmotic pressure is sufficient to increase the rate of ADH release. Changes in the blood volume have a similar effect, a supposition that has been reemphasized recently in connection with studies on obese patients (58). There is a significant increase of ADH discharge in obesity states, but no difference could be demonstrated between the serum osmolarity of obese and normal persons. The former state is, however, associated with hypovolemia (low circulatory minute-volume, low circulatory blood volume, low renal blood flow, reduced extracellular fluid). Interestingly, in obese subjects, enhanced aldosterone secretion is observed and it was suggested that the increased ADH secretion is associated with the activation of the so-called Henry-Gauer reflexes (58, 482). Electrolyte changes also influence the release of this neurohormone, but hyponatremia and renal salt-wasting may be secondary to the sustained production of ADH, as is seen in neurologic disorders (181). Stressful emotional stimuli (e.g., noise, pain) induce increased ADH release by direct action upon the central nervous system. For example, it was observed that psychic agitations in immediately preoperative periods result in an increase of serum antidiuretic activity (371). Similarly, oxytocin release may also be governed by direct neural reactions activated through a variety of emotions (Lit.: Heiman [278]).

The main physiologic importance of vasopressin undoubtedly lies in its ability to regulate water reabsorption in the renal tubule, though, phyletically speaking, it is not the only antidiuretic hormone of the neurohypophysis (281, 283, 339, 493, 557). The mechanism by which ADH regulates water metabolism has not been completely elucidated. As noted, it certainly exerts an effect upon the distal tubules of the kidney, to promote the reabsorption of water. Studies with labeled vasopressin indicated that it acts on tubular cell-receptors by -SS-interchange, probably forming two mixed hormone-receptor disulfide bridges (573). Such interaction could account per se for the effect of -SS- containing peptide hormones, such as ADH, oxytocin and insulin, on the permeability of cell membranes. Interestingly, the neurohypophyseal hormones increase the water permeability of frog bladder wall essentially independently of their actions on net sodium transport. Oxytocin is more active than vasopressin in this respect (556). It may be postulated that the antidiuretic effect of posterior lobe hormones results from a similar action on the water permeability of the distal renal tubule. Pasqualini *et al.* (186) think, furthermore, that ADH has a direct effect on the distribution of body water and/or on the nervous centers regulating thirst sensations. Concerning the metabolism and fate of ADH, it is well established that a great portion of the hormone is destroyed in the body; liver and kidney tissues are particularly effective in inactivating it. Hypothalamic homogenate also inactivates ADH, but this process is reversible, the antidiuretic activity being restored by acetic acid extration (323). The possible binding of vasopressin to proteins of hypothalamic origin may have importance in its regulatory functions.

New-born animals and infants are unable to concentrate their urine to the same extent as are adults and there is evidence that at the time of birth the neurosecretory system is not completely differentiated to produce a sufficient amount of ADH (280, 526). It is also true that in an early period of life the renal tubules do not react to ADH in the adult manner, because of morphologic or functional immaturity. Experiments of Heller and Lederis (282) showed that the amounts of ADH and oxytocin in the neurohypophysis of infant rats is very low when compared with adults; however, it seems that the release-mechanism of ADH by dehydration already operates shortly after birth. The finding that the pituitary of infant animals deprived of milk for 24 hours contained 10–30% less ADH activity than did those of litter-mate controls could be thus interpreted. This would mean, actually, that ADH is released at an age when the kidney is unable to respond to it. The alternative explanation would be that the neurohormonal reflexes responsible for ADH secretion are not activated, but the withdrawal of milk at so early an age somehow inhibits the hormone synthesis in, or transport from, the hypothalamic secretory center. In adult rats, withdrawal of food and water for the same period stimulates both the release and—as is shown by the concomitant increase in hormone storage—the rate of synthesis of ADH. Blindness is usually associated with irregularities of water metabolism, but Rodeck's (528) studies on blind animals clearly indicate that the maturation of the neurosecretory system is independent of the development of photo-vegetative reflexes. Notably, during embryonic life the supraoptic nucleus maturates earlier than the paraventricular (766); another study on the maturation of neurosecretory centers was recently performed by Duchesne (136). An excellent review has just been published, showing that the final adjustment of the 24-hour daily cycle of water metabolism is the sum of the influence of many voluntary and involuntary factors originating from cortical and subcortical centers and exerting a continuous influence on the function of the hypothalamic neurosecretory system (527, 528). The recent work of Jahn *et al.* (326) and of Montastruc (450) is of interest in connection with interactions between ADH regulation and the activity of other endocrine systems.

It has been repeatedly proposed that vasopressin may be one of the main factors responsible for the activation of the adenohypophysis and the release of ACTH (see p. 63–65). It now seems to be established that although this neurohypophyseal hormone has ACTH-releasing activity, it exerts also a direct stimulatory effect on the adrenal cortex. Studies have shown that this cortisol-stimulating activity and its pressor effect are independent of each other and that the former seems to be highly specific. Perfusion of isolated adrenals with other polypeptides, such as oxytocin, insulin and glucagon, or such pressor amines as adrenaline and noradrenaline did not result in augmented cortisol output in these studies (295). But, while ACTH causes continuous stimulation of cortisol secretion during prolonged perfusion of the adrenals, vasopressin produces only a transient effect under similar conditions. On the other hand, vasopressin causes a greater increase in secretion rate of corticoids than do supramaximal doses of ACTH.

It is widely accepted that the other neurohypophyseal hormone, oxytocin, is of physiologic significance in the milk-ejection reflex, but its role as a humoral mediator stimulating prolactin secretion is still open to question (see also p. 76–79). It is also a matter of controversy as to whether oxytocin plays any physiologic role in renal or cardiovascular functions or in the transport of sperm after mating. There is some evidence accumulating that the antidiuretic and chloruretic activity of posterior lobe extracts are not linked to the same substance. That the oxytocin fraction is entirely responsible for the chloruretic actions is still questionable (733, 734).

### *Adenohypophysis*

*Corticotrophin (ACTH)*.—The release of ACTH from the adenohypophysis is usually associated with stimuli (collectively known as stressors) that affect the homeostatic equilibrium of the organism. There is no longer doubt concerning SELYE's fundamental concept: the ACTH discharge is a nonspecific character of the pituitary response (597). The primary physiologic function of ACTH is to stimulate the adrenal cortex.

Whether or not the hypothalamus is in the focal point of convergence of the neural pathways mediating ACTH release is not definitely established. KIVALO AND RINNE (354) found no relationships between the activity of the supraoptic and paraventricular nucleus of the hypothalamus and the release of ACTH. The transverse nerve fibers occurring in the region of the median eminence, which terminate around the capillary loops of the portal vessels and contain neurosecretory materials, seem to cross the fibers of the supraoptic-hypophyseal tract and may, therefore, have a different site of origin from those of the actual tract. Another interesting finding shows that, in short-term experiments, ACTH-overdosage does not exert any demonstrable effect on the neurosecretory picture of the hypothalamic nuclei; prolonged administration of ACTH, nevertheless, may produce hypotrophy of the cellular nuclei and nucleoli, but here again, the neurosecretory material in the cytoplasm remains unaffected (372). In this connection, we can also cite the observation of STIGLIANI (730) that the choroid plexuses in man contain PAS- and Gomori-positive substances in the form of droplets localized in the layer immediately beneath the epithelium and sometimes also in the central villous region; this material may also represent BARGMANN's neurosecretion.

In common with a number of processes in the organism, the regulation of ACTH secretion has an inhibitory as well as an excitatory component. Recent critical reviews by SAYERS *et al.* (552) and by SAFFRAN (544) emphasize the possibility that the inhibitory and excitatory influences can both be mediated through the hypothalamus. However, there are studies that strongly suggest the governing role of the cerebral cortex and limbic system in both excitatory and inhibitory aspects of the pituitary-adrenocortical function. For example, dogs respond to burns with increased corticoid output, even after the brain above the inferior colliculus is removed and the pituitary left in situ but isolated from nerve impulses (170). This finding was interpreted to mean that higher areas of the brain tonically inhibit lower areas, which presumably produce ACTH-releasing neurohormones. EGDAHL (170) believes that a center located in the hind brain is responsible for regulation of ACTH secretion, while the center essential for adrenal medullary activation following burns or peripheral nerve stimulation is located in the medulla oblongata. OKINAKI *et al.* (477, 478) showed, furthermore, that stimulation of the posterior orbital surface, the amygdaloid nuclear complex, and the reticular formation of the midbrain transiently facilitated the pituitary-adrenocortical function, while stimulation of the hippocampus resulted in prolonged suppression. Using similar electrical stimulation techniques, but in the upper posterior hypothalamic area and in the area preoptica, SUZUKI *et al.* (735) observed an initial slight increase in 17-dehydroxycorticoid secretion followed by a marked and prolonged decrease below the prestimulating level. It remains to be established whether all these findings indicate the existence of several inhibitory centers or of simply pathways of inhibitory fibers for ACTH secretion. It should be always kept in mind that the secretion of ACTH is inversely related to blood levels of corticoids under certain conditions, such as adrenalectomy or injection of large amounts of these hormones. Such evidence supports the existence of humoral mechanisms in the inhibition of ACTH release and it was suggested by McCANN *et al.* (428) that the adrenal steroids block the discharge of ACTH from the pituitary by 1. a direct action on the adenohypophysis, and 2. by decreasing the release of vasopressin, a neurohormone presumed to stimulate ACTH release.

On the other hand, as many forms of stress are associated with strong emotional stimuli, the participation of nervous pathways in the activation of the anterior lobe was obvious early on. Even moderate emotional reactions due to discomfort or nervous stimuli of very short duration provoke significant adrenocortical hyperactivity (183, 211). But if the organism is exposed to a stressor agent without emotional content or if the psychosomatic factors are eliminated (e.g., by anesthesia), the pituitary is still known to be activated. In other words, more mechanisms must exist for regulating ACTH secretion. In fact, as we see today, the release of ACTH is a property shared by a great number of substances, rather than the property of a single neurohormone. Consequently, a discussion of neural influences on the pituitary-adrenal axis is presented here, not with the view that humoral and neural mechanisms of endocrine regulation are in any way mutually exclusive, but rather to show that the ultimate pattern of endocrine secretion represents the participation of either or both types of regulatory mechanisms. It might be expected, furthermore, that the extent and complexity of neural influences on endocrine functions increase in more highly developed animals, roughly in proportion to the striking overgrowth of the neocortex.

Among others, three peptide materials found in the neurohypophysis, ADH, oxytocin and the so-called corticotrophin-releasing-factor (CRF)—which may be products of the hypothalamic system that produces the stainable NSM—were found to stimulate ACTH release. Not only are ADH, oxytocin, and the CRF very similar in amino acid composition, but they share to some extent each other's major biological activities (560), just as ADH has weak but definite oxytocic properties, the purified CRF, itself, possess antidiuretic activity. ADH, the neurohormone earliest suggested as the releaser of ACTH, still receives support in this respect (116, 295, 365). Notably, it was demonstrated by means of direct arterial perfusion of the adrenals that synthetic vasopressin stimulates the secretion of cortisol (295). This effect is not mediated via the adenohypophysis or any other organ but is rather the result of direct stimulation of the adrenal cortex by vasopressin itself (see also p. 60). On the other hand, several recent attempts have been made by various groups of workers to prove that

CRF obtained from neurohypophyseal and posterior hypothalamic extracts is a different substance from ADH and oxytocin (258, 389, 425, 541, 554, 559). In rats with hypothalamic lesion, crude extracts from the stalk-median-eminence region produced a marked release of ACTH, which cannot be accounted for by their content of vasopressin (429). LIPSCOMB *et al.* (399) also showed that, in animals with hypothalamic lesions or pharmacologic blockade (Nembutal + morphine, cortisol), CRF preparations stimulate the release of ACTH, at doses where pressor equivalents of highly purified lysine vasopressin were inactive. ROYCE AND SAYERS (540) obtained a fraction of crude brain extracts that was substantially free from corticotrophic and pressor activities but induced adrenal ascorbic acid depletion. However, the precise chemical structure of CRF is still inknown; also many justified criticisms have been made or can be applied to assay techniques used in these studies if one correlates the findings (208, 209, 224, 705). However, on re-evaluating their pituitary incubation method, GUILLEMIN AND SCHALLY (257) claimed that the effect of CRF in this system cannot be explained on the basis of inhibition of ACTH inactivation; CRF does not act either by potentiating ACTH at the adrenal level or by an inherent adrenocorticotrophic activity. Notably, crude hypothalamic extracts increase the activity of acid phosphatases in pituitaries, in vitro (115,568). Proof that this effect is specific for CRF would be most helpful to future research. At any rate, it would be fruitful to collect more data concerning biochemical changes that occur in the pituitary itself as a result of the actions of hypothalamic products.

It was demonstrated, furthermore, that vasopressin- and ACTH-release can be independently influenced by pharmacologic means. In the studies of GEORGE AND WAY (231) lesions of the median eminence completely blocked the adrenal acid depletion that normally occurs following morphine administration. Lesions of the hypothalamus that produced diabetes insipidus blocked the antidiuretic response of a small dose of morphine (0.1 mg/kg), but failed to inhibit the response to larger doses (1.0 to 10 mg/kg). Thus, the release of vasopressin is not necessarily accompanied by proportionate release of ACTH, at least by morphine. Interestingly, in a series of post mortem studies, age, sex and stress (as assessed by the lipid pattern in the adrenal cortex), the disease state, and steroid therapy, had no obvious influence on the yield of vasopressin and oxytocin in the posterior lobe (138).

In *summary,* the nature of the anterior-pituitary-activating factor(s) has not yet been clearly established. It seems reasonable to believe that CRF and vasopressin share the role of ACTH-releasing neurohormone: CRF may be the chief ACTH-releasing factor(s) from the stalk-median eminence, while vasopressin is probably the mediator in the neural lobe. It should be kept in mind, furthermore, that the principal substance responsible for ACTH release may vary according to the species (136, 331, 702).

*Pituitary-Adrenal-Activation*

The close relationship between emotional responses to environmental factors and pituitary-adrenocortical activity is illustrated by the substantial elevation of plasma 17-hydroxycorticosteroid (17-OH-C) levels observed in psychosomatic stress situations by MASON (420). It was demonstrated that the pituitary-adrenocortical system is remarkably sensitive to psychologic influences in both man and monkey. The ACTH-release occurs, not in association with a specific emotional state, but rather with a wide variety of emotional disturbances that may have relatively undifferentiated elements of distress or arousal. These conclusions have been derived from the results of three general experimental approaches; studies 1. of rather gross environmental influences (transfer, handling, housing conditions) on 17-OH-C levels in the monkey, 2. of conditioned emotional responses (avoidance procedure) and 17-OH-C levels in the monkey and 3. of 17-OH-C levels in human subjects during stressful life situations (sleep-deprivation, preoperative state, etc.). There is a diurnal rhythm of the plasma 17-OH-C level, and the neural-mediated effects of stress upon ACTH release are either superimposed upon or act intimately through the same mechanisms that govern the diurnal oscillations. If confirmed, this would point to the importance of secondary or compensatory regulations that probably influence the response to prolonged or repeated psychosomatic stress.

The reticular-activating system may be involved in the tonic effects of the nervous system regulating the adenohypophysis (553) and this assumption is compatible with the current ideas of HARRIS (271) and MAGOUN (408), who claim that that excitation of the reticular system would be the route by which stressful stimulation leads to hypothalamico-pituitary activity and consequently to ACTH elaboration. Electrophysiologic studies (191) indicating similarities between the hypothalamus and midbrain reticular formation are in keeping with the above anatomical and endocrinologic investigations, findings that emphasize a close relationship of these two structures. It may be assumed, therefore, that the afferent impulses reaching the hypothalamus directly from the midbrain reticular formation play an important role in modifying the autonomic and neuroendocrine activity of this region of the brain and supply the information for elaboration and integration of emotional reactions. Additional evidence is needed, however, to support the contention that in emotional stress the activation of the reticular formation results in a stimulation of the adrenal medullary secretion (e.g., in the release of adrenergic hormones), which on its turn causes ACTH discharge (707). Psychosomatic reactions are known to induce adrenaline and noradrenaline discharge (183) and it is indeed likely that the elevated blood level of adrenergic mediators contributes to the concurrent activation of the pituitary-adrenocortical axis. But the latter can occur independently, as has been shown in the past by experimental techniques involving exclusion of the sympathetico-adrenal system by surgical or pharmacologic means, and, more recently, by BEAULNES AND POIRIER's finding that monkeys treated with tranquilizers show a loss of the hyperglycemic response to immobilization but retain normal eosinopenic and lymphopenic reactions (70). The participation and importance of the sympathetic system in certain stress reactions remain obscure at present, since almost all aspects of adrenergic transmission (from synthesis of the neurohormones to their destruction) are still clouded with unanswered questions and unresolved conflicts of observation and opinion (470).

'Denervated' pituitary synthesizes and secretes ACTH at a lowered basal rate and is unable to respond to acute stressor stimuli with increased ACTH discharge; but it retains a partial ability to respond to chronic influences, such as adrenalectomy, with increased synthesis and release of ACTH. Assuming that the hypothalamic lesions produced in the median eminence in these studies by MCCANN AND HABERLAND (427) completely eliminated the neural control of the pituitary, another mechanism of control must account for the residual effect. DEAR AND GUILLEMIN (148) also showed such residual ACTH secretion after lesioning of the median eminence; more precisely, they detected circulating free corticosteroids in the peripheral plasma of hypothalamic-lesioned animals. However, this residual ACTH secretion was found to be diminished with time and had almost disappeared by the 60th post lesion day. This additional finding was interpreted to mean that in such animals the hypocorticoid state is unable to elicit the well known reciprocal hypersecretion of ACTH. The reason for the obvious discrepancies outlined above is not clear. Progressive degeneration around the lesioned areas may affect receptor sites for the circulating corticoids; but the results obtained by SCHAPIRO AND KATZ (563) with cortisol $C^{14}$ are more compatible with the hypothesis that the pituitary is relatively richer in such receptor sites than are the hypothalamic structures.

From SLUSHER's (706) studies concerning the influence of brainstem lesions on stress-induced corticoid release it was concluded that the ability of the adrenal to release additional corticosteroids to stressor influences appears to be related to the intactness of those areas of the central nervous system most probably concerned with facilitatory release mechanisms of ACTH. The importance of such neuroendocrine integrity is reflected by ARVAY *et al.* (17). On the other hand FORTIER (210, 212) showed that the pituitary ACTH-content reflects a balance between synthesis, release, and possible destruction of ACTH, in situ. His studies confirmed that the ACTH-releasing effect of stress is markedly influenced by the level of circulating adrenocortical hormones, and that the withdrawal of these hormones enhances both the release and synthesis of ACTH, but has a predominant effect on the latter. The complexity of the problem may be stressed by the observation obtained by splanchnic nerve stimulation by OKINAKA *et al.* (479), which suggested that a neural factor modifies the function of the adrenal cortex apart from the regulation through ACTH. HALÁSZ AND SZENTÁGOTHAY (261), furthermore, pointed out the existence of an afferent neural link between the adrenal cortex and the nucleus ventromedialis hypothalami, through which the actual functional state of the adrenocortical cells may influence diencephalic activities. If confirmed this observation may have great significance, since the group of TONUTTI (782) attributed importance to the role of the nuclei ventro- and dorso-medialis in the control of ACTH-release.

Investigations employing different hypothalamic lesions give very limited information concerning the localization of pituitary-regulating centers, because the interpretation of such experiments is rather complicated. Lesion techniques always destroy a number of hypothalamic nuclei and tracts in addition to certainly interrupting a great many pathways whose functions are incompletely understood. Nevertheless, lesions in the anterior hypothalamus (365), in the mid-hypothalamus, and in the posterior region were all shown to result in pituitary-adrenal inertia (552). On the other hand, similar lesions are reported to potentiate the ACTH-releasing effect of at least some of the stimuli studied (140, 363). Marked adrenal hyperactivity subsequent to lesions of the paraventricular nucleus has also been observed (369). In order to overcome these discrepancies, SMELIK (707) puts forward the assumption that the hypothalamic centers are involved in different ways in the mechanism of ACTH release, depending upon the nature of the stressor agent. He observed that anterior lesions diminish the effect of 'somatic' stimuli and abolish the activity of 'psychic' stimuli. Psychic stimuli were also abolished by posterior lesions, but not somatic ones, while tuberal lesions blocked the ACTH-releasing effect of both types of stressor agent. Consequently, it was concluded that the anterior and posterior lesions interrupt different axons that normally conduct the stimuli from higher centers to the tuberal area. But in the final analysis, 'somatic' and 'psychic' agents would have the same lower pathways, obviously through the ventral mid-hypothalamus. However, as previously stated, the complexity of the diencephalic centers precludes selection of any single structure as being responsible for ACTH discharge, on the basis of ablation studies only. Furthermore, objections may be directed against the view that any stressful stimulation invariably evokes, via an unknown first mediator, the release of a hypothalamic neurohumor (ADH or CRF) into the portal circulation, which then stimulates pituitary ACTH secretion. This is certainly an oversimplified generalisation that cannot account for a number of observations.

We note that the above differentiation between 'somatic' and 'psychic' stimuli resembles a former categorization of FORTIER (207), which distinguishes between 'metabolic' and 'neurotropic' stressor agents. A similar recent attempt was made by ROCHEFORT *et al.* (526), by carrying out ACTH depletion experiments. However, there is still doubt concerning the correctness of distinguishing between 'psychic' (or 'neurotrophic') stressors, which would elicit ACTH-discharge through neural pathways, and 'systemic' ('somatic' or 'metabolic') stressors, which would act by releasing some hypophysiotrophic material of extrahypothalamic origin into the circulation or by producing metabolic changes. The findings of CASENTINI *et al.* (108) suggest that all stressors invariably act through the excitation of some nervous pathway. MARTINI *et al.* (419) demonstrated that 'systemic' stressors, i.e., laparotomy and unilateral adrenalectomy, are ineffective in stimulating ACTH secretion after midbrain transection. On the other hand, SMELIK (708, 709) postulates that the 'psychic' stress stimuli act on ACTH-release by the mediation of endogenous adrenaline, whereas in the case of 'somatic' stress, neither the posterior lobe nor adrenaline is involved.

Interestingly, there is an initial biphasic response to stressor agents, consisting of a brief elevated secretion of ACTH followed by a period of lower or less than normal output. This phenomenon is not due to secretory exhaustion, but to the inability of the pituitary to release ACTH at a given time during stress situations. A sustained rate of hormone secretion is usually observed over a prolonged period, after the initial biphasic response. Treatment of stressed animals with reserpine or production of lesions in certain hypothalamic sites interferes with the suppression period and results in continuous elevated ACTH secretion (360). Thus, some neural mechanism is most likely involved. Other studies on time relationships, however, lead to the conclusion that the rapid increase of the blood-ACTH concentration may be under neural control, while the second phase is regulated by the plasma level of ACTH (301). Even adrenalectomized rats react with a fall of the pituitary ACTH concentration when subjected to stress, a response that can be prevented by pretreatment with cortisone or ACTH (353). This is obviously further evidence that the circulating level of both ACTH and corticoids influences the ACTH release from the hypophysis (see also p. 63). The complexity of the problem may be stressed by the observations that exogenous ACTH raises the pituitary-ACTH content in adrenalectomized animals (probably through inhibition of the endogenous ACTH discharge), but in intact animals steroid-induced depletion of pituitary-ACTH concentration is neither prevented nor ameliorated (308, 309, 353). Rats treated with large doses of $\triangle^1$-hydrocortisone do not exhibit a decrease in the ascorbic acid concentration after exposure to painful stimuli, injection with histamine or nicotine, but large doses of vasopressin elicit the adrenocortical response (779). The data may be interpreted to indicate that whereas the treatment with corticoids does not affect the responsiveness of the hypothalamus, it markedly decreases the reactivity of the adenohypophysis and neurohypophysis of animals exposed to noxious stimuli.

Neuroleptic phenothiazine derivatives (chlorpromazine and cyamepromazine) counteract the cardiac-necroses-eliciting effect of stressors, such as forced immobilization, bone fracture, or noradrenaline overdosage. Continuous anesthesia with Nembutal protects against the pathogenic action of restraint, but not against that of noradrenaline and bone fracture (52). These findings may imply that the phenothiazine compounds block some common, presumably neural, pathways through which various stressors elicit cardiac lesion in the suitably conditioned animal. However, the possibility has also been considered that the action of neuroleptics in this regard is not specific, but simply a secondary consequence of starvation caused by the drug administration. It was observed that adaptation to diverse stressors is similarly active in preventing this type of experimental cardiac damage (45), while, on the other hand, PREMACHANDRA AND TURNER (497) revealed that the depression of thyroid activity by reserpine is secondary to depression in food intake. Psychodepressant drugs (e.g., chlordiazepoxide and meprobamate) and psychostimulant agents (e.g., iproniazid and imipramine) may also alter stress responses; it was also shown that their primary site of action is in the limbic system, the area involved in emotional responses (558). Diphenylhydantoin (Dilantin) is another drug known to exert an inhibitory influence on pituitary-adrenocortical activation. BONNYCASTLE AND BRADLEY (88) observed that rats treated with diphenylhydantoin fail to show the expected depletion of adrenal ascorbic acid following unilateral adrenalectomy, vasopressin, noradrenaline, or histamine injection. This blockade seems to occur in two stages: 1. a presumably central initial phase, in which the adrenal cortex maintains its ability to respond in a normal manner to exogenous ACTH, and 2. a more prolonged phase, in which there is a reduction in the responsiveness of the adrenal itself to ACTH.

*Aldosterone.*—It appears that aldosterone secretion is relatively independent of the pituitary-adrenal axis. The secretory rate of this corticoid can vary independently of that of corticosterone or cortisol. Thus, a physiologic mechanism acts specifically to stimulate aldosterone secretion in response to environmental changes that call for increased levels of this mineralocorticoid.

Changes in the body fluid volume and the levels of sodium or potassium are well established regulating factors, but obviously ACTH is also a potent stimulator in this respect. This latter observation indicates that the functional maintenance of the zona glomerulosa is not exclusively controlled by extra-pituitary factors. The effect of ACTH may be independent of sodium intake or of cortisol secretion, and appears to be self-limited in that it may be lost even if administration of ACTH is continued (63). ACTH was constantly found to increase aldosterone secretion when perfused through the adrenals of hypophysectomized animals (296). This ACTH effect was also observed in earlier acute experiments, but it cannot be reproduced by chronic administration of ACTH; the reason for this disparity is not clear. After complete hypophysectomy in the dog, atrophy is seen, not only in the inner cortical zones, but in the glomerulosa also, to a certain extent (20). Reimplantation of a portion of the pars distalis resulted only in partial maintenance of the mass of each of the adrenocortical zones, which would suggest that some factors other than the pars distalis play a role in this regard.

Afferent pathways are, as yet, unknown; probably the vagus is involved (186). In this regard BARTTER *et al.* (63) reported that constriction of the inferior vena cava leads to an increase of aldosterone secretion, whether or not the vagus nerves are intact. Release of such constriction lowers aldosterone secretion when the vagi are intact, but not after they have been sectioned. Constriction of the common carotid artery leads to an increase of aldosterone secretion in the normal animal, but is ineffective when the carotid arteries are partially deprived of their nerve supply. The assumption that the integration of this complex regulatory mechanism would be at the brain stem level, specifically in the central gray substance of the rostral midbrain (186), deserves further investigation. Psychosomatic factors are certainly involved in all these experiments, and consequently the cerebral cortex may exert an influence at the brain stem level to alter aldosterone secretion, a possibility that has to be included.

FARRELL's (185, 186) studies suggest the existence of atrophic hormone analogous to ACTH but specific for aldosterone secretion. This so-called adrenoglomerulotrophin has not as yet been chemically characterized, except that it behaves in many respects as a lipid and is extremely potent: 8–10 µg are required for maximal steroidogenesis (187). Ablation studies pointed to the importance of the midbrain and epiphyseal area; indeed, certain lesions (mostly involving the pineal gland) lead to increased output of aldosterone, suggesting disruption of an inhibitory system. Furthermore, in pinealectomized, sodium depleted dogs, not only aldosterone but also the cortisol secretion rates are higher (187). Therefore, FARRELL and his group are now attempting to prove the hypothesis that: 1. the epiphysis cerebri elaborates an anti-corticotrophin that competes with pituitary ACTH and with adrenoglomerulotrophin to restrain adrenal activity, and 2. the quantitative relationship between these three substances in any given situation may determine the final rate of steroidogenesis.

Another interesting concept was recently introduced by HILL *et al.* (292) concerning the hormonal regulation of adrenal glomerulosa and its mineralocorticoid production. Activation of the glomerulosa corresponds to changes in the leukocytes and the lymphoid tissues, which are the opposite of those found during the glucocorticoid phase of stress. Taking into account the mutual antagonism between mineralocorticoids and glucocorticoids, the assumption has been derived that the activation of the glomerulosa is elicited by the ascendant glucocorticoid effects, especially their influence on electrolyte and water exchanges through the cell membranes. Hence, the hyperactivity of the glomerulosa counterbalances the glucocorticoid effects by abolishing them. A unitive theory is now needed to correlate all the factors explored (i.e., the relative participation of nervous pathways, neurohumors, pituitary, glucocorticoids, electrolyte levels, and intravascular volume changes) in order to establish the physiologic system regulating aldosterone secretion.

### *Regulation of Trophic, Adaptive Hormones Other than ACTH*

*Thyrotrophin (TSH)*.—Despite a number of evidences concerning a central nervous participation in the regulation of TSH release, the nature of this control mechanism and its relation to other visceral regulatory functions of the brain remain uncertain.

It was demonstrated by Yamada and Greer (794) that thyroxine injected into either the anterior pituitary or the anterior hypothalamus inhibits thyroidal release of radioiodine. This suggests that an increased level of circulating thyroid hormone might act at both the pituitary and hypothalamic levels to suppress TSH secretion. Mess (438) assumes from ablation experiments that the nuclei habenulae of the epithalamus plays an important role in the nervous pathways regulating TSH secretion, but he does not exclude the existence of humoral mechanisms. Lesions of the anterior hypothalamus produce 'goiter block' in the guinea pig, preventing not only the thyroid weight increase but also the microscopic manifestations of goitrogenesis (86). These findings were interpreted to mean that neither the synthesis nor the release of TSH can reach high levels in the absence of appropriate hypothalamic structures. In other experiments, the development of propylthiouracil-induced goiters of rats was studied in relation to this hypothesis (793). Systematically ineffective amounts of thyroxine injected into the anterior hypothalamus inhibited goiter formation. Since the adrenal and testicular weights were not affected, Yamada concluded that intrahypothalamic thyroxine specifically inhibits TSH secretion without interfering with other trophic hormones.

Additional ablation studies repeatedly suggested that the region involved in TSH regulation lies in the anterior hypothalamus, in the midline between the paraventricular nucleus and the infundibulum (515). On the other hand, physiologic and neuroanatomic data indicate that this thyroid regulating region of the anterior hypothalamus is distinct from that responsible for temperature regulation. REICHLIN (515), therefore, advanced the hypothesis that this brain area serves to integrate short term heat loss, heat conservation, and heat mobilization reactions, with long-term metabolic control by the pituitary-thyroid axis.

BLANQUET AND TOBIAS (85) carried out interesting studies on the thyroid function after radiation of the median eminence. They succeeded in radiating localized sections of the rat hypothalamus by means of a focused beam of high energy particles from the cyclotron: the uptake of $I^{131}$ determined in vivo was normal or slighly elevated; however, the amino acid content of the thyroid gland was greatly altered. The concentration of diiodotyrosine and monoiodotyrosine (precursors of the hormone) was normal, but that of thyroxine was low. Thus, it is possible to obtain selective effects on thyroid metabolism even in the absence of pituitary lesion, a finding that suggests that the median eminence area exerts a control over the synthesis of thyroxine. Interestingly, cases of congenital goiter have been reported in children in whom the uptake of $I^{131}$ was generally elevated and the circulating iodine was chiefly in the form of monoiodotyrosine and diiodotyrosine to the exclusion of thyroxine. According to ALBRIGHT (6), some of these patients perhaps represent a previously unrecognized syndrome, hypothalamic goiter, in which the primary lesion is in the diencephalic structure. In fact, the clinical features of hypothyroidism in man are suggestive of a disordered TSH regulation possibly resulting from a functional disturbance of the central nervous system. MCCULLAGH *et al.* (431) reported on patients in whom hyperthyroidism developed after section of the pituitary stalk. Assays for TSH in the blood at the time when signs of pituitary deficiency existed showed the presence of a thyroid-activating substance similar to that found in other cases of hyperthyroidism. In this connection, it is worthy of note that the data of VOLPE *et al.* (763) failed to provide any evidence that the function of the normal thyroid gland is readily affected by severe mental and physical stresses, a clinical finding that is in sharp disagreement with experimental observations (94, 272).

Although appropriate hypothalamic lesions reduce baseline thyroid activity, the hormonal feedback regulation of the pituitary-thyroid axis operates despite extensive diencephalic damage (514). This and similar findings suggest that while the anterior lobe itself is responsible for both increased and decreased blood concentration of thyroid hormone, the 'setting' at which the pituitary reacts is governed by nervous system mechanisms involving the hypothalamus. The extensive studies of HARRIS and his associates (101, 272, 273) also indicate that both a diencephalic neural mechanism and the pituitary itself are responsible for the regulation of thyroid function, but the central nervous system takes priority over the influence of the servo-mechanism in regulating TSH release.

It appears, furthermore, from observations following long-term TSH administration that the acceleration of synthesis and release of thyroxine and the hypothalamic neurosecretory phenomena, especially in the paraventricular nucleus, are related to each other (4). In partially thyroidectomized rats, histologic signs of enhanced neurosecretion were observed in the fibers leading from the supraoptic and paraventricular nuclei, during the compensatory enlargement of the residual thyroid tissue (700). SCHREIBER *et al.* (567) prepared a protein-free fraction from hypothalamic extracts that increased the acid phosphatase activity of the adenohypophysis, and further studies give rise to the assumption that the same, as yet unidentified, neurohumor would be responsible for the stimulation of TSH output (569). The existence and role of the so-called TRF (Thyroid-Regulating-Factor), a neurohormone considered to be present in the anterior hypothalamus by Japanese workers (697, 698), and which has been recovered even from urine (699), also needs confirmation. Indeed, SAITO AND TANI (545) claim that they partially purified this material after extraction from hypothalamic tissue and urine. The TRF (a peptide) obtained had no ACTH-releasing, vasopressor, or oxytocic activity, but exhibited a very weak antidiuretic property, and acted only on the thyroid. On the other hand, GREER *et al.* (251) obtained no consistent effect on TSH release with intrahypothalamic or intrahypophyseal injection of a variety of hypothetical 'neuro-humoral' substances or hypothalamic extracts.

In contrast with the above views, PURVES (499) believes that the maintenance of normal levels of thyroid hormone depends primarily on a desensitization of the anterior lobe to the action of the circulating hormone. This may be ascribed to the destruction or modification of thyroid hormone in the median eminence and stalk, or to the secretion by these nervous tissues of a substance binding the hormone in a concentration that is ineffective on the anterior lobe. A neuroendocrine transmitter substance with a direct stimulating action on the TSH producing cells is considered by him to be less likely. Thus, according to this alternative hypothesis, the secretion of TSH is mainly, if not entirely, controlled by the level of circulating thyroid hormone. CHRISTENSEN (117) presented, furthermore, evidence that it is actually not the total content of thyroid hormone in the plasma, but the content of free, non-protein-bound thyroxine that regulates the pituitary influence on the thyroid.

The investigations of FLORSHEIM (199) may be cited also to indicate that the thyroid-pituitary feedback system controlling TSH release is independent of the hypothalamus. In rats with anterior hypothalamic lesions, the maximal circulating TSH levels after goitrogen feeding were lower than in controls, as measured by bioassay techniques. However, the discharge of the labeled hormone from the thyroid of lesioned and control rats was inhibited by equal doses of exogenous thyroxine. The observation that a tranquilizing agent (reserpine) inhibits thyroid function probably through suppression of TSH secretion (83, 451, 452) cannot be quoted to contradict the above conclusion. The secretion of at least two other pituitary trophic hormones (ACTH and gonadotrophin) is also inhibited by reserpine, but the primary site of the pharmacologic actions of tranquilizers remains controversial (358, 552). In fact it was shown by PREMACHANDRA AND TURNER (497) that the depression of thyroid activity by reserpine is secondary to depression in food intake and not a result of inhibition of some hypothalamic endocrine function.

Interestingly, electrical stimulation of cervical sympathetic fibers enhances the hormonal secretion of the thyroid, even in hypophysectomized dogs bearing pituitary autographs (318); the significance of this observation awaits clarification. It is also known that, curiously, the thyroid gland may continue to function even in the absence of the pituitary, thus without any intervention. Such persistent thyroid function after hypophysectomy was reported in patients whose thyroid proved histologically normal, and showed that autonomous function is not necessarily associated with recognizable alterations of the thyroid epithelium (488).

The difficulties in the design and interpretation of experiments studying the regulation of TSH release have been recently discussed by

Rose *et al.* (537). It was emphasized that many of the conclusions concerning various aspects of TSH release are based on suggestive rather than on definite data. Linquette (398) reviewed some clinical aspects of hypothalamico-pituitary-thyroid interrelation that may be of interest concerning conditioning actions of thyroid hormone.

*Gonadotrophins (GTH)*.—Much experimental data have been presented during the past few years supporting the participation of nervous reflexes and especially the hypothalamus in the regulation of GTH (16, 134, 555, 718). Reviews of Harris (273) as well as Benoit and Assenmacher (78, 79) reflect the generally accepted opinion that, while the secretion of follicle stimulating hormone (FSH) and luteinizing hormone (LH) are under hypothalamic control, that of prolactin, or luteotrophic hormone (LTH), is less under nervous influence. Pituitary transplanted to the kidney can still maintain LTH secretion (433, 550). Investigations on the participation of higher regions of the central nervous system in GTH regulation has only just begun, but evidence is already accumulating that the limbic system probably plays a fundamental role.

Destruction of the paraventricular gray area and the median eminence, in the rat, induces profound atrophy of reproductive organs, while lesions in the preoptic and anterior hypothalamic areas produce persistent estrus, hypertrophied uteri, and inhibition of corpus luteum formation, in the ovary. D'Angelo (141) showed, furthermore, that the adenohypophysis of lesioned rats in persistent estrus loses its capacity to augment secretion of FSH under conditions of enhanced demand (e.g., unilateral oophorectomy). In such animals with hypothalamic constant estrus, the hypophyseal LH content is also subnormal; after ovariectomy, the LH content increases in the pituitary, but not in the plasma (741). Studies of Davidson and Ganong (146) showed that destruction of the posterior median eminence resulted in testicular atrophy of dogs, without there being evidence of adrenocortical or thyroid inhibition. Lesions in other parts of the median eminence were not effective in this respect.

Thus far, the areas and central nervous pathways specifically involved in the control of each of the gonadotrophic activities have not been accurately defined. Lesions placed in the median diencephalon of ovulating hens inhibit ovulation, regardless of the precise site of the lesion (507). On the other hand, lesions in the anterior hypothalamus or in the medial portion of the amygdaloid complex were associated with precocious ovarian stimulation (174). This latest observation suggests the inclusion of the amygdaloid complex in this regard, an assumption supported by the observation of YAMADA AND GREER (795) that testicular atrophy occurs in amygdalectomized rats, a finding that may be related to the absence of functioning amygdaloid structure necessary for adequate secretion of GTH. The existence of an influence originating from still higher centers was proposed by some South American workers (133, 444, 532) who claim that hemidecortication releases the hypothalamus from some restraining action exerted either by the cerebral cortex or by subcortical structures, and thus, resulting in an increased GTH secretion from the hypophysis.

The opinions are also controversial concerning the possible localization of inhibitory and excitatory centers regulating ovulation: SAWYER (555) points to the importance of the reticular activating system of the midbrain tegmentum and basal diencephalon, whereas CRITCHLOW (134) favors centers located ventro-medially in the mesodiencephalic junction.

It appears from recent experiments that progesterone does not cause a release of ovulation-inducing hormone by direct stimulation of the pituitary, but it acts upon certain regions of the brain. RALPH AND FRAPS (509) showed that progesterone regularly induces premature ovulation in the hen, when injected into certain regions other than the hypothalamus or the caudal neostriatum of the forebrain. Lesions placed in these areas within 2 hours after systemic injection of progesterone prevent the expected ovulation (508). Thus, progesterone-induced release of LH is mediated through some neural pathways. Such neuroendocrine-mechanism-producing changes in the reproductive activity of birds (see review of NALBANDOV: [467]) and mammals (196) can be activated by continuous lighting and there is some indication suggesting that the pineal gland is here involved.

Oxytocin was again proposed as the neurohormone affecting GTH release (13), but the evidence is not yet convincing. In fact, any posterior polypeptide may play a role in GTH regulation, since injections of neurohypophyseal preparations (Pitressin, Pitocin, lysine-vasopressin and oxytocin) were all shown to induce a significant rise in the secretion of GTH (18); however, MOORE's (453) data may indicate that in most instances the release of ACTH by the adenohypophysis is accomplished at the expense of ovulating hormone secretion. It is probable that in these complex processes, just outlined, the nature of the hypothalamic mediation may be neurohumoral in character: extraction of stalk-median eminence tissue resulted in a substance producing LH release. The nature of this material has not been established; however, McCann *et al.* (426) claim that it is not identical with any known hypothalamic constituent.

The changes in the pituitary that occur at puberty are also initiated by some extrapituitary mechanism that is probably mediated through the central nervous system. Gellert and Gagnong (229) showed that electrolytic lesions involving the acruate nucleus in the posterior tuberal region result in precocious puberty of the rat. Similar observation was presented by Bogdanove and Schoen (87). According to Donovan and Werff-Bosh (158) destruction of the area situated basally behind the optic chiasma may also result in advanced puberty of rats. It is also known that small tumors of the posterior hypothalamic tissues are often associated with accelerated sexual maturation. However, the mechanism by which hypothalamic lesions accelerate the onset of puberty remains undetermined. The two possible explanations would be that such lesions 1. interfere with suppressor mechanisms or 2. act by irritating GTH stimulation, probably through unspecific effects. Neither of these arguments can be excluded. On the other hand, it was also shown by Corbin and Schottelius (131) that bilateral lesions of the area from the mamillary body to the ventromedial nucleus result in delayed puberty. These authors note the similarity between the characteristic signs of Fröhlich's syndrome and the delayed puberty, sexual infantilism, and obesity resulting from posterior hypothalamic destruction. A logical conclusion would be that delayed puberty is sometimes due to differential immaturity of certain hypothalamic regions; however, there are certain discrepancies even in the reports just outlined.

Increased interest has been focused on the nervous pathways regulating lactogenic responses. A detailed review with some original observations was recently presented by Denamur and Martinet (155); this concerned the role of the nervous system in the development of mammary glands and in the initiation and maintenance of lactation. It is known that, following parturition, the nursing stimulus elicits a reflex release of lactogenic hormone; and it is probable that some neural stimulus arising from the pregnant uterus is instrumental in causing a similar discharge during late pregnancy. The experimental data of Grosvenor and Turner (255) suggest that a progressive accumulation of lactogenic hormone occurs during the period of mammary gland development, and is then suddenly discharged to initiate secretory activity of mammary gland alveoli.

That adrenergic blocking agents (Dibenamine) and anticholinergic drugs (atropine) effectively inhibit pituitary lactogen discharge suggests that cholinergic and adrenergic links are both involved in the reflex arc responsible for the secretion of lactogenic hormone (254). The importance of sympathetic and hypothalamic pathways was indicated also by the observation that electrical stimulation of the uterine cervix can initiate and maintain lactation (434). Such stimuli probably evoke a reflex release of oxytocin and lactogen.

PURVES AND AVERILL (500) found that lesions placed slightly lateral and ventral to the paraventricular nucleus selectively affect lactation; the mammary gland of such rats, although well developed, contained no milk. They postulated that such lesions diminish the secretion of lactogenic hormone to an extent that is still sufficient for luteotrophic action but not for lactogenesis. According to YOKOYAMA AND OTA (796) lesions in the medial hypothalamic area (e.g., in the nucleus ventromedialis and dorsomedialis) also inhibit lactation, and it was concluded that these nuclei participate in the milk ejection reflex, probably being linked to the secretion of oxytocin. On the other hand, however, GROSVENOR AND TURNER (254) observed that physiologic doses of oxytocin injected into anesthetized lactating rats fail to alter pituitary lactogen from the control prenursing level. This result would mean that oxytocin has no stimulatory effect upon pituitary lactogen release in the lactating animals, and is contrary to the recent hypothesis that oxytocin is a humoral link involved in the discharge of lactogenic hormone. There are also other observations suggesting that the suckling stimulus causes prolactin secretion without mediation by oxytocin (797). In fact, numerous drugs (e.g., acetylcholine, serotonin, reserpine), stressful stimuli, and other factors can induce mammary growth and lactation in estrogen-primed rats and other mammals (435, 436); it is believed that all these agents induce the release of prolactin and ACTH, since the initiation of lactation requires ACTH or glucocorticoids (as conditioning factors) in addition to prolactin.

*Somatotrophin (STH)*.—The somatrophic function of the adenohypophysis is relatively free of hypothalamic influence. It appears that the general metabolic state of the organism, the activity of the pituitary, and its STH content are interrelated in a complex manner that may govern the rate of STH secretion. In accordance with this view are the observations of SOLOMON AND GREEP (713) suggesting that the STH content of the pituitary is influenced either by the circulating level of thyroxine or by some metabolic action of the thyroid hormone.

Lesions destroying the median eminence, primary hypophyseal portal plexus, or pituitary stalk all induce moderate to marked, but never complete, growth failure in rats. The STH content of the pituitary of the animals with such lesions was significantly lower than normal as was the content of TSH (513). The endocrine changes observed were multiple (thyroid, adrenals and gonads were all affected); however, appropriate replacement therapies did not restore the growth to normal. Experiments of HINTON AND STEVENSON similarly showed that ablation in the region of the supraoptic nucleus retards growth, probably through impairment of production or release of TSH or STH (298). In another study performed by REICHLIN (514) no special neural localization of the lesion responsible for poor growth could be made, but it was noted that the most striking effects occurred following large lesions of the median eminence that involved the primary portal plexus and stalk. The question whether or not these findings provide evidences of a specific hypothalamic function for the regulation of STH cannot be answered with certainty. In addition to any specific effects on STH regulation, indirect effects on growth may be exerted through lesion-induced thyroid inhibition, gonadal atrophy, adrenocortical dysfunction, chronic fever, diabetes insipidus, or simply through disturbed pituitary blood supply. It should be considered, furthermore, that the animals with such hypothalamic lesions are under considerable stress: thus nonspecific factors may also play a role in the development of growth disturbance. In summary we can state that there is still no direct evidence that STH secretion is regulated by the hypothalamus or some other neural pathway and nothing certain is known concerning any possible relationship between neurohypophyseal function and growth.

### *b) Actions of Stress and Corticoids at Cellular Level*

After having reviewed the neuroendocrine relationships in adaptive reactions as well as the pathways through which various stimuli may lead to increased secretion of adaptive hormones, the question arises as to how stressors and corticoids alter the susceptibility of various tissues. In this connection it is important to distinguish between *'corticotypic' and 'non-corticotypic' action of stress* because it is often difficult to establish whether the changes observed are due to some extra-adrenal mechanism elicited by stress or are simply secondary consequences of an increased corticoid secretion.

Interestingly, most of the effects of stressors are 'corticotypic' in that they increase such typical actions of corticoids as thymolysis, eosinopenia, catabolism, or the inhibition of inflammation. On the other hand, the corticoid itself fails to accentuate the actions that are typical of the particular stressor used—for example, the vasoconstriction of cold, the vasodilatation of heat, or the hypoglycemia of insulin. The mechanism through which stress thus sensitizes for corticoids has not yet been elucidated, although decreased hepatic detoxification or diminished excretion of the hormones may be involved (625). Yet conditioning by stressors is not necessarily 'corticotypic'. A clear-cut case in point is the aggravation of osteolathyrism that can be reproduced by virtually any systemic stressor. This phenomenon is even more interesting because the glucocorticoids that are produced during stress (e.g., cortisol) actually inhibit osteolathyrism, so that here stress and glucocorticoids exert opposite effects upon the development of a morbid lesion (611). Similarly, the most diverse stressors sensitize the rat for the production of convulsions by the oral administration of $NaClO_4$, although glucocorticoids (e.g., cortisol, triamcinolone) exhibit an extraordinarily pronounced protective effect against these perchlorate convulsions (41, 43).

ACTH may also exert extra-adrenal effects and consequently some of the 'non-corticotypic' actions of stress may be due to an increased ACTH secretion. For example, recently MARKS *et al.* (414) demonstrated that the renal juxtaglomerular apparatus is an extra-adrenal target of ACTH. It was observed that ACTH produces hypergranulation of the juxtaglomerular cells even in the absence of pituitary and adrenals, while absence of ACTH depletes juxtaglomerular granules. The renal effect of stressor agents (e.g., toxic doses of vasopressin and hydralazine), which usually produce hypergranulation of juxtaglomerular cells, is blocked by hypophysectomy. Thus, these findings clearly revealed that, here, ACTH mediates the responses to stress of some renal tissue.

Little is known concerning any extra-adrenal *action of stress at the cellular level,* which may explain the diverse pathologic changes observed following acute stress situations. The shock-phase of the A-R is accompanied by changes in enzyme activities in liver, heart, brain, as well as in many other organs. PACKER *et al.* (484) have demonstrated uncoupling of oxidative phosphorylation, as well as shifts in concentrations of phosphate, sodium, potassium and calcium, accompanied by swelling of mitochondria in shock states. The intracellular changes suggest that the permeability of some cells is probably changed.

Otomo and Michaelis (483) showed that following trauma the permeability of the blood-brain barrier is increased to penetration of $P^{32}$. Similar damage at the blood-brain barrier may result in increased penetration of toxic metabolites and consequently in alterations of control mechanisms governed by the central nervous system. It is also known from the observations made by Selye (589) that stress can render the gut permeable for substances present in the alimentary tract but which normally do not transverse it. Compounds such as adrenaline or histamine, which under normal conditions are only poorly adsorbed after oral ingestion, readily enter the blood stream and thus cause intoxication in guinea pigs or rats exposed to cold or muscular exercise. Recently it was claimed that soldiers suffering from various injuries in the Korean war, and therefore under considerable stress, presented an impaired water absorption from the gastro-intestinal tract (313, 314); similar observation was made in dogs submitted to acute hemorrhage (234).

As early as in 1923, thus prior to the formulation of the stress concept, it was demonstrated by McClure and Aldrich (430) that the disappearance time of intradermally injected NaCl-solution is reduced in several pathologic conditions. This procedure was even considered as a test of the 'resistance of the terrain' that may help the physician in the treatment of the patient or to determine the operability of elderly people. Such shortening of the disappearance time was seen in patients with scarlet fever and diphtheria (56, 402), lobar pneumonia (274), toxemia of pregnancy (385), cardiac diseases (481), thyrotoxicosis (454), jaundice (455) and tuberculosis (189), the extent of shortening being roughly proportional to the severity of the illness. The same modification in the rate of absorption was seen when NaCl was injected into patients in shock (380). It was shown, on the other hand, in animal experiments that physiologic saline is absorbed more quickly from the small intestine in dogs submitted to anoxic anoxia (757, 758), or after intensive bleeding (759), than in the controls. However, some other authors claimed that such intestinal water absorption is not clearly affected until the advanced stage of shock is reached (234). Experiments of Moyson and Toussaint (460) performed with phosphate salts in guinea pigs demonstrated that the stress of trauma or of visceration is able to bring a clear diminution in the intestinal absorption of these salts.

Another related and interesting question is the action of stress on carbohydrate metabolism; however, it is still uncertain how much of this is due to the increased corticoid activities. Continuous exposure of rats to certain damaging agents, such as cold, exercise, various drugs, X-rays, was shown to induce a marked increase in the hyperglycemic action of orally administered glucose (422). HOWARD (313) described a similar striking elevation in the blood sugar concentration following various types of injuries, while the same phenomenon was observed by MARKS AND BISHOP (415) in patients with neoplastic diseases. However, the results obtained by testing the absorption of glucose do not give proof of any effect of stress in this regard. In fact, when glucose absorption was determined directly in the intestine, a lowered absorptive capacity for glucose could be measured in stressed animals (132). There is presently no reason to believe that stress has any specific effect on the metabolism of carbohydrates, but rather the alterations observed are due to the excesses of glucocorticoids and adrenergic hormones.

The apparently opposite actions of stress on the absorption of certain drugs were discussed in a recent paper of MALEK AND KOLC (410) in which they also described experiments concerning the absorption of several drugs following tourniquet trauma in the rabbit. Based on the finding that under these conditions the absorption of insulin and potassium thiocyanate injected intramuscularly was decreased, while that of Congo red, dextran or microbial suspension was significantly accelerated, the authors concluded that a dissociation occurs. Certain drugs are absorbed via the blood capillaries and venous circulation, and in this case the rate of absorption is slowed down. On the other hand, the rate at which other compounds are absorbed through the lymphatic system is increased by stress. If further confirmed, this observation would be extremely important in order to understand the opposite actions of stress on the toxicity of various chemicals.

Diuresis is diminished during a severe A-R. However, pretreatment with the same or even another stressor changes the response, so that the antidiuretic effect of stress is not only blocked but sometimes even reversed. This observation was taken as evidence in support of the view that an A-R produced by one stimulus raises the resistance of the organism against both this stimulus and any other stressor agent (337).

It is well established, furthermore, that animals exhausted by chronic exposure to stressor agents are unable to dilute their blood by mobilizing the water and salt in cells and tissues for transfer to the vascular system to maintain a volume of circulating fluid compatible with life. However, these disturbances of water metabolism are mainly due to lack of sufficient amounts of cortical hormones and, in fact, these early experiments indicated the regulatory influence of the adrenal cortex over the internal distribution of water and certain electrolytes (597).

It is also still uncertain at *which level of cellular function corticoids* exert their activity, although a great deal of work has been done along these lines. In general, it seems to be likely that steroids may act by 1. altering the permeability of target cells, 2. acting as carriers in ion transport and 3. modifying specific tissue enzyme systems. Presumably, any mechanism, or a combination, may be responsible.

It has been postulated that, since the steroid molecule consists of a lipid nucleus and superimposed centers of unsaturation and oxygen functions, it would be oriented at a lipid-water interface such as the cell membrane (178). In this strategic position corticosteroids could govern intracellular biochemical activity by regulating the ingress and egress of key metabolites. The same influence could be effected at other phase boundaries within the cell structure. This hypothesis seems reasonable, since it is known that plasma protein binds these hormones and thus could carry them from the adrenal cortex to the peripheral cells, there they may compete with the intracellular nucleotide coenzymes and thus regulate the rate of enzymatic reaction. There is little question, furthermore, that the corticoids influence renal regulation of electrolyte balance and basically affect carbohydrate utilization in tissues (783).

It is, of course, not a new idea that the fundamental mechanism of hormone action at a cellular level is concerned with *regulation of the permeability processes* in target cells. In this regard, perhaps the most important was the demonstration by LEVINE and his associates (394) that insulin has a definite effect on cell permeability that appeared to be a primary action of insulin, adequate to account for most, if not all, of the physiological effects of this hormone. More recent studies of SCHWARTZ *et al.* (573) with labeled vasopressin indicated that it acts as tubular cell-receptors by -SS- interchange, probably forming two mixed hormone-receptor disulfide bridges. Such interaction could account per se for the effect of -SS- containing peptide hormones, such as insulin, oxytocin and vasopressin, on the permeability of cell membranes.

The possibility that permeability processes in the adrenal cortex might be subject to regulation by ACTH has also been considered (276). It was, in fact, demonstrated that in intact cellular preparations ACTH has effects upon cell permeability to sugars and amino acid (277). These permeability effects could account for most of the secondary consequences of ACTH administration; nevertheless, evidence exists that this hormone has metabolic effects in vitro (in preparations with altered or destroyed cellular permeability) that cannot be explained in terms of a hormone action to facilitate substrate entry into the cells. Thus, if we consider the cell membrane as the exclusive determinant of cellular permeability processes, and hormone action is also to be localized at the cell surface, it would appear to be necessary to give up the hypothesis that hormone action involves a single primary reaction with the cell. However, it is now recognized that certain enzymes are organized as multienzyme sequences, localized in semi-isolated compartments within the cell; for example, the enzymes of the tricarboxylic acid cycle and systems involved in electron transport and ATP generation are compartmentalized in the mitochondria (246). Consequently, if cell permeability is considered to encompass not only transfer across the cell surface, but also diffusion of substrate through intracellular barriers enclosing compartmentalized multienzyme sequences, the difficulty of accounting for the effects of ACTH on cell permeability disappears. This is, however, only a speculative possibility; there is no definite agreement in the literature concerning this question.

Mineralocorticoids (e.g., DOC) are well known to influence electrolyte balance in mammals, promoting sodium retention and increasing potassium excretion. These effects are generally believed to be the result of DOC action on cation transport processes in the membranes of the renal tubules. The functional complexity of the kidney make detailed analysis of the mechanism involved in DOC action extremely difficult. However, DOC action is not restricted to the kidney; a definite effect of DOC on cation distribution has been reported in a variety of in vitro systems ranging from heart muscle (263, 731) to yeasts (128). These observations raise the possibility that DOC-responsive sites involved in cation permeability may be present in cells of diverse origin. Studies of HECHTER AND LESTER (277) strongly suggest that DOC (and probably also other mineralocorticoids) acts to modify a cytoplasmic system for cation transport.

It is also known that corticoids can alter the permeability of connective tissue. Most methods for demonstrating such an effect are based on spreading reactions showing deviation from the normal spread of injected dyes or collodial materials. The effects usually demonstrated are acute and do not necessarily indicate what may occur on chronic administration of steroid hormones. For example, BAKER AND WHITAKER (54) as well as HAYNES (275), among others, have demonstrated that a single injection of cortisone has definite antipermeability effect, while a chronic administration of the same hormone increases the permeability of the ground substance. RAGAN *et al.* (505) and EKMAN *et al.* (172) demonstrated that short-term administration of cortisol results in the production of a more viscous synovial fluid. It was concluded that the increased viscosity presumably reflects a higher degree of polymerization of the mucopolysaccharides present in the connective tissue and thereby influences permeability. On the other hand, it has also been demonstrated that administration of corticoids suppresses the synthesis of mycopolysaccharides, particularly chondroitin sulfate (169). Consequently, the hypothesis was advanced that this suppression of synthesis can effect a depletion of mucopolysaccharides in connective tissues and result in enhanced permeability (576). Thus, there are various concepts supported by experimental findings concerning therole of corticoids in permeability changes, but the mechanisms involved have not yet been elucidated.

In reviewing briefly the action of corticoids on *electrolyte metabolism,* it will be recalled that $Na^+$, the principal cation of extracellular fluid, is filtered by the glomerulus and then reabsorbed by the renal tubule by means of a cation-exchange process in which $K^+$ and $H^+$ are secreted from the tubular cell to tubular urine. Hence, steroids that promote $Na^+$ retention also cause $Cl^-$ retention (to preserve electroneutrality) and increase excretion of $K^+$ and $H^+$. The net effect of a given corticoid on sodium excretion will vary directly with the degree to which it increases glomerular filtration rate (GFR) and inversely with the extent to which it enhances tubular reabsorption. Thus the naturally occurring corticosteroids, cortisone, cortisol, DOC and aldosterone, when given in large doses, increase tubular reabsorption to a greater extent than GFR and induce sodium retention and potassium loss (96). Synthetic corticoids, such as prednisone and prednisolone, on the other hand, increase GFR to a greater degree and, therefore, in small doses do not lead to the electrolyte imbalance observed with the natural steroids. When, however, a fluorine atom is added to carbon 9 of the cortisol or even to the prednisolone nucleus, the resulting compounds exercise an aldosterone-like effect on the renal tubule and cause marked retention of sodium and loss of potassium. Yet when carbon 16 of the 9α-fluoroprednisolone molecule is either hydroxylated (triamcinolone) or methylated (dexamethasone) its aldosterone-like effect on tubular reabsorption of $N^+$ is considerably, if not completely, overcome. In fact, triamcinolone may produce a slight increase in sodium excretion, apparently as a result of increased GFR (162, 166).

It is important to point out that, when given in massive doses, both the mineralocorticoids and glucocorticoids seem to exert some effect on the electrolyte metabolism. Moreover, there are observations to indicate that glucocorticoids are apparently a vital part of the mechanism which maintains the internal water and electrolyte balance of vertebrate organisms although the precise role they play in this important function is unknown. For example, it is known that stressor agents (e.g., electroshock) induce circulatory failure in fasted adrenalectomized dogs maintained on mineralocorticoid (DOC). SWINGLE *et al.* (737) observed that treatment with glucocorticoids (e.g., cortisol or triamcinolone) results, under these experimental conditions, in rapid return of normal activity and vigor accompanied by increased arterial pressure, plasma volume, and decreases in hemoconcentration. SELYE (597) also noted that although both glucocorticoids and mineralocorticoids can prolong the life of adrenalectomized animals, the former are much more effective than the latter in raising resistance to stressor agents.

Although the effect of corticoids on excretion of sodium and potassium by the kidney has been extensively studied, there is relatively little information concerning their effect on the elimination of cations via the gastrointestinal tract. BERGER *et al.* (80) showed that administration of DOC to rats or humans decreases fecal excretion of sodium, thereby indicating an increase in the gastrointestinal absorption of this cation. In their studies, an effect of DOC on potassium transfer in the gut was not conclusively shown. POUTSIAKA *et al.* (496) found, furthermore, that 9α-fluorocortisol, when given in large doses to intact dogs, results in a chronic state of polydipsia and polyuria with gross evidence of dehydration. With fluorocortisol treatment the fecal excretion of sodium was reduced and that of potassium enhanced but the converse was true for urinary excretion. The serum sodium was elevated and there was a negative potassium balance. Thus, although an atypical urinary pattern of cations was observed in these experiments, it may be considered that the effect of fluorocortisol on cation transfer in the kidney is anologous to its effect on cation transfer in the gut; with both organs functioning to lower sodium and augment potassium excretion.

The electrolyte changes observed in the blood and urine do not reflect always the actual intracellular electrolyte alterations, however, usually hypokalemia and hypernatremia ensue during acute stress situations and/or consequent to the administration of corticoids. The degree of the alteration in tissue electrolytes may vary not only according to various corticoids, but also with many other conditions. For example, while most of the stressor agents produce sodium and chloride retention and accordingly result in alterations of the extra- and intracellular ion components, exposure to cold results in marked sodium retention, without concomitant chloride retention (55). In rats, injected with cortisone, regardless of the sodium content of the diet, a severe potassium depletion was observed in various tissues, however this was not accompanied by significant alterations in intracellular sodium. Under similar experimental conditions the administration of DOC resulted in impressive increase in sodium as well as significant decrease in potassium of tissues (361, 126). In another series of experiments by the same experimenter, analyses of skeletal muscle from adrenalectomized rats given cortisone in amounts sufficient to induce severe hypertension revealed no impressive alterations in sodium or potassium content. In contrast, skeletal muscle from adrenalectomized rats given comparable amounts of DOC and with comparable degrees of hypertension showed marked increase in sodium and reduction in potassium content. According to WOODBURY AND KOCH (788) aldosterone appears to be capable of enhancing electrolyte transport in all tissues, while DOC is devoid of direct effect on muscular tissue. Thus the changes in muscle electrolyte composition which are observed following DOC administration would be the passive result of actions of this steroid at other sites.

It is now also clear that many factors other than the rate of secretion by the adrenals determine both the peripheral blood level and cellular action of corticoids. The *role of the liver* should be especially stressed, since hepatic steroid inactivation is a main factor in the regulation of adrenal function. Increased thyroid activity, for example, accelerates the rate of reduction of the steroids by the liver and hence indirectly may cause adrenal hypertrophy (572). Such secondary conditioning influence of organs may result in fundamental alterations of bodily reactions. The ameliorating effect of hepatitis and pregnancy on certain diseases well illustrates this.

As known, during pregnancy there often occurs a suppression of the manifestations of a number of diseases. This effect has been noted in migraine, asthma, angioneurotic edema, primary fibrositis, intermittent hydrarthrosis, psoriatic arthritis, rheumatoid arthritis and rheumatoid spondylitis. A similar suppressive effect in rheumatoid arthritis and several others of the diseases listed may occur in the course of hepatitis and jaundice (293). In fact, these suppressive effects of both pregnancy and jaundice were the basis from which HENCH (284, 286) successfully reasoned his way to the discovery of the anti-rheumatic action of cortisone. Although the mechanism of the beneficial effect of pregnancy on the rheumatic diseases is not entirely solved, careful studies on the metabolism of corticoids in patients with liver disease have revealed subnormal levels of conjugated 17-hydroxycorticosteroids in the blood, and a delay in the removal of cortisol but not of tetrahydrocortisol from the plasma (93). Thus, the apparent impairment of 17-hydroxycorticosteroid conjugation in patients with liver disease was not observed following the infusion of tetrahydrocortisol. It appears, therefore, that there is no detectible impairment of glucuronide conjugation, provided the proper substrate for conjugation is supplied. The delay is in the enzymatic transformation of cortisol to reduce 17-hydroxycorticosteroids, which are then readily conjugated (180). As the non-reduced hormones are active biologically, whereas the reduced forms are inactive, it is possible that this might explain, in part, the anti-rheumatic effect of liver disease.

That stress may alter the pathway of intermediary metabolism of cortisol has been suspected for a long time. Evidence that patients with liver disease metabolize this hormone abnormally (357) might be directly applicable to many individuals with serious injury such as war wounds, multiple fractures, burns, and hemorrhagic shock, in all of which alteration of liver function is readily demonstrable. Clear experimental demonstration that stress alters the intermediary metabolism of corticoids was presented by STEENBURG AND GANONG (723). These authors showed that the adrenalectomized dog undergoing trauma on a constant dose of hormone has a higher rise in the free hormone than does the untraumatized control, and that the post-surgical patient has a markedly increased level of corticoids in response to a standard ACTH infusion. Another piece of evidence is that reported by GOLD *et al.* (233) showing that the ratio of tetrahydrocortisone to tetrahydro-hydrocortisone in the urine, as separated by paper chromatography, is altered after trauma. Finally, evidence was provided by SANDBERG *et al.* (549) who found an increased blood level of 17-hydroxycorticosteroids following standard cortisol infusion in stress situations.

It would be, of course, impossible to analyze separately each of the factors that possibly alter the synthesis and metabolism of corticoids, or even to enumerate simply the experimental findings showing the great many alterations in metabolic, enzymatic and other vital activities, consequent to stressful experiences and/or administration of corticoids. However, the basic question still remained to be answered: *'how do stress and corticoids act at cellular level'*; how may one explain the physiologic and pathologic effects of these agents in the light of the modern concepts of cellular function? On the basis of the shortly summarized observations as well as by considering the fundamental work of SZENTGYÖRGYI (738, 740), FLECKENSTEIN (198) and LABORIT (379) and their groups on cellular function, the following hypothesis may be advanced:

The pituitary-adrenal axis is activated by any stressor stimulus either external or internal in origin. We can understand the physiologic role of stress only if we accept the view that the reason for this endocrine mobilization (which takes place at the expense of all regulatory and metabolic functions intended for anabolic purposes and therefore momentarily only of secondary importance for survival purposes), is a release of energy by some specialized cell groups in order to permit struggle or defense. These cell groups, to be able to release the amount of energy needed for this complex response to stress, will require that sodium penetrate into them, and carbohydrates insure their metabolic supply following the rapid exhaustion of the reserves. The adrenal corticoids, in view of the sodium retention and the gluconeogenesis which they bring about, make this response possible. The fact that the gluconeogenesis is the mean biochemical process which must be controlled by the pituitary-adrenal axis during stress was repeatedly confirmed in experiments, this axis remaining at rest following exposure to stressor agents if a massive supply of glucose is given (177). On the other hand, it was demonstrated also in in vitro experiments that any stimulation of an excitable structure is accompanied by a penetration of sodium into the cell and migration of potassium toward the extracellular space.

Thus, we have arrived at a point where it may be stated that the endocrine glands, whose functional state depends on environmental stimuli but are governed by neurohumoral control, are capable, in turn, of regulating the functions of some tissues and organs by their direct influence on cellular metabolism. Namely, it seems that in final analysis the metabolic rate of cells is controlled by an ionic concentration ratio between the intracellular and extracellular space. On the other hand, the degree of intensity of cell metabolism is related to the variations in cell membrane permeability. Consequently, it is only a secondary question whether the corticoids act directly on the cell membrane or indirectly alter the membrane potential through influencing ionic balance: at any rate, they can basically influence the metabolism of cells, tissues and organs.

But how does this same cellular function become harmful? We have seen that when the organism is called upon to release more energy following exposure to stress, the means which it brings into play (e.g., increased secretion of corticoids) appear to achieve this objective by a process identical to that observed on the isolated organ, namely an entry of sodium and an outward migration of potassium. Now, the restoration shifts of ions (re-entry of potassium and sodium elimination) again require energy. When there is sufficient supply of glucose, the normal metabolic processes within the cell insure the constant ejection of sodium and re-entry of potassium which are essential to the maintenance of a differential ionic concentration between the cell and the interstitial space, in other words, to the maintenance of normal membrane permeability. During severe stress, however, the carbohydrate reserves are quickly destroyed. Consequently, the energy will be not sufficient to keep the restorative metabolic function activated. New biochemical mechanisms come into play; gluconeogenesis occurs at the expense of proteins, creating a nitrogen catabolism. Schematically, this metabolic function leads to the increased release of $H^+$ ions at the end of the oxidation-reduction chains. The ratio between the intracellular and extracellular $H^+$ion concentration will be reduced as well as the membrane permeability further increased. This will result in continuous migration (instead of re-entry) of potassium from the cell while sodium penetrates into it (instead of the necessary outward migration). Finally as the result of the electrolyte imbalance, the death of the cell ensues.

## V. Conditioning as Applied to Cardiovascular Pathology: Stimuli Influencing the Resistance of the Heart Muscle

It was pointed out on the previous pages that certain agents produce disease under any circumstances. The effect of such primary pathogens does not depend upon a special condition of the organism. On the other hand, it was shown previously that potential pathogenic agents produce disease only under conditioning influences. In applying this categorization to cardiovascular pathology, one finds only very few agents or conditions that invariably produce cardiovascular lesions in man or animals. Reports of clinical cases as well as the variable results obtained in animal experiments suggest that most of the cardiotoxic agents are potential pathogens, whose cardiotoxic effect most likely depend upon conditioning factors capable of sensitizing the elements of the cardiovascular system.

*Primary cardiotoxic agents and conditions.*—It was observed by HICKS (291) and WACHSTEIN AND MEISEL (765) that multiple myocardial necroses occur in rats treated with high doses of *plasmocid* (a rather toxic and now obsolete antimalarial). The necrotizing effect of plasmocid upon the heart seems to be independent of conditioning factors, since under normal conditions necroses always ensue when the doses given are large enough. Thus, based on these observations, plasmocid would be a classical example of a primary cardiotoxic agent. However, the investigations described in this monograph as well as the findings already published earlier revealed that even the action of this presumably primary pathogen can be modified by dietary means (44, 48, 639, 642, 644), stressors (641, 659), pregnancy (663) and corticoids (660).

Extensive focal myocardial necroses can be produced in various experimental animals by a single intravenous injection of certain proteolytic enzymes, particularly *papain,* trypsin, ficin and crude streptokinase (346, 347, 485). It is generally believed—although not definitely proven—that proteolytic enzymes, such as papain, produce necroses by acting directly upon the tissue proteins. However, as will be seen in more detail later, our experiments do not support the assumption that papain would be an unconditionally acting pathogen. For example, when rats are restrained for 17 hours, just prior to the intravenous injection of an otherwise fatal dose of papain, they not only survive, but their cardiac muscle shows an almost complete resistance to the necrosis-producing effect of this proteolytic enzyme (48). On the other hand, if a stressor such as noradrenaline is given or forced restraint is applied concurrently rather than prior to the papain injection, the cardiac lesions are greatly aggravated (26, 641).

It was also observed by several investigators that large doses of *cardiac glycosides* and their aglycones produce cardiac necroses in animals (368, 387, 396). There is no uniformity of opinion regarding the mechanism through which cardiac glycosides produce morphologic changes in the heart. However, during the last years it has become evident that the actions of digitalis are intimately associated with the intracellular concentration of potassium ions (377). Thus, one would expect that digitalis produces cardiac lesions through direct metabolic effects. Yet, recently it was recognized that the toxic actions of cardiac glycosides (e.g., digitoxin, digitalis) can be greatly aggravated by the concurrent administration of thyroxin (149) and $NaH_2PO_4$, and prevented by KCl, $MgCl_2$ (437) and aminophylline (375). It may be concluded, therefore, that cardiac glycosides are also rather potentially cardiotoxic agents than unconditionally acting pathogens.

Myocardial lesions have been noted in experimentally produced *potassium deficiency* in animals (205, 215, 367, 406); similar cardiac changes have been found in humans dying from conditions associated with potassium deficiency (236, 348, 423). The earliest changes consist of swelling and loss of striations of muscle fibers. The fibers gradually become necrotic and finally disappear, leaving the containing sarcolemma. Associated with these changes there is an immigration of leukocytes into the area of necrosis. A deficit of body potassium is apparently essential for the production of the cardiac necrosis. Potassium is the major intracellular cation, and, as such, plays a key role in the interrelationships between cell structure and function. It is, therefore, not surprising that a deficit of this mineral is accompanied by alterations in cellular activity and anatomic integrity. Although there are multiple structural alterations in the various organs (kidney, liver, skeletal muscle, etc.) of potassium deficient animals, it is generally believed that the cardiac lesions are not secondary consequences of the functional and structural abnormalities observed in other organs (776).

Yet, it was early recognized that this type of cardiopathy may also be influenced in its development. For example, FOLLIS (263) observed that the cardiac lesions are much more extensive in potassium-depleted rats which are violently exercised. Other features of the potassium-deficiency syndrome were not aggravated; no changes were observed in the voluntary muscles. This is even more interesting, since the potassium content of the muscles of potassium deficient animals is lowered and it would be expected that exercise, by causing a further reduction of this cation, might lead to necroses not only in the heart but also in voluntary muscles. The experiments of FOLLIS indicate that the aggravation of the cardiac lesions by exercise cannot be explained so simply. It has been stated by CANNON *et al.* (103) that the addition of sodium to the diet enhances the severity of cardiac necroses. Although this effect was attributed to an increased sodium content of the cells, it might simply be the consequence of a more intense deficit of potassium due to sodium load. PERDUE AND PHILLIPS (492) observed that a potassium deficient diet with a 20% content of corn oil induces more marked cardiac lesions than a diet with only 5% oil. MORRISON (459) observed that subtotal nephrectomy aggravates the cardiac necrosis normally produced by potassium deficient diet. Many additional examples will be presented during the description of our own experiments that the development of potassium-deficiency cardiopathy can be significantly influenced (enhanced or prevented) by treatment with electrolytes, exposure to stressor agents, etc.

The cardiac manifestations of other dietary deficiencies are also influenced by various agents: the choline-deficiency cardiopathy is greatly enhanced by STH (780), the cardiac necrosis due to magnesium deficiency is aggravated by corticoids, dihydrotachysterol and certain Na-salts (448).

*Secondary or indirectly acting cardiotoxic agents.*—Interstitial myocarditis with focal myocardial necroses and calcification has been observed after treatment with various *sulfonamide compounds,* such as sulfaguanidine, sulfathiazole and Na-acetylsulfathiazole (14, 214, 392). It seems from the investigations of LEHR (391) that sulfonamide drugs are secondary cardiotoxic agents, since the cardiac damage is a secondary consequence of renal injury. However, the parathyroid and the adrenals also participate in the complex mechanism through which these nephrotoxic compounds elicit cardiac damage. The hyperfunction of the parathyroid is a consequence of the breakdown of renal function rather than stimulation by toxic substances released by the damaged kidney; it could be idunced not only with sulfonamides, but also by bilateral nephrectomy. According to this hypothesis an excess of parathyroid hormone would be primarily responsible for the cardiac lesions. SELYE (628) recently reviewed his extensive work on uremic cardiopathies and by discussing earlier findings he pointed out that it is important to distinguish clearly between: 1. the calcifying parathyroid type of cardiopathy, and 2. the miliary myocardial necroses and myocarditis. Both can be elicited by either nephrectomy or sulfa drugs, but the two types of changes do not necessarily run parallel and only the former is prevented by parathyroidectomy. Therefore, he feels that the parathyroids are not the only ultimate pathway through which renal deficiency produces cardiovascular lesions, although they are indispensable for the calcification.

It is well known that there is a causal relationship between arteriosclerosis and occurrence of cardiac necrosis; spontaneous infarcts tend to develop with the greatest frequency in middle-aged or older men, in whom some degree of coronary sclerosis has already developed (790). Consequently, *agents influencing the onset of arteriosclerosis* may be regarded as secondary predisposing factors for cardiac necroses. Supporting this view, we note that experimental observations also revealed that 'artificial aging' of the arterial system greatly sensitizes the heart to the necrotizing effect of subsequent treatment with electrolytes and corticoids (617). Rats were pretreated with dihydrotachysterol (DHT), during 10 days, so as to produce Mönckeberg-sclerosis of the coronary arteries. After this, no further treatment was given until all the animals had recovered, as judged by their growth and clinical appearance. Then, a combined electrolyte-steroid treatment was initiated (Me-Cl-COL + $NaH_2PO_4$) at a dose level that, in non-pretreated animals, caused only occasional microscopic foci of myocardial necrosis. It was found that, in the DHT-pretreated rat, this dose level of Me-Cl-COL + $NaH_2PO_4$ produces particularly extensive, macroscopically visible patches of necrosis throughout the heart. It was, furthermore, quite unexpectedly noted that after sensitization with DHT, intense, proliferative, and eventually obstructive changes develop in all part of the coronary tree during the electrolyte-steroid treatment.

Subsequent experiments showed that the development of the DHT-sclerosis is basically influenced by a great variety of external and internal conditioning factors, some of which are also known to affect myocardial metabolism (e.g., corticoids, electrolytes, stress). SELYE (613, 628) recently extensively discussed the problems of experimental atherosclerosis and the work performed in this Institute, so we will enumerate only some additional data showing the multiplicity of possible interactions in this regard.

The conditioning action of the neuroendocrine system apparently bears some relationship to development of arteriosclerosis and related cardiovascular diseases (538, 712, 755, 777). MYASNIKOV (465) found evidence in rabbits that drugs acting directly upon the central nervous system exert a modifying influence on serum cholesterol and on the development of atherosclerosis. RAAB (502) recently reviewed literature showing relationship of neurohormones (e.g., adrenaline and noradrenaline) to atherogenesis, while SCHAPIRO AND MARMORSTON (564) demonstrated that dogs maintained on an atherogenic diet exhibit greater responses to stress produced by electric shock or by cold than the normal-diet fed controls, as measured by corticoid output. MCALLISTER *et al.* (424) observed, furthermore, that the elevation of serum cholesterol values and atherosclerosis are apparently intensified by intense muscular exercise in dogs fed cholesterol and thiouracil. Of 10 dogs fed a supplemented ration for about fifteen months, 5 were made to run five miles daily on a treadmill. The controls were allowed virtually no exercise. For the exercised dogs, average cholesterol concentrations were significantly higher. Extensive atherosclerotic lesions, especially in the terminal aorta and iliac and femoral vessels, were noted in specimens dissected from these exercised animals. In some, the coronary arteries were also affected. Only slight atherosclerosis was observed in vessels from controls. It seems that excessive overexertion can condition for potentially angiotoxic agents, and RAAB (501) postulated that intense exercise as well as other stressor stimuli may likewise upset the neurovegetative adrenergic-cholinergic balance in cardiovascular tissue metabolism by promoting a local overaction of catecholamines.

These experimental observations tending to implicate the neuroendocrine system in cardiovascular pathology are supported by statistical data which suggest a higher incidence of arteriosclerosis in social and occupational situations involving greater mental tensions, responsibilities, anxieties and frustrations (Lit.: RAAB [501, 502]). However, such clinical observations cannot be evalutated simply on the basis of psychic stress alone without consideration of other interfering factors, e.g., physical activity or inactivity, respectively. The importance of local unspecific reactions affecting the vascular system was suggested by animal experiments (712) and by observations concerning a limitation of arteriosclerotic lesions to extremities that had performed strenuous work over long periods of time (364, 374). An asymmetrical development of arterial tickening in the radial arteries has been ascribed to right- and left-handedness respectively, and in persons who did a great deal of stair climbing a significantly higher incidence of peripheral arteriosclerosis was claimed to exist by comparison with non-stair climbers (382).

Numerous investigators have shown, furthermore, that stressful life experiments are capable of evoking hypercholesterolemia also in man. Several workers have studied the serum concentration of cholesterol and lipids in students before, during and after the stress of examinations. All of them, including THOMAS AND MURPHY (740), WESTLAKE *et al.* (777), GRUNDY AND GRIFFIN (256) as well as DREYFUSS AND CZACZKES (161), found higher values during the stressful periods than otherwise. DREYFUSS and his associate also measured the clotting time and found it accelerated in 36 medical students the morning of an examination. The studies of FRIEDMAN AND ROSENMAN (218, 219) have given evidence that the lipid regulating mechanisms are responsive to situational stresses. The authors found higher serum cholesterol concentrations, a far greater incidence of arcus senilis and a vastly increased incidence of coronary artery diseases in subjects classified as oriented toward competitive activities with deadlines, as compared with anxious but noncompetitive people or with more passive subjects. RUSSEK (542) reported similar findings among coronary patients, while DREYFUSS (160) and WEISS *et al.* (772) observed special situational stresses as antecedent events to episodes of coronary occlusion. On the other hand, the large statistics of MORRIS (458) and LUONGO (404) concerning coronary morbidity and cardiac deaths among different occupational groups provided an impressive argument in favor of an anti-atherogenic efficacy of steady moderate exercise.

Of course, the possibility that any such conditioning actions are actually related to the mechanisms of atherosclerosis is mostly speculative. Moreover, it should be kept in mind that not only are the mechanisms regulating the concentration of serum lipids and cholesterol unknown at present, but the significance of the relation of serum concentration of these substances to integrity of arteries is equally obscure. Indeed, the extent to which the presence of atherosclerosis determines vascular accidents is also uncertain.

*Potential cardiotoxic agents.*—Among the great variety of potentially cardiotoxic agents, *corticoids, electrolytes and stress* appear to be the most common factors in the pathogenesis of necrotizing cardiopathies.

Recent experimental observations (613) showed that among 49 steroids tested as regards their cardiotoxicity, DOC, cortisol and halocorticoids are particularly active in sensitizing the heart for the production of cardiac necroses with certain Na-salts (especially $NaH_2PO_4$, $Na_2SO_4$ and $NaClO_4$). The administration of a combination of both mineralo- and glucocorticoid substances, or of a single compound possessing both these activities (e.g., Me-Cl-COL) is extremely effective in producing an electrolyte-steroid-cardiopathy characterized by necroses (ESCN), as well as sensitizing the heart to a great variety of essentially different agents. For example, after pretreatment with Me-Cl-COL, pentamethylentetrazol, Na-fluoroacetate, and diisopropylfluorophosphate all consistently elicited cardiac necroses in the rat, although neither these compounds nor the steroid showed any cardiotoxic properties when given alone (635). It was observed, furthermore, that among the halogenated corticoids tested, only triamcinolone (a pure glucocorticoid) failed to condition the cardiac muscle to the toxic effect of Na-salts. On the other hand, however, this synthetic hormone was found to be especially active in the production of 'spotty myolysis', when given simultaneously with noradrenaline to intact or adrenalectomized animals (646).

Investigations dealing with the participation of electrolytes in the production of cardiopathies give a number of interesting results. Like Me-Cl-COL, $NaH_2PO_4$ greatly predisposes the cardiac muscle to the necrotizing effects of proteolytic enzymes (e.g., papain, ficin) as well as to that of arsphenamine, while the cardiotoxic actions of other agents (noradrenaline, vasopressin) are not significantly influenced by this electrolyte (613, 633, 645). Only certain Na-salts (phosphates, sulfates, sulfites and perchlorate) were effective in inducing an ESCN; therefore it was concluded that both the anion and the cation are important factors in the pathogenesis of this type of experimental cardiac disease. It was also noted that the same steroid can predispose the rat for the production of qualitatively dissimilar cardiac lesions, but different electrolytes are necessary to elicit one or another type of change. For example, administration of $NaH_2PO_4$ or Ca-acetate can alter the calcifying and slight necrotizing actions of DHT, so that a suppurative, acute myocarditis results. While the concurrent administration of DOC + $Na_2HPO_4$ produces large patches of infarctlike necroses (ESCN) in the rat, the same steroid when given with NaCl elicits quite a different type of lesion: instead of necroses, a typical hyalinizing myocarditis (ESCH) occurs (for lit. see: 613, 628).

It is especially interesting that NaCl—which usually exerts a definite, though mild, desensitizing effect upon the production of an ESCN—greatly augments the sensitivity of the heart to the production of necroses by stressor agents, such as forced restraint (42, 638). It is important to note here, that simple exposure to stress in the absence of any special conditioning factors only occasionally produces cardiac lesions in animals. Usually small, scattered necroses of individual muscle fibers are seen in histologic sections of hearts in such animals. Disseminated necrosis (or at least fuchsinophilic degeneration) of individual muscle fibers is more common and the occasional formation of minute foci of necroses in the myocardium appears to be merely a somewhat more advanced stage of the same phenomenon. The miliary necroses produced with a number of different agents by various authors (e.g., adrenaline, vasopressin, thyroxin, acetylcholine, dinitrophenol, malononitrile) may well depend upon the simple stressor, rather than the specific, actions of such pathogens (613, 628). On the other hand, it will be shown later by some original experiments that adaptation to stress can even protect the animals against the most diverse cardiotoxic agents.

It is obvious, therefore, from the previous pages that stress can affect the heart through 1. the excessive production of corticoids (as well as of adrenergic hormones) and 2. extra-adrenal neural pathways.

Only few conclusive studies have been carried out on the *direct effects of corticoids* upon isolated cardiac tissue. The first report intimating that the secretion from the adrenal cortex directly affected cardiac behavior was published in 1926 by ROGOFF AND STEWART (533) who noted a diminution in heart rate due to adrenal insufficiency. With the availability of cortisone and its use as therapeutic agent, reports were published by HENCH *et al.* (285), PERERA *et al.* (491), SOMERVILLE (716) and others, describing a return to normal in the electrocardiogram (ECG) of patients being treated with cortisone for adrenal insufficiency. On the other hand, the first observation showing that organic cardiovascular lesions can be regularly produced by DOC was published by SELYE as early as 1940 (591).

In 1951, ABRAMS AND HARRIS (2) reported ECG changes in rabbits following the administration of cortisone, and concluded that this was the result of a direct action upon the heart. Later HOFFMANN (302) perfused isolated guinea pig and frog hearts with cortisone and observed that with low concentrations (1 to 10 μg/ml) a positive inotropic action. This finding was confirmed by EMELE AND BONNYCASTLE (175) using the hypodynamic cat papillary preparation. In reports of other workers, however, only a negative inotropic action is mentioned as elicited by cortisone on the rabbit Langendorff preparation (89, 102, 696). Apparently, this can be explained by the high doses employed because LACROIX AND LEUSEN (381) reported a depression in myocardial oxygen consumption following large doses of cortisone.

The result of TANZ (742) may be quoted as evidence of the protective or normalizing action of small amounts of cortisone on the whole isolated cat heart preparation and histological preservation on the papillary muscle preparation. This action is not surprising in view of the fact that adrenal insufficiency is often characterized by cardiac impairment. Moreover, the protective action of certain glucocorticoids on skeletal muscle has been demonstrated by BAJUSZ AND SELYE (43), and NASMYTH (469) was able to show that a perfusion of 0.1 μg/ml of corticosterone through isolated rat hearts (taken from animals that had been adrenalectomized 72 hours previously) causes a slight increase in the amplitude of contractions. SOLOMON *et al.* (714) demonstrated, furthermore, that the addition of corticosterone to the heart-lung preparation of adrenalectomized rats restored cardiac work capacity. Several studies on dogs also showed this 'normalizing' ability of glucocorticoids on the heart. For instance, NAHAS (466) observed that the administration of cortisol will prevent the onset of acute acidotic heart failure and CROSSFIELD and co-workers (135), using adrenalectomized dogs, have been able to demonstrate the disappearance of asystoles following the injection of certain glucocorticoids.

These results tend to support the belief that certain naturally occurring corticoids (especially glucocorticoids) are necessary for normal cardiac function by virtue of a direct effect upon the myocardium.

As another important characteristic of corticoids it may be considered their possible dual actions. This is suggested by TANZ (743) who showed that small doses (1 μg/ml) of cortisone tend to restore the amplitude of contractions to control levels in the isolated heart preparation, while 'toxic' doses (40 μg/ml) often result in abnormal contractile pattern. According to experimental observations of BAJUSZ (28–31) cortisol exerts somewhat similar dual action on peripheral nerve regeneration and on the development of muscle atrophy. These experiments indicated that the beneficial or adverse effect of cortisol administration is largely dependent on the amounts injected daily. A dose level of cortisol was demonstrated to significantly facilitate the recovery of sensory and motor function, and through enhancement of the nerve regeneration, to beneficially alter the final degree of muscle atrophy. Compared with this therapeutically active dose, smaller quantities proved to be ineffective, while a larger dose even exerted an opposite effect (i.e., it delayed the rate of recovery of nerve function and subsequently increased the degree of atrophy in the triceps surae muscle). Dual conditioning actions of hormones other than corticoids are also known. For example, in sub-totally pancreatectomized rats, early treatment with estrogens produces a biphasic effect: the incidence and severity of diabetes is first increased, but later reduced or even definitely suppressed. In alloxan-diabetic rats, prolonged estradiol administration may result in a similar effect, in that the diabetes is first intensified but subsequently suppressed. Thus, these and other experiments revealed that estrogens can either exacerbate or ameliorate diabetes (Lit.: DANOWSKI [143]). Small amounts of these hormones aggravate diabetes, while the administration of larger doses may decrease hyperglycemia and insulin needs. The mechanism of this dual action of estrogens in obscure. The protective action is probably due to stimulation of beta cell growth in the islets of Langerhans and consequently to increased insulin production.

Such dual actions of hormones may have a basically important role in the variability of results obtained at different laboratories and in different sizes of animals. It may explain, furthermore, why some investigators obtained beneficial results from the administration of corticoids to patients with cardiac disease (e.g., cardiac infarcts), while others were unable to confirm these findings (Lit.: KAISER [334]). Studies on the cardiotonic activity of a highly active synthetic corticoid, fluorocortisol, in a concentration of 0.5–1.0 μg/ml result in a positive inotropic action, an increased uptake of intracellular sodium and loss of potassium. In a concentration of 10–20 μg/ml, fluorocortisol gives rise to a negative inotropic action, loss of intracellular sodium and increased uptake of potassium. Small doses of fluorocortisol result in partial recovery of failing heart preparations, while larger doses added to the 'normally' functioning heart bring about failure quite rapidly. This latter functional alteration was found to be accompanied by morphologic abnormalities (743).

There are observations indicating that some extra-adrenal, presumably *neural pathways* also participate in the mechanism through which various stressors elicit cardiac necroses in the suitably conditioned animals. In rats treated with $NaH_2PO_4$ and maintained on small amounts of corticoids after adrenalectomy, stressor agents elicit cardiac necroses just as in intact animals (686). It was also noted that the fatal cardiac damage which normally ensues in the fluorocortisol + Na-acetate-sensitized animals upon exposure to stressors (e g., restraint, noradrenaline, bone fracture) is prevented by a single dose of chlorpromazine and cyamepromazine injected just before exposure to stress. In these experiments continuous anesthesia with Nembutal protected only against the cardiac necrosis-eliciting effect of restraint, but not against that of noradrenaline and bone fracture. These findings were interpreted to imply that the phenothiazine compounds block some common, presumably neural pathways, through which various stressors elicit cardiac lesion (52).

It is well known that stressful physical and emotional stimuli may alter cardiovascular function. Briefly, expected changes include temporary tachycardia and increase in the cardiac output with each beat (stroke volume), followed by return to resting levels at a rate depending upon the intensity of the stimulus (e.g., amount of exercise). In healthy subjects, changes in the pattern of the ECG do not ordinarily occur from the influence of moderately acting stressors; when they do, they are thought to indicate a degree of cardiac insufficiency and a reduction of the reserve capacity of the heart (786). HICKAM *et al.* (290) established that variations in stroke volume and cardiac output correspond to changes in emotional stresses. STEVENSON *et al.* (727) related them to some of the symptoms of neurocirculatory asthenia. The possible importance of such alterations in cardiac function to patients with already damaged hearts has not been assessed.

Arrhythmias, including paroxysmal atrial tachycardia, extrasystoles, atrial fibrillation, and even the more serious paroxysmal ventricular tachycardia may occur in association with stress of individuals who have no other detectable evidence of heart disease (787). Ordinarily, when there are changes in the pattern of the ECG during stressful situations, the assumption is made that there is a disturbance of cardiac nutrition. In the study of STEVENSON *et al.* (728), 19 patients displayed changes in S-T segments or T waves to a degree considered significant, when exercise was performed during a period of stress. The same exercise on a day of relative security and relaxation produced less change in the ECG, or none at all. In all but one of the 19, it was possible to produce ECG changes during an interview covering pertinent personal problems and without exercise or conscious anticipation of muscular effort. This information is in keeping with the general concept that man and animal during stress may react with his cardiovascular apparatus as if he were about to engage in strenuous muscular activity without any actual awareness of anticipating exercise (167). Although the functional changes may be quickly reversible, the possibility that repeated or sustained stress situations may lead to irreversible changes must be taken in consideration (785). The question, whether or not these functional abnormalities resulting from stress contribute to the development of morphologic lesions of the heart muscle, cannot be answered, however, on the basis of the data in hand.

Information as to precisely what circulatory patterns and cardiac activities are subject to influence from neural centers—which neural pathways also participate in adaptation reactions in general—is still only fragmentary, but it tends to indicate that the cerebral cortex and the hypothalamus must be considered along with the pituitary and adrenal glands as potentially controlling cardiovascular responses (60). The influence of the cerebral cortex upon the cardiovascular system is documented by anatomical, physiological and psychological data. The cortical areas that control cardiac activities are located in the anterior half of the brain and include the tip of the frontal lobe, the orbital cortex, the motor and premotor cortex, the anterior part of the temporal lobe, the insula and the cingulate gyrus (151). Above the medulla oblongata, the region which appears to be more concerned with cardiovascular control than any other is the hypothalamus. The great number of evidence which supports this statement had its origin in the work of KARPLUS AND KREIDL (338). In spite of the considerable amount of work done in this field, the physiology of the hypothalamic areas which influence cardiovascular function is rather obscure. For example, according to the views adopted by GELLHORN (230) the hypothalamus can be functionally divided into a rostal 'parasympathetic' portion and a caudal 'sympathetic' area. Others, however, claim that such distinction cannot be made and there is a complex hypothalamic mechanism of cardiac control that goes into action during the display of agressive or defensive behavior (Lit.: BARD [60]). Obviously much more work is needed in order to understand the role of the nervous system in the cardiovascular adjustment reactions activated by emotional and physical stresses.

In *summary* it may be simply stated that the participation of higher neural structures in adaptive cardiovascular regulation is suggested by the following observations:

1. cardiovascular changes result from anticipation of exercise, of eating or of an emotional situation (711);

2. experimentally induced cardiovascular changes, such as those following injection of adrenaline and noradrenaline, do not mimic cardiovascular changes typical of stress (59);

3. the latency of the cardiovascular response to stress is too short to result from hormonal mechanism (200).

Unfortunately, no data are available as yet concerning the conditioning influence of such nervous mechanisms upon the development of necrotizing cardiopathies.

Having discussed the participation of stress in the pathogenesis of cardiopathies we note that another interesting example of conditioning was established during studies on the cardiovascular effects of *nicotine* and smoking. Ever since FAVAGER in 1887 (188) claimed that excessive tobacco smoking produced coronary constriction which, repeated over many years, gradually resulted in organic heart disease, nicotine has been considered an important cause of coronary heart disease. This view has been generally maintained, especially by German authors (Lit.: AHN [3]), but also American investigators presented evidence suggesting that intensive smoking could account for certain clinical syndromes, including extrasystoles, tachycardia and angina pectoris (269). Hence, several clinicians considered tobacco smoking to be a direct precipitating cause of myocardial infarction.

However, experimental findings failed to support the concept that nicotine administration or cigarette smoke inhalation causes coronary artery constriction in the normal heart. Moreover, it was adequately demonstrated that cigarette smoke inhalation by the healthy person results in a significantly increased coronary blood flow with no significant change in myocardial substrate or oxygen utilization (61). An increase in coronary blood flow following administration of nicotine has also been observed in the intact dog (349, 565), in the heart-lung preparation (412), and the isolated perfused rabbit heart (386).

Some explanation of the discrepancies between the clinical and experimental findings was offered by the observation of RINZER *et al.* (523). These authors showed that while nicotine causes an increase in coronary flow in the normal heart, it produces a marked diminution of coronary flow in the atherosclerotic heart. Similar observations were described also by BELLET and his associates (76). In these experiments, following the production of coronary insufficiency by coronary artery ligation and narrowing of the lumen of the coronary arteries, the pattern of response of the coronary blood flow was significantly different from than that observed in the normal dog, following nicotine administration. Tobacco smoke on dogs with coronary insufficiency showed effects that were similar to those of exposure to stress. More precisely, the findings obtained in the electrocardiogram, namely RT segment elevation and the production of ectopic rhythm, were similar to those that are observed in the experimental animal and in the human subject resulting from emotional stress and/or exercise in the presence of coronary insufficiency. Thus, when the ability of the coronary arteries to compensate for an increased workload is impaired, such as in the atherosclerotic heart, or in the heart with ligated coronary arteries, administration of cigarette smoke or nicotine elicits on adverse change in the dynamics and in the electrical activity of the myocardium. In other words, vasculatory deficiencies condition the effect of nicotine upon the heart muscle in an adverse way.

It is probable that the conditioning interactions described are even more complex, since it is known that the cardiovascular response to nicotine is due, at least partially, to the liberation of adrenergic hormones (139). Van Slyke and Larson (760) have clearly shown that the pressor response to nicotine in dogs is significantly reduced after adrenalectomy. It is also well established that ordinary doses of cigarette smoke can liberate antidiuretic hormone from the posterior pituitary, presumably by activation of the supraoptico-hypothalamic system (127). Adrenaline, vasopressin and corticoids may all serve as sensitizing or desensitizing agents to the vascular effects of smoking. Thus, differences in the reactivity of the hypothalamo-hypophyseal-adrenal system may be a main factor that determines the varying reactions to smoking found even in healthy individuals (747).

It is interesting to note that production of coronary insufficiency may alter the response of the heart not only to nicotine, but also to other potentially cardiotoxic compounds. For example, in rats, following occlusion of the left coronary artery near its origin, the myocardium outside the resulting infarct becomes unusually resistant to the production of diffuse cardiac necroses by isoproterenol (694). The mechanism of this protection is unknown. Perhaps, when in the state of compensatory hypertrophy (such as occurs after infarction), the cardiac muscle becomes insensitive to toxic actions of isoproterenol. On the other hand, the resistance may also be due to hemodynamic changes within the myocardium and its vessels, or to absorption of chemical compounds from the infarcted muscle.

*Miscellaneous agents and conditions.*—Notoriously, there are agents or conditions that are difficult to fit into either of the previous categories in a satisfactory manner, mainly because of our inadequate knowledge on their cardiotoxic actions. For example, there are currently two major theories regarding the role of *factors that provoke cardiac changes characteristic of rheumatic fever.* These hypotheses relate the disease either to a hypersensitivity mechanism or to direct action of biologically active materials. In an attempt to elucidate this problem, many investigators have tried to reproduce the pathological process in animals. A variety of experimental systems has been devised utilizing the following agents:

1. horse, bovine duck and pig sera, and fractions thereof (171, 359, 456, 519, 784);
2. living and killed streptococci and various fractions and products thereof (125, 346, 347, 409, 525);
3. various materials from patients suffering from rheumatic fever (447, 736);
4. combinations of normal organ extracts and the above-listed materials (109);
5. histamine, mineralocorticoids, various Gram-negative endotoxins such as Escherichia coli lipopolysaccharide and meningococcal endotoxin (287, 675, 750, 768, 769).

Although the direct acute effects of these agents have been studied, most experiments have employed the delayed hypersensitivity or anaphylactic shock mechanism. The majority of the observations involved the myocardial changes noted in rabbits (400, 475, 750), but also in other animals including the guinea pig (330), rat (109), mouse (347), monkey (525), swine (769) and dog (485).

The finding of Rich and Gregory (519) that experimental vascular and cardiac lesions can be produced in animals by repeated injections of horse serum has suggested to the above as well as to several other groups of workers (376, 405, 524) that this condition may be somewhat similar to rheumatic carditis and periarteritis nodosa in the human being. However, the results obtained were extremely variable; positive results observed with certain agents by one investigator could not be confirmed under the experimental conditions used by other workers. For instance, Kirschner and Howie (351) reported that they had produced comparable cardiac lesions in 7 of 12 rabbits similarly injected. Norlin (475), under similar circumstances, obtained cardiac lesions only in 7 of 32 test animals. Murphy and Swift (463) reported to have successfully induced rheumatic-like cardiac lesions in rabbits by intracutaneous injections of living streptococci. But since only a small percentage of the rabbits developed the lesions after many repeated infections, they concluded that some host factor may play a basic role in the pathogenesis of these tissue alterations. On the other hand, ROBINSON (525) failed to reproduce the results of MURPHY AND SWIFT. CHAR AND WAGNER (114) produced carditis in rabbits by several biologically active agents (e.g., extracts prepared from streptococci, human serum protein, bovine serum albumin). The morphologic alterations noted differ sharply from human rheumatic fever; there is an apparent closer resemblance to those lesions seen in acute streptococal myocarditis (289, 411). Significant alteration in the heart was observed in 49 of the 58 animals, and it was noted that different rabbits reacted differently to a given agent even when the dosages administered were equal.

The data obtained by other investigators are not less confusing. CAVELTI (109, 110) in 1947 first presented evidence favoring heart tissue as a source of autoimmunizing antigen. He reported that repeated intraperitoneal injections of rats with a mixture of homogenized rat heart tissue and killed group A streptococci over a period of 1 to 3 months resulted in the production in the serum of agglutinins for collodion particles coated with a saline extract of heart tissue in 45 to 80% of the animals, lesions involving endocardium, myocardium and epicardium were produced. Confirmation of these results has never been reported. However, in the same year JAFFE AND HOLZ (325) independently described myocardial lesions in rats and rabbits immunized for 9 months with a mixture of homologous heart tissue and killed streptococci. The pathological description of the lesions and the published illustrations do not correspond with the lesions described by CAVELTI. In their illustrations the lesions appeared to involve the myocardium chiefly and the connective tissue to a lesser degree, and were characterized by the authors as consisting primarily of muscle degeneration with secondary inflammation.

The Japanese investigators MECKAWA (407) and SHOJI (701) have presented work suggesting that a cephalin fraction of mammalian heart tissue injected in admixture with foreign serum or other protein serving as carrier may induce interstitial myocarditis. The lipoid fraction was regarded as organ-specific. The brief descriptions and illustrations are chiefly of an interstitial myocarditis, although myofiber degeneration and vascular lesions were also noted. Finally, we may cite here the experiments of FRICK (216) who showed lesions in rats following repeated intraperitoneal injections of homologous heart in FREUND's adjuvant plus tuberculin. These were not described in detail, but revealed connective tissue damage in perivascular distribution, myocardial hemorrhages and, in a small minority of animals (0.78%), focal areas of myocardial degeneration.

Based on the experimental observations just outlined numerous hypotheses have been proposed in attempts to explain the pathogenesis of rheumatic heart lesions. None of these has been entirely satisfactory, as is suggested, for example by a further variety of experimental and clinical studies published within recent years dealing with the possible mechanisms of cardiac damage. These have concerned:

1. the pathological effects on the heart of enzymic substances (26, 106, 346, 347, 633, 640);
2. cardiac lesions, especially of myofibers, resulting from repeated focal streptococcal infections, and the morphologic resemblance of such lesions to those observed in rheumatic carditis (351, 462, 463);
3. cardiac lesions following establishment of focal infection of pharyngeal tissue (232);
4. the demonstration of the localization of specific antigens in the heart, as a possible focus for allergic reaction (336);
5. the demonstration of leukocyte-platelet thrombi in rheumatic hearts and studies of the possible relationship of this finding to the Shwartzman phenomenon type of hypersensitivity (725);
6. finally, studies on the participation of an autoimmune reaction in pathogenesis of cardiac lesions (109, 110).

The mechanisms responsible for these strikingly comparable tissue changes are as yet completely unknown. However, the production of the 'rheumatic-like' myocardial lesions in such diverse ways and with such a wide variety of agents throws doubt upon the specificity of the mechanisms involved. The different reactivity of various animals may indicate that some internal conditioning factors play an important role in the development of this type of cardiac damage. Notably, according to several investigators (82, 120, 240), adrenal cortical extracts, 17-hydroxycorticosterone and ACTH have been found of value in preventing of the myocarditic lesions of repeated serum injections. As already noted, the experimental arthritis (produced by the injection of formalin into the paw of a rat) as well as the so-called 'anaphylactoid inflammation' (that ensues in rats, following the intraperitoneal or intravenous administration of macromolecular substances), are similarly conditioned by the same types of hormones. On the other hand, the investigations of SELYE showed furthermore that heavy overdosage with DOC can, under certain conditions, produce a facsimile of 'rheumatic' diseases in animals. Using DOC, it was possible to induce nephrosclerosis with hypertension, periarteritis nodosa, and a myocarditis with intense hyalinization; but the development of this cardiovascular syndrome depends upon certain conditioning factors (673, 675, 683, 685). Unilateral nephrectomy and an excess of dietary NaCl proved to be especially effective in increasing sensitivity to this particular effect of the mineralocorticoid. Essentially the same changes will appear after treatment with STH or with crude lyophilized anterior pituitary tissue (LAP). The syndrome can also be duplicated by exposing sensitized animals to a variety of stressors, such as cold and infections (592, 598, 600). It may be concluded, therefore, that acute and/or chronic stress reactions probably play some conditioning role in the development of 'rheumatic-like' cardiac lesions produced by diverse means, since, utilizing toxic doses of various drugs, bacterial toxins and other damaging stimuli, similar lesions were observed in acute studies.

As another completely unsolved problem, the *relation of the pancreas to cardiovascular disease,* may be discussed here (see also: General Introduction, pp. 1–9). The well-substantiated observation that degenerative cardiovascular disease occurs more frequently in persons with pancreatic disease than in the general population has prompted inquiry into the nature of this association. According to Joslin (332) cardiorenal-vascular complications may account for about 75% of total deaths in diabetics. In this disease virtually all components of the vascular system are involved, including the arteries, arterioles, capillaries, and venules. There appears to be general agreement that diabetes or a related factor not only accelerates the onset but also increases the incidence and severity of arteriosclerosis and cardiac abnormalities (521). It is interesting, furthermore, that although coronary occlusion in the nondiabetic occurs several times more frequently in males than in females, diabetes obliterates this sex difference, in addition to increasing the over-all incidence (121, 535).

Some investigators have presented evidence that poor control of the diabetic state favors a high incidence of cardiovascular disease (324, 536, 778), but equally impressive reports show no correlation between the level of control and protection against vascular complications (75, 767). The biochemical abnormalities in diabetes have been studied extensively with regard to their possible causal relationship to the genesis of cardiovascular disease. There seems to be no valid reason to implicate hyperglycemia per se as an etiological agent for arteriosclerosis in diabetics, but it has been suggested that wide fluctuations in blood sugar level may be harmful (350). The presence of mucopolysaccharides in the ground substance and basement membranes of normal blood vessels raises the question of the importance of altered metabolism of these substances in increasing the susceptibility to vascular disease (770). McManus (432) has suggested that mucopolysaccharides might be deposited from the blood stream into the vascular wall. However, protein-bound polysaccharides and glucosamine have been found by Keiding and Tuller (343) to be elevated in diabetic subjects regardless of the presence of vascular alterations. The higher levels of these substances in the blood may be the result rather than the cause of degenerative changes in the diabetics.

As was already discussed (p. 95), the relationship of lipid levels to atherosclerosis has received considerable attention in both the diabetic and the nondiabetic. The observations of Hirsch *et al.* (299) point to a direct relation between hyperglycemia and hyperlipemia in the diabetic and emphasize the importance of good control of the blood sugar level. Available evidence, however, does not demonstrate consistent differences in blood lipids between normal and diabetic persons (126, 268). Ricketts (520) has pointed out the failure of evidence thus far available to indicate that the increased incidence of atherosclerosis in diabetics is related to a disturbance in lipid metabolism or to an elevation of any of the serum lipid fractions.

Because of the association in man between diabetes and cardiovascular disease, many experimental studies have been conducted in animals to determine the influence of the pancreas on atherogenesis. It is important to note the marked species differences in susceptibility to arteriosclerosis and the divergent opinions regarding the degree of similarity of experimental lesions to those found in man. Methods employed to induce pancreatic deficiency in animals include total or partial pancreatectomy, arterial and pancreatic duct ligation, toxic destruction of islet cells, and administration of anterior pituitary hormones and corticoids.

Dragstedt (159) observed a twelvefold greater incidence of arteriosclerosis in totally depancreatectomized dogs that were controlled with insulin and fed a relatively high-fat diet than in the controls. The lipid levels of the affected dogs were within the normal range or reduced. Allen and Lisa (7) failed to find vascular alterations in partially depancreatectomized dogs. Insulin-maintained diabetic dogs fed a diet low in fat did not develop atherosclerosis, according to Chaikoff and Kaplan (111). Stamler *et al.* (721) observed, furthermore, that neither choline nor inositol, both known to be nutritional factors in pancreas, prevent the hypercholesteremia or hyperlipemia in cholesterol-fed chickens, nor do they reduce the incidence or severity of atherosclerotic lesions. In the studies of STAMLER AND KATZ (722), the addition of pancreatic factors to the mash of depancreatized, cholesterol-fed chicks was without influence on the development of atherosclerosis.

Attempts to induce atherosclerosis in alloxan diabetic rats by feeding of cholesterol have been unsuccessful (340), but it is well known that this species is usually resistant to vascular sclerosis. Of considerable interest is the fact that the presence of alloxan diabetes in rabbits retards atherogenesis due to cholesterol feeding (165). Treatment of such rabbits with insulin ameliorates the diabetic state and counteracts the inhibitory effect on atherogenesis due to the diabetes (164). In the guinea pig, alloxan does not produce atherosclerosis or even permanent diabetes. It has been thought that the guinea pig is resistant to this diabetogenic agent because of the ability of pancreatic islets to reform from ducts and acinar tissue (329).

Finally, a possible relationship of elastase to cardiovascular disease was suggested by the finding that the pancreatic elastase content is diminished in atherosclerotic humans (57). BALÓ AND BANGA (57) have further demonstrated in the pancreas the presence of an elastolytic enzyme that they term elastase. Evidence has been reported that this enzyme is produced by the pancreatic alpha cells (107, 384), however, more recently COHEN *et al.* (123) point to the acinar cells as the source of this enzyme. At any rate, experimental studies revealed that whereas elastase retards the development of atherosclerosis in cholesterol-fed rabbits (383), its oral or intramuscular administration to cholesterol-fed chickens fails to reduce either the incidence or severity of artherosclerosis (744).

This short review of the literature pertinent to the role of the pancreas in the development of cardiovascular disease shows that although the pancreatic disease, diabetes mellitus, is associated with an increased incidence and relatively early onset of arteriosclerosis, studies have not revealed any adequate explanation for this association. Investigations in animals also suggest that the pancreas may in some manner be involved in the genesis of cardiovascular lesions, but, here again, the pathogenic relationship remained obscure.

In *summary* we may say that a survey of the literature shows that most, if not all, of the agents capable to elicit necrotizing cardiopathies are potential pathogens, whose cardiotoxicity largely depends upon other factors or conditions. Causes that lead to the development of cardiac necroses are often likely to derive from the environment. However, the characteristics of a situation acting as a potential cardiotoxic agent may activate, but do not determine, the nature of the response of the organism. The response will depend upon the state of the cardiovascular system at the time of stress and on the organisms' defense reactions in general. Thus, the effect of a cardiotoxic agent or situation may depend mainly on conditioning interactions that sensitize or desensitize the cardiac muscle on the one hand, and alter the general adaptation reactions, on the other hand. The great ability of stressor agents to participate in the pathogenesis of cardiac necroses seems to depend upon the fact that the elements of the cardiovascular system are not only connected with, but extremely responsive to impulses reaching them via autonomic and endocrine pathways from the highest integrative centers of the nervous system. Although the role of the autonomic nervous system and the hypothalamo-pituitary-adrenal axis in response to stress has received intense study, the interrelations between these systems and cardiovascular pathology are virtually unexplored.

## VI. Conclusions and Outline of Problems

The fact that stress—no matter how produced—elicits a rather stereotyped response, the G-A-S, has now been widely accepted. It is also clear that at least some reactions of the G-A-S do possess a defensive value, i.e., they facilitate adaptation to various stressor agents. A survey of the literature showed, furthermore, that by suitable humoral conditioning, disease susceptibility can be markedly altered; not only is it possible to increase or decrease resistance to stress (e.g., influence survival), but we can selectively focus the effect of stress upon certain organs. It was illustrated on many experimental models and clinical findings that not only hypersensitivity reactions, inflammatory processes, and the so-called collagen diseases, but also other non-endocrine maladies are markedly influenced (enhanced or prevented) through conditioning influences (e.g., diet, exposure to stress, corticoids, age).

Humoral and nervous mechanisms help to adjust the activity of different organ systems to changing conditions in the organism or its surroundings. In the humoral mechanism, the pituitary-adrenocortical system plays a particularly important role. However, the adaptive reactions of the organism are governed by complex neuro-endocrine interactions. Developments of the last decade have made it clear that the nervous system itself is, in a sense, a complex endocrine system producing humoral substances for the control of endocrine functions and, probably also, of a number of other bodily activities. Thus, chains of alternating neural, neurohumoral, and conditioning processes are enormous.

Also, it is clear that inadequate adaptation to stress as well as an excess of 'adaptive hormones' (corticoids, STH, ACTH, etc.) can, under certain circumstances, become the cause of disease or, at least, can condition the body to the production of morbid changes. Unfortunately, the actions of stress and corticoids at the cellular level are not yet understood. Stress may exert extra-adrenal action on cell permeability, enzyme activities, water and electrolyte metabolism, renal function, etc. Corticoids also influence the permeability of target cells. They may act as carrier in ion transport and certainly modify the activities of specific tissue enzyme systems. There is little question, furthermore, that the corticoids influence renal regulation of electrolyte balance and basically effect carbohydrate utilization in tissues. Currently some of the major problems of adaptation and maladaptation are related to questions of how integration and control of metabolism, particularly hormonal control, are achieved at the molecular level.

Among this great variety of possible actions of stress and corticoids are, as a part, those affecting the elements of the heart or more precisely the cardiovascular system as a whole. It was long suspected that inability to adapt successfully to stressful situations may be a factor in the development of necrotizing cardiopathies. Although the role of the autonomic nervous system and the hypothalamo-pituitary-adrenal axis in response to stress has received intense study, the interrelations between these systems and cardiovascular pathology are virtually unexplored.

Stressful circumstances can influence the cardiovascular system through trans- and extra-adrenal neural and humoral pathways. For instance, the vascular reactions subserved by neural mechanism may range from the altogether peripheral axon reflex through a variety of autonomic effector functions mediated via the spinal cord, and reflexes at the level of the brain stem brought about through afferents from specialized receptors in the blood vessels and in the brain. These are sensitive to minor changes in the composition of the blood, especially to reductions in oxygen tension or alterations in blood pH, etc. It is known that the efferent impulses activated thereby may result in widespread and often disabling bodily changes. Information as to precisely what circulatory patterns and cardiac activities are subject to influence from neural centers—which also participate in adaptation reactions in general—is still only fragmentary, but already impressive enough to indicate that the cerebral cortex and the hypothalamus must be considered along with the pituitary and adrenal glands as potentially controlling cardiovascular responses in man and animals. Thus, the relationship of adaptive reactions to cardiovascular pathology is extremely complex.

To gain fundamental information about the nature of any complex biological interaction, we have to develop techniques that permit us to analyse it by breaking it down into its constituent elementary units. By re-evaluating the scattered literature concerning the experimental production of cardiac necroses we may conclude that most of the agents tried elicit cardiac lesions only under certain circumstances. If this is true, it would mean actually that the organism possesses natural defensive mechanism with which to defend itself against the potential cardiotoxic action of various agents. Furthermore, it would be possible to conclude that changes in the external or internal environment could significantly participate in the pathogenesis of cardiac necroses.

Consequently our experimental work is concerned with the two following basic problems:

1. To what extent do systemic stress reactions participate in the development of various experimental cardiopathies? Does exposure to stress influence the potential cardiotoxic effect of other agents? Which are the factors that determine the susceptibility of the heart muscle to the pathogenic actions of stress?

2. Are there conditioning factors capable of selectively sensitizing or desensitizing the heart to the effect of various agents known to be partially cardiotoxic? Could agents became cardiotoxic under certain circumstances, which usually never produce cardiac necrosis even in lethal doses?

Let us merely point out here that for the purpose of these comparative studies, we employed as pathogens:

1. noradrenaline and vasopressin as agents capable of producing 'spotty myolysis' with disappearance of muscle-fiber segments, without extensive necroses or inflammation;

2. stressor agents, such as forced restraint, quadriplegia, hot and cold baths, or surgical trauma, which likewise produce, but only occasionally, small necrotic foci in otherwise untreated animals;

3. papain, because this proteolytic enzyme preparation elicits acute, miliary, disseminated myocardial necroses;

4. plasmocid, since it produces large, patchy myocardial necroses and myocarditic lesions;

5. dihydrotachysterol (DHT), a steroid of the vitamin D group, because it causes intense calcium deposition in the heart and in the coronary arteries;

6. methylchlorocortisol (Me-Cl-COL) + $NaH_2PO_4$, since this combined treatment is highly effective in producing a typical electrolyte-steroid-cardiopathy (ESCN), characterized by massive, infarct-like cardiac necroses with secondary inflammation, but without any demonstrable histological change in the structure of the coronary arteries.

In addition to those enumerated above, several other agents were also tried. Some (for example, Na-fluoroacetate, pentamethylentetrazol, Na-arsenate) were used particularly because of contradictory reports in the literature concerning their ability to produce cardiac necroses; others (for example, diisopropylfluorophosphate, pseudomonas aeruginosa infection), because they were not known to produce this type of cardiac damage.

We felt that comparative studies with such a wide variety of potentially cardiotoxic agents would give us some information concerning common features in the pathogenesis not only of cardiac necroses in general, but especially of those spontaneous diseases that are not accompanied by acute occlusion of the coronary vessels.

PART II

Personal investigations:

# Conditioning Factors for Cardiac Necroses

# I. General Methodology and Glossary

The materials and special techniques employed for the study of experimental cardiopathies are detailed in each original experiment (see section: *Materials and Techniques*). However, in order to avoid unnecessary repetition, in the following we describe the technical procedures that were generally applied. The inclusive Glossary is designed only to define the sense in which certain technical terms and abbreviations are used in the next part of this monograph.

*Assessment of organ lesions.* The diagnosis of cardiac necroses, nephrocalcinosis, and hepatic necroses was made with the aid of a dissecting loupe at autopsy. The diagnosis so obtained was checked in most instances with histologic sections. The severity of the lesions (necrosis, calcification) was expressed in the form of an arbitrary scale of 0 to 3: 0 designating no lesion; 1 just detectable lesion; 2 moderate lesion; 3 marked lesion. It is important to note that sometimes the cardiac lesions (which are easily visible as yellowish or grayish patches between the darker healthy muscle tissue) can be graded more accurately by inspection of the whole heart than by studying a few histologic sections through each specimen. Therefore, as specified in each experiment, the readings were obtained by inspection with the dissecting loupe in some cases, while in others the grading was based on histologic studies. The incidence (per cent positive animals within the group) and the severity of the cardiac lesions (the latter with the standard error of the mean grade), as well as the mortality rates and other findings of special interest, are summarized in the tables. When it seems necessary in order to evaluate the results, the means of the final weights are also indicated in separate columns with the corresponding standard errors.

*Cold baths.* Among the various stressor agents that are capable of eliciting acute stress situations, cold baths were often used. The rats were placed in a large pail of water, the temperature of which was kept just at the freezing point by the addition of ice-cubes. Usually, the animals were subjected to this treatment for 1–3 minutes, twice during one day, care being taken to lift their heads above the water line when the rats became too numb to swim.

*Diets.* In all standard experiments, the rats received the normal laboratory diet, 'Purina Fox Chow' (obtained from the Ralston Purina Co. of Canada) and tap water, throughout the period of observation.

However, for the production of certain cardiopathies, special synthetic diets were used. Therefore, in the following we shall describe the standard rations for the induction of K-, Mg-, Cl- and Na-deficiency.

*K-deficient diet.*—As a rule, we used the following K-deficient diet (supplied by Nutritional Biochemicals Corporation, Cleveland, Ohio):

*Chief ingredients (g/100 g diet)*

| | |
|---|---|
| Corn starch | 64.2 |
| Casein | 30.0 |
| Butter fat | 3.5 |
| Calcium carbonate | 1.3 |
| Sodium chloride | 1.0 |

*Vitamin mixture (g/100 pound diet)*

| | |
|---|---|
| Vitamin A conc. (200,000 U./g) | 4.5 |
| Vitamin D conc. (400,000 U./g) | 0.25 |
| Alpha tocopherol | 5.0 |
| Ascorbic acid | 45.0 |
| Inositol | 5.0 |
| Choline chloride | 75.0 |
| Menadione | 2.25 |
| p-Aminobenzoic acid | 5.0 |
| Niacin | 4.5 |
| Riboflavin | 1.0 |
| Pyridoxine HCl | 1.0 |
| Thiamine HCl | 1.0 |
| Calcium pantothenate | 3.0 |
| Biotin | 0.01 |
| Folic acid | 0.09 |
| Vitamin $B_{12}$ | 0.00135 |

*Mg-deficient diet.*—As a rule, we used an Mg-deficient diet of the following composition (supplied by General Biochemicals, Inc., Chagrin Falls, Ohio):

*Chief ingredients (g/100 g diet)*

| | |
|---|---|
| Casein, high protein | 25.00 |
| Choline chloride | 0.25 |
| Corn oil | 5.00 |
| Dextrose (Cerelose) | 58.28 |
| Gelatin | 5.00 |
| i-Inositol | 0.10 |
| dl-Methionine | 0.30 |
| Salt mixture (see below) | 5.99 |

*Vitamin mixture (g/100 pound diet)*

| | |
|---|---|
| Biotin | 0.0140 |
| Calcium pantothenate | 1.1340 |
| Folic acid | 0.1132 |
| Menadione | 0.2268 |
| Nicotine acid | 3.1748 |
| Pyridoxine hydrochloride | 3.1748 |
| Riboflavin | 0.2720 |
| Thiamine hydrochloride | 0.2720 |
| Vitamin $B_{12}$ | 0.0020 |
| Alpha tocopherol | 0.9200 |
| Vitamin A conc. (200,000 U./g) | 9.0800 |
| Vitamin D conc. (400,000 U./g) | 0.9200 |

*Salt mixture (g/100 pound diet)*

| | |
|---|---|
| Calcium carbonate | 904.84 |
| Calcium phosphate | 226.44 |
| Copper sulfate | 0.92 |
| Iron citrate | 84.52 |
| Manganous sulfate | 12.08 |
| Potassium iodide | 2.40 |
| Potassium phosphate | 981.16 |
| Sodium chloride | 507.20 |
| Zinc carbonate | 0.76 |

The casein used for this and other mineral-deficient diets was highly purified and did not contain heavy metals (e.g., copper) in excess of 0.003%. Its maximum bacterial count was 5,000/g. The Mg-content of this diet is usually analyzed at various times during the course of the experiment to safeguard against contamination. Calculated by the EDTA-method, employing 10% trichloracetic acid extract of ashed samples, the Mg-content varied between 0 and 0.145 mg/100 g of diet. By contrast, Purina Fox Chow, used as a control diet, was found to contain approximately 144–300 mg/100 g diet, when the same analytic procedure was followed (448).

*Cl-deficient and high-Cl diets.*—In experiments designed to study the effect of low or high Cl-rations, the composition of the *basic diet* (supplied by General Biochemicals, Inc. Chagrin Falls, Ohio), was:

*Chief ingredients (g 100/g diet)*

| | |
|---|---|
| Sucrose | 70.65 |
| Vitamin-free test casein GBI | 18.30 |
| Butter fat (salt-free) | 5.00 |
| Vitamin mixture (see below) | 1.05 |
| Salt mixture (see below) | 5.00 |

*Vitamin mixture (g/100* pound diet*)*

| | |
|---|---|
| Alpha tocopherol | 10.215 |
| Calcium pantothenate | 2.043 |
| Carotene in oil, 3,333 U./g | 150.000 |
| Choline dihydrogen citrate | 272.400 |
| i-Inositol | 13.620 |
| Menadione | 0.102 |
| Niacin | 27.240 |
| Pyridoxine phosphate | 0.953 |
| Riboflavin | 0.953 |
| Thiamine monophosphate | 0.953 |
| Viosterol 400,000 U./g | 0.125 |

*Salt mixture (%)*

| | |
|---|---|
| Calcium lactate | 20.400 |
| Calcium gluconate | 12.000 |
| Potassium phosphate (monobasic) | 11.200 |
| Potassium chloride | 31.200 |
| Sodium phosphate (dibasic) | 2.500 |
| Sodium chloride | 4.974 |
| Sodium bicarbonate | 2.500 |
| Ferric citrate | 9.500 |
| Magnesium chloride | 3.800 |
| Copper sulfate | 1.900 |
| Zinc acetate | 0.026 |

The *composition of the low-Cl diet* differed from the basic diet only as regards the salt mixture, which was (in %):

| | |
|---|---|
| Calcium lactate | 20.400 |
| Calcium gluconate | 12.000 |
| Potassium phosphate (monobasic) | 11.200 |
| Potassium bicarbonate | 31.200 |
| Sodium phosphate (dibasic) | 2.500 |
| Sodium bicarbonate | 7.474 |

| | |
|---|---|
| Ferric citrate | 9.500 |
| Magnesium oxide | 3.800 |
| Copper sulfate | 1.900 |
| Zinc acetate | 0.026 |

The total Cl-content of the low-Cl diet was 0.035%, while that of tha basic diet was 0.935% and that of the high-Cl diet, 1.62%.

The *composition of the high-Cl diet* differed from the basic diet only as regards the salt mixture, which was (in %):

| | |
|---|---|
| Calcium chloride | 32.400 |
| Potassium phosphate (monobasic) | 11.000 |
| Potassium chloride | 31.200 |
| Sodium phosphate (dibasic) | 2.500 |
| Sodium chloride | 7.474 |
| Ferric chloride | 9.500 |
| Magnesium chloride | 3.800 |
| Copper chloride | 1.900 |
| Zinc chloride | 0.026 |

*Na-deficient diet.*—For these experiments the *composition of the basic diet* (supplied by General Biochemicals, Inc., Chagrin Falls, Ohio) was:

*Chief ingredients (g/100 g diet)*

| | |
|---|---|
| Sucrose | 70.65 |
| Vitamin-free test casein GBI | 18.30 |
| Butter fat (salt-free) | 5.00 |
| Vitamin mixture (see below) | 1.05 |
| Salt mixture (see below) | 5.00 |

*Vitamin mixture (g/100 pound diet)*

| | |
|---|---|
| Biotin | 0.0140 |
| Calcium pantothenate | 1.1340 |
| Folic acid | 0.1132 |
| Menadione | 0.2268 |
| Nicotine acid | 3.1748 |
| Pyridoxine HCl | 3.1748 |
| Riboflavin | 0.2720 |
| Thiamine HCl | 0.2720 |
| Alpha tocopherol | 0.9200 |
| Vitamin A conc. (200,000 U./g) | 0.0800 |
| Vitamin D conc. (400,000 U./g) | 0.9200 |

*Salt mixture (%)*

| | |
|---|---|
| Calcium carbonate | 32.4 |
| Potassium phosphate (monobasic) | 21.2 |
| Potassium chloride | 21.2 |

| | |
|---|---|
| Ferric citrate . . . . . . . . . . . . . . . . . . . . . . . . | 9.5 |
| Magnesium oxide . . . . . . . . . . . . . . . . . . . . . . . | 3.8 |
| Copper sulfate . . . . . . . . . . . . . . . . . . . . . . . . | 1.9 |
| Sodium chloride . . . . . . . . . . . . . . . . . . . . . . . | 5.0 |
| Sodium phosphate (dibasic) . . . . . . . . . . . . . . . . . . | 5.0 |

Rats show approximately the same growth-rate whether they are kept either on this basic diet or on the normal laboratory food, 'Purina Fox Chow'.

The *composition of the Na-deficient diet* differed from the basic diet only as regards the 'salt mixture'. In the Na-deficient diet, 5.0% 'vitamin-free test casein CBI' and 5.0% sucrose were substituted for the Na-salts; therefore, the percentage of the remaining salts was not changed.

*DHT*. Dihydrotachysterol.

*DOC*. Desoxycorticosterone acetate.

*Electrocardiogram (ECG)*. The ECG was registered in unanesthetized animals on a Sanborn Polygraph in the 3 standard and in precordial leads, corresponding to $V_2$, $_4$ and $_6$. The rats were fastened to a board. Their paws, smeared with an electrode jelly, were wired to the patient cables. Round copper-tin-zinc electrodes 1 mm in diameter, fixed to an isolating band, were used for precordial leads, after the jelly had been applied to exactly the desired location. Speed of the paper was 100 mm/sec and the sensitivity 1 mV = 15 mm.

*ESCH*. *E*lectrolyte-*S*teroid-*C*ardiopathy characterized by *H*yalinization in the walls of coronary arteries and the myocardium itself. This lesion is most readily induced by an excess of NaCl, after conditioning by mineralocorticoids.

*ESCN*. *E*lectrolyte-*S*teroid-*C*ardiopathy characterized by *N*ecroses of the myocardium. This change is induced, for example, by an excess of $Na_2HPO_4$, $Na_2SO_4$ or $NaClO_4$, after sensitization with corticoids.

*F-COL*, or fluorocortisol. 9α-fluoro-hydrocortisone acetate.

*Fuchsin stain*. A special staining technique, which is especially suitable for the demonstration of early, prenecrotic changes (i.e., the accumulation of a strongly fuchsinophilic material) of the myocardium. For the detailed description of the method see p. 131.

*Infarctoid cardiopathy*, or infarct-like cardiac lesions. Large circumscribed patches of cardiac necrosis, which tend to develop suddenly, especially during stress, but are not due to organic obstructions of the coronary arteries.

*Microcrystal suspension.* All the steroids used in the original experiments were injected in the form of microcrystal suspension. This was prepared as follows: Materials: Tissue grinder (Fisher 16 × 150); Motor (Palo Laboratory Supplies, 110 v); Rheostat Autotransformer (Superior Electric Co. range: 0–135 v); Tween-80 Detergent (BRICKMAN), which helps to maintain the microcrytals in aqueous suspension. Procedure: we place a small quantity (no more than 500 mg) of the steroid-powder at the bottom of the homogenizer tube. One drop of Tween-80 is added to each 10 ml of water. We homogenize at a moderate speed, moving the tube up and down, until the suspension is homogeneous (approx. 10 minutes).

*Me-Cl-COL,* or methylchlorocortisol. 2α-methyl-9α-hydrocortisone acetate.

*Muscular exercise.* Forced muscular exercise was used as a stressor agent, while gradual muscular exercise (conducive to adaptation) was applied in order to study the effect of slowly increasing work upon the development of cardiac lesions. The rats exercised in a motor-driven revolving drum-cage, 12 inches in diameter and subdivided by metal partitions into 12 compartments, each 3 inches wide. One rat was placed in each compartment and the drum allowed to turn at the rate of 18 revolutions per minute. When rats with a body weight of 100 g were used, 2.5 to 3 hours continuous exercise was sufficient to produce severe alarm reaction and to elicit cardiac necrosis after suitable electrolyte-steroid conditioning.

*Papain.* Papain is a proteolytic enzyme contained in the dried latex of Carica papaya. The papain solution used in our experiments was prepared as follows: 5 g of crude papain powder (Fisher Scientific Co.) were added to 50 ml of distilled water; this turbid suspension was mixed in a Waring blendor for 10 minutes and then passed through a No. 40 Whatman filter paper. The resulting opalescent, amber-colored filtrate was injected into the jugular vein of the rats, under light ether anesthesia. In some of our experiments (as specified later), instead of the filtrate, the crude papain powder suspension was injected. Essentially similar cardiac lesions can be obtained by both solutions; however, when the crude solution is used, somewhat smaller doses are required.

*Plasmocid.* Two chemical variations of this cardiotoxic and now obsolete antimalarial agent were used: 1. 8-(3-diethylaminopropylamino)6-methoxyquinoline (supplied by the Lilly Research Laboratories) and 2. 6-methoxy-8-(3-diethylaminopropylamino)-quinoline dihydroiodide (supplied by Dr. R. C. ELDERFIELD, Department of Chemistry, University of Michigan, Ann Arbor). The former has been found to be somewhat more active, but the cardiac lesions produced by both preparations were essentially similar.

*Rats.* Unless otherwise specified, female Sprague-Dawley rats were used in all experiments.

*Restraint,* or forced immobilization. Restraint is an especially active stressor agent in eliciting cardiac lesions; it is applied by strapping the rats with adhesive tape to a board, in the prone position, usually for 17 hours. During this time, the animals struggle in an effort to free themselves and hence are under considerable stress.

*Quadriplegia.* The standard procedure (referred to in the text simply as 'quadriplegia') consists in bilaterally transecting both the cervical plexuses as well as the femoral, sciatic, and obturator nerves. The operation is performed under ether anesthesia. The cervical plexuses are approached through small incisions in the axillae, while the femoral, sciatic and obturator nerves are all exposed through a single, suprapubic, midline incision.

## II. Sensitization of the Heart Muscle: Positive Conditioning Actions

### A. Stress, Corticoids, and Steroids of the Vitamin-D Group

#### *a) Sensitization with Me-Cl-COL for the Induction of Cardiac Lesions by Diverse Stressor Agents*

In previous studies, it was demonstrated that sudden exposure to stressor agents—e.g., cold, muscular exercise, restraint, trauma, noradrenaline—elicited large infarct-like patches of myocardial necrosis in rats pretreated with certain corticoids (e.g., 2α-methyl-9-α-fluorocortisol, Me-Cl-COL) and $NaH_2PO_4$ (689). Even pretreatment with less active steroids (such as cortisol or DOC) in combination with $NaH_2PO_4$ sensitized the rat and rhesus monkey to the production of myocardial necroses by stress (616, 691). However, it is important to distinguish between the cardiac lesions (ESCN) that are produced gradually by the persistent actions of corticoids and sensitizing Na-salts and the infarctoid cardiopathies that are elicited by the sudden effects of stress. When rats were briefly treated with small amounts of Me-Cl-COL plus $NaH_2PO_4$, this pretreatment caused little or no cardiac damage, yet subsequent exposure to stress immediately elicited severe and extensive cardiac necroses in all animals.

A review of the literature showed, furthermore, that many drugs and food constituents can produce focal myocardial necroses, at least under certain experimental conditions (see pp. 92–112). All these observations suggested that there may be some common pathway in the mechanism through which various agents can produce cardiac necroses in animals. It was tempting to assume that the cardiotoxic activity can be ascribed to the stressor action of the agents used, but this hypothesis was not proven by the previous experiments. In fact, in most of the previous studies, the rats were sensitized to the action of stressors with corticoids plus sodium phosphates. Although the necrosis-eliciting effect of various stressors in these experiments was significant, some of the control animals sometimes showed heart lesions which resulted from the Me-Cl-COL plus phosphate pretreatment alone (689).

The possibility of precipitating infarct-like, myocardial lesions by sudden exposure to stressors is especially important, in view of its obvious clinical implications. It was felt that the precipitating effect of stress could be most clearly demonstrated in rats sensitized only by a corticoid. The concurrent administration of sodium-salts may obscure the results, since it is possible that stress itself might act largely through metabolic changes that make sensitizing sodium-salts more readily available. In view of these considerations, our task was to establish the necrotizing ability of a great variety of noxious agents in the rat conditioned for this non-specific type of response by pretreatment with a highly active corticoid (Me-Cl-COL), a steroid that never produces cardiac necroses when given alone.

*Materials and Techniques*

Four hundred and eighty rats with an average initial body weight of 100 g (range 90–110 g) were divided into 48 equal groups. Twenty-four groups received no treatment until the eighth day of the experiment and served as controls, to show the eventual myocardial-necrotizing effect of the various agents (or stressors) used. The remaining groups were treated from the beginning until the termination of the experiment with Me-Cl-COL as described below: these showed the ability of corticoid (Me-Cl-COL) overdosage to condition for the cardiotoxic effect of the most diverse stressors. After this preparatory period all groups (e.g., controls and Me-Cl-COL-pretreated groups) were treated with various agents, in doses verified (by preliminary experiments) to be definitely damaging to rats of this sex, strain and size. Some of the stressors used (e.g., Na-fluoroacetate, dinitrophenol, diphtherotoxin, muscular exercise) were selected particularly because of contradictory reports in the literature concerning their ability to produce cardiac necroses when these agents are administered without conditioning. Others (for example, diisopropylfluorophosphate, cold baths, or pseudomonas aeruginosa infection) were not previously known to produce this type of cardiac damage.

All stressors were applied during 24 hours only, between the eighth and ninth days of the experiment; in addition, as diphtherotoxin is slow-acting when given subcutaneously, it was also administered on the sixth day. Unless otherwise indicated, single interventions (e.g., spinal-cord transection) were performed at 4. P.M., on the eighth day while double interventions (e.g., hemorrhage, injections of drugs) took place at 4 P.M., on the eighth, and at 9 A.M. on the ninth days. All drugs were injected subcutaneously. The stressors used were:

*Cold bath* (immersion in icy water at 1 °C, during three minutes, twice);

*Hot bath* (immersion in water at 48 °C, during five minutes, twice);

*Muscular exercise* (two and one-half hours in the morning and three hours in the afternoon, in a drum, 12 inches in diameter, revolving at 18 revolutions per minute);

*Restraint* (the animals were strapped to a board by adhesive type, in the prone position, once during 17 hours);

*Motor denervation* of extremities (both cervical plexuses, as well as the femoral and sciatic nerves, were severed, like all other surgical operations, under ether anesthesia);

*Spinal-cord transection* (with a thermocautery, at the height of the seventh cervical vertebra);

*Vagotomy* (transection of both vagi, at the height of the thyroid);

*Crushing of intestines* (stomach, ileum and cecum, each crushed three times with a hemostat);

*Hemorrhage* (removal of 3 ml of blood from the jugular vein, twice);

*Adrenaline or Noradrenaline* (200 µg, in 0.2 ml of oil, twice);

*Vasopressin* ('Pitressin', 10 I.U., in ml of water, twice);

*Pentamethylenetetrazol* ('Metrazol', 6 mg, in 0.2 ml of water, twice);

*Table I*

Stress and Cardiac Necroses

| Group | Treatment* | Total doses of the stressor agents | Final body weight (g) | Cardiac necrosis | Mortality |
|---|---|---|---|---|---|
| 1 | None | — | 122 ± 2.8 | 0 | 0 |
| 2 | None + Me-Cl-COL | — | 83 ± 3.8 | 0 | 0 |
| 3 | Cold bath | — | 126 ± 2.0 | 0 | 40 |
| 4 | Cold bath + Me-Cl-COL | — | 86 ± 3.2 | 2.6 ± 0.23 | 0 |
| 5 | Hot bath | — | 122 ± 3.0 | 0 | 0 |
| 6 | Hot bath + Me-Cl-COL | — | 76 ± 3.8 | 1.3 ± 0.20 | 0 |
| 7 | Muscular exercise | — | 126 ± 2.5 | 0 | 0 |
| 8 | Muscular exercise + Me-Cl-COL | — | 89 ± 3.4 | 1.7 ± 0.36 | 10 |
| 9 | Restraint | — | 112 ± 3.5 | 0.6 ± 0.20 | 0 |
| 10 | Restraint + Me-Cl-COL | — | 83 ± 2.0 | 2.8 ± 0.10 | 10 |
| 11 | Motor denervation of extremities | — | 110 ± 2.5 | 0 | 10 |
| 12 | Motor denervation of extremities + Me-Cl-COL | — | 89 ± 3.8 | 1.0 ± 0.27 | 10 |
| 13 | Spinal-cord transection | — | 115 ± 3.0 | 0 | 0 |
| 14 | Spinal-cord transection + Me-Cl-COL | — | 81 ± 2.9 | 0.2 ± 0.15 | 20 |
| 15 | Vagotomy | — | 113 ± 3.5 | 0 | 80 |
| 16 | Vagotomy + Me-Cl-COL | — | 75 ± 2.5 | 1.7 ± 0.27 | 80 |
| 17 | Crushing of intestines | — | 125 ± 1.4 | 0 | 0 |
| 18 | Crushing of intestines + Me-Cl-COL | — | 89 ± 1.5 | 0.2 ± 0.15 | 20 |
| 19 | Hemorrhage | — | 117 ± 4.2 | 0 | 20 |
| 20 | Hemorrhage + Me-Cl-COL | — | 83 ± 3.5 | 1.7 ± 0.27 | 50 |
| 21 | Adrenaline | 600 µg | 127 ± 4.9 | 1.0 ± 0 | 0 |
| 22 | Adrenaline + Me-Cl-COL | 400 µg | 82 ± 3.5 | 2.1 ± 0.32 | 0 |
| 23 | Noradrenaline | 600 µg | 131 ± 3.8 | 0.4 ± 0.40 | 0 |
| 24 | Noradrenaline + Me-Cl-COL | 400 µg | 80 ± 2.5 | 2.9 ± 0.10 | 0 |

| | | | | | |
|---|---|---|---|---|---|
| 25 | Vasopressin | 30 I.U. | 128 ± 2.0 | 0 | 0 |
| 26 | Vasopressin + Me-Cl-COL | 20 I.U. | 81 ± 3.0 | 1.5 ± 0.40 | 0 |
| 27 | Pentamethylenetetrazol | 18 mg | 134 ± 3.2 | 0 | 0 |
| 28 | Pentamethylenetetrazol + Me-Cl-COL | 12 mg | 94 ± 2.5 | 0.6 ± 0.40 | 0 |
| 29 | Diisopropylfluorophosphate | 1.8 mg | 105 ± 2.9 | 0.4 ± 0.40 | 20 |
| 30 | Diisopropylfluorophosphate + Me-Cl-COL | 1.2 mg | 73 ± 2.6 | 1.9 ± 0.32 | 30 |
| 31 | Na-fluoroacetate | 0.15 mg | 121 ± 2.5 | 1.2 ± 0.20 | 0 |
| 32 | Na-fluoroacetate + Me-Cl-COL | 0.10 mg | 78 ± 2.8 | 2.0 ± 0.10 | 0 |
| 33 | Na-iodoacetate | 7.5 mg | 131 ± 2.5 | 0 | 0 |
| 34 | Na-iodoacetate + Me-Cl-COL | 5 mg | 84 ± 3.6 | 0 | 0 |
| 35 | Dinitrophenol | 18 mg | 125 ± 2.6 | 0 | 0 |
| 36 | Dinitrophenol + Me-Cl-COL | 12 mg | 91 ± 3.0 | 0 | 20 |
| 37 | Picrotoxin | 0.6 mg | 136 ± 1.9 | 0 | 0 |
| 38 | Picrotoxin + Me-Cl-COL | 0.4 mg | 93 ± 3.0 | 0.8 ± 0.32 | 0 |
| 39 | Na-arsenite | 1.8 mg | 136 ± 2.9 | 0.2 ± 0.20 | 0 |
| 40 | Na-arsenite + Me-Cl-COL | 1.2 mg | 92 ± 2.4 | 0.6 ± 0.35 | 0 |
| 41 | Na-arsenate | 7.5 mg | 129 ± 4.4 | 0 | 0 |
| 42 | Na-arsenate + Me-Cl-COL | 5 mg | 92 ± 3.0 | 0.4 ± 0.27 | 0 |
| 43 | Digitoxin | 2.25 mg | 110 ± 3.5 | 0 | 0 |
| 44 | Digitoxin + Me-Cl-COL | 1.5 mg | 70 ± 1.9 | 0 | 0 |
| 45 | Diphtherotoxin | 1.5 ml | 143 ± 3.0 | 0 | 0 |
| 46 | Diphtherotoxin + Me-Cl-COL | 1.0 ml | 94 ± 1.9 | 0.2 ± 0.15 | 0 |
| 47 | Pseudomonas aeruginosa infection | 2.4 ml | 125 ± 4.2 | 0.2 ± 0.17 | 40 |
| 48 | Pseudomonas aeruginosa infection + Me-Cl-COL | 1.6 ml | 92 ± 3.7 | 1.0 ± 0.36 | 20 |

* The daily dose of Me-Cl-COL (when given) was 500 µg.

*Diisopropylfluorophosphate* (0.6 mg in 2 ml of oil, by stomach tube, twice);
*Na-fluoroacetate* (2.5 mg in 0.2 ml of water, twice);
*Na-iodoacetate* (2 mg in 0.2 ml of water, twice);
*Dinitrophenol* (0.6 mg in 0.2 ml of water, twice);
*Picrotoxin* (0.2 mg in 0.2 ml of water, twice);
*Na-arsenite* (0.6 mg in 0.2 ml of water, twice);
*Na-arsenate* (2.5 mg in 0.2 ml of water, twice);
*Digitoxin* (750 μg, in 0.2 ml of water, twice);
*Diphtherotoxin* (1:2.5 dilution in 0.9% NaCl; 0.5 ml, once on sixth day, 1 ml once on eighth day);
*Pseudomonas aeruginosa infection* (1:100 suspension in 0.9% NaCl (turbidity, 50) into a subcutaneously prepared air-pouch, once on sixth day).

Me-Cl-COL administered in the form of microcrystals of its acetate in 0.2 ml of water, subcutaneously, 500 μg/day, to the Groups indicated in Table I.

The doses listed above were given to the Me-Cl-COL-treated groups. However, by the eighth day, under the influence of this potent corticoid the body-weight of the rats had dropped from 100 to 80 g while that of the controls without pretreatment had risen to 110–113 g; to compensate for this difference, the dose of the stressors had to be adjusted accordingly, in these controls. Hence, the amounts of all drugs given to the animals not pretreated with Me-Cl-COL were higher, by one half, than those given to the pretreated animals (see Table I). The hemorrhage was similarly adjusted, in that one-third more blood was removed in the controls. No such correction was deemed necessary as regards heat, cold, muscular exercise, restraint, motor denervation, spinal-cord transection, vagotomy or crushing of the intestines.

For further safety, two additional types of controls (10 rats for each) were used for each stressor agent, namely: 'weight controls' (younger rats, whose mean body-weight, like that of the Me-Cl-COL pretreated animals, was 80 g at the time of exposure to stress), and 'age controls' (animals of the same age as those of the principal experiment, but whose body weight was diminished to 80 g by partial starvation). These control groups received the same treatment as did the Me-Cl-COL-pretreated groups. However, the findings in these additional weight and age controls were essentially the same as in the not Me-Cl-COL-treated animals of the principal experiment and, hence, they are not listed in Table I.

During the experiment, the animals were fed exclusively on 'Purina Fox Chow' and received tap water to drink.

On the 10th day, all survivors were killed with chloroform; their hearts were fixed in formalin and stained with the fuchsin-technique:

1. fix, for 48 hours, in 10% formaldehyde solution neutralized by calcium carbonate; 2. dehydrate in dioxane; 3. embed in paraffin; 4. deparaffinize in xylol; 5. two changes of alcohol 95%; 6. a few seconds in alcohol 70% and in alcohol 50%; 7. wash in running water, 5 minutes; 8. rinse in distilled water; 9. stain 15 minutes in solution A (50 ml of cresyl truly violet [stock solution = lg in 500 ml water and filtration after 1 hour] + 150 ml distilled water + 0.8 ml oxalic acid 1% solution. [Must be prepared just before use.]); 10. rinse in distilled water; 11. stain 8 minutes in solution B (20 ml of phosphomolybdic acid 10% + 20 ml of phosphotungstic acid 10% + 10 ml of acid fuchsin 2% + 0.8 ml aniline hydrochloride 1% + 2 ml glacial acetic acid + 150 ml distilled water); 12. rinse in glacial acetic acid 0.5%; 13. differentiate in glacial acetic acid 0.5%, 12 minutes; 14. rinse in distilled water; 15. dehydrate in alcohol 70% and 2 changes absolute alcohol; 16. clear in xylol and mount in balsam (613).

The diagnosis of cardiac necroses was based upon the histologic findings. This is important, because, under these particular circumstances (Me-Cl-COL conditioning and subsequent exposure to stressors), even extensive necroses are often difficult to see by mere inspection with the dissecting loupe. The reason for this occasional indistinct macroscopic appearance of histologically advanced and extensive necroses is not clear. Perhaps the decomposition products that usually endow dead muscle fibers with a characteristic yellow color do not form rapidly, or perhaps they are too quickly removed, under certain conditions of experimentation. In any event, the possibility of a marked discrepancy between histologically detectable and macroscopically obvious necroses must always be kept in mind.

## *Results and Conclusions*

It is evident from the findings given in Table I that Me-Cl-COL alone failed to produce any cardiac necroses; however, it significantly increased the cardiotoxic effect of numerous, quite unrelated agents, particularly that of cold (Group 4) and hot baths (Group 6), muscular exercise (Group 8), restraint (Group 10), motor denervation (Group

12), vagotomy (Group 16), adrenaline (Group 22), noradrenaline (Group 24), vasopressin (Group 26), diisopropylfluorophosphate (Group 30), Na-fluoroacetate (Group 32), picrotoxin (Group 38), and pseudomonas aeruginosa (Group 48). In many of the other groups, Me-Cl-COL likewise increased the incidence of cardiac necroses (Groups 18, 28, 40, 42, 46), but the difference between the corticoid-treated and the corresponding control groups was less striking and not statistically significant. In the remaining groups Me-Cl-COL produced no necrotic foci, but merely an increase in individual fiber necroses and fuchsinophilia; such minor effects have been disregarded in our grading.

It is possible that some of the agents failed to produce myocardial necrosis because they did not produce sufficiently severe stress at the dose levels tested. On the other hand, excessive systemic damage does not favor the production of this necrosis. In severe shock (produced in this experiment by spinal-cord transection) the pulse is weakened and the peripheral resistance is lowered to such a degree that necroses are not elicited even when the animal is pretreated with Me-Cl-COL. Despite the failure of the coronary blood supply that occurs in 'artificial hibernation' induced by cold, or during cardiac arrest with K, for example, the myocardium does not show a marked tendency for necrosis.

In any event, we may conclude from the results summarized in Table I that, after Me-Cl-COL conditioning, cardiac necroses can be induced by a great variety of essentially different agents; hence, the lesions are largely a nonspecific effect of stress.

The general conclusion that can be drawn from our investigations is that the myocardial necroses which occur without any morphological evidence of a vascular obstruction are largely, but not totally, nonspecific, in that they can be produced by many, but not by all, stressors. The concept of relative nonspecificity receives further support from the observation that certain factors sensitize (e.g., corticoids, Na-salts), while others desensitize (e.g., $MgCl_2$, KCl), the cardiac muscle for the production of necroses by a great variety of agents (Lit.: 613, 802). In view of the facts just mentioned we assumed, as a working hypothesis, that nonspecific stress occupies a key position in the pathogenesis of the necrotizing cardiopathies, and that the latter could consequently be regarded as 'diseases of adaptation' caused by some derailment of the general adaptation syndrome.

Our observations suggest that, during stress, an excessive production of corticoids or the undue activation of such steroids by certain electrolyte shifts may produce irreversible metabolic derangements in the cardiac muscle fibers, and thereby induce necrosis. The 'fuchsinophilic degeneration' appears to be one of the earliest morphologically detectable manifestations of such biochemical disturbances in the myocardium. Inflammation is a secondary consequence of this same derangement and, hence, an integral part of the lesion. Since any sizeable focus of myocardial necrosis is secondarily invaded by inflammatory cells, it would be only misleading to distinguish sharply between cardiac necrosis and necrotizing myocarditis. Of course, inflammation may occur in the heart, as in any other organ, without being preceded by necrosis, but no matter how a necrotic focus is produced in the myocardium (e.g., by coronary occlusion, or thermocoagulation), even in the absence of any exogenous chemical or microbe, the dead tissue is destroyed and removed by inflammatory cells. We emphasize these points because they suggest that whatever may be learned about the pathogenesis and prevention of cardiac necroses will also be applicable to at least some types of myocarditis, especially to the so-called 'nonspecific chronic myocarditis' that eventually develops in everybody who lives long enough.

As it stands today, our hypothesis has two severe flaws: first we have seen that several stressors (e.g., spinal-cord transection, bleeding, dinitrophenol) do not produce a necrotizing cardiopathy, even when the rats are optimally conditioned by corticoids and/or electrolytes; second the postulated, common, metabolic derangement in the cardiac-muscle fiber, which we believe is induced by stress under certain conditions, has not yet been identified.

Our concept is not offered as a final solution, but, despite its admitted weaknesses, it seems to be the working hypothesis most compatible with all the known facts. There is overwhelming evidence in support of the view that certain conditioning factors (corticoids, Na-salts) can predispose to the production of necrotizing cardiopathies by wholly unrelated stressors. As some agents capable of producing severe stress nervertheless fail to elicit pronounced myocardial necroses, this may be a promising lead for further investigations. For example, this fact suggests experimentation to verify whether there exist adaptive mechanisms that can protect the heart against necrosis when stress of a certain intensity is produced in a certain way. The same attitude must be taken with regard to the second point, namely, our present ignorance of the fundamental biochemical derangement that causes myocardial necroses. It would be gratuitous, at present, to elaborate a detailed biochemical theory of the necrotizing cardiopathies. It is obvious from the data summarized briefly in this paper that electrolyte shifts are important and it may be that the corticoids condition the cell by altering its affinity for certain ions—perhaps through changes in cell permeability. Our histologic observations suggest, furthermore, that some strongly fuchsinophilic material tends to accumulate in the myocardial fiber, just before necroses occur. Whether the accumulation of the substance is the cause or the consequence of damage, we do not know, but these are avenues for future reasearch.

The question arises whether this type of biochemical conditioning, which we recently established, could play a part in the pathogenesis of the cardiac infarcts that occur in man. It has long been known that in many cases of clinical cardiac infarcts (about 30–40%) even careful examination of the coronary vessels failed to reveal any evidence of an acute obstruction. But some atheromatosis does commonly occur, and this may produce a partial occlusion or, at least, a rigidity of the vascular wall. Such changes could interfere with the vasodilatation necessary to supply increased amounts of blood to the heart when its requirements for oxygen and nutrients suddenly rise (e.g., during neuromuscular stress). It is conceivable, therefore, that, at times of stress, this increase in demand could cause myocardial infarction, despite the absence of an acute coronary occlusion. This view is further substantiated by previous observations showing that systemic stress can precipitate an ESCN (electrolyte-steroid-cardiopathy with necrosis) in animals suitably conditioned by a corticoid plus $NaH_2PO_4$, just as it can cause cardiac infarcts in predisposed human beings (Lit.: 613, 628, 802).

*Summary*

Experiments are described that demonstrate the ability of diverse agents to elicit manifestations of cardiac necrosis, in rats specifically conditioned for this type of nonspecific response by treatment with Me-Cl-COL.

The results obtained from these studies showed that:

1. Me-Cl-COL alone failed to produce any cardiac necrosis.
2. Pretreatment with Me-Cl-COL significantly increased the cardiotoxic effect of numerous, quite unrelated agents.

3. As myocardial necroses can be elicited by such diverse agents, it may be concluded that this type of cardiac damage is a result of non-specific stress.

### *b) Interactions Between Steroid Hormones in the Production of the ESCN*

As already noted, simultaneous treatment with certain Na-salts ($Na_2HPO_4$, $NaH_2PO_4$, $NaClO_4$ or $Na_2SO_4$) and highly active synthetic corticoids, such as Me-Cl-COL, elicits massive necrotic patches in the cardiac muscle. This type of cardiac damage is now referred to in the literature as the ESCN (Lit.: 613, 802). It was felt that the newly discovered interactions between electrolytes and steroid hormones may help to elucidate some fundamental problems of cardiac physiology and pathology; hence extensive studies were undertaken concerning the role of the electrolyte component and the participation of the steroids in the pathogenesis of the ESCN.

The ESCN was accidently discovered in rats injected with Me-Cl-COL and treated simultaneously with $NaH_2PO_4$ by stomach tube. On the other hand, even fatal doses of the steroid or the sodium phosphate alone failed to produce myocardial necroses. As Me-Cl-COL possesses both mineralo- and glucocorticoid properties, the question arose whether the cardiotoxic effect is more closely related to the mineralocorticoid or the glucocorticoid action.

Among 49 steroids that have been tested as regards their cardiotoxicity so far, Me-Cl-COL proved to be most effective in producing the ESCN. However, 2α-methyl-9α-fluorocortisol and the two corresponding non-methylated steroids (9α-chlorocortisol and 9α-fluorocortisol) are likewise very effective in this respect. The only halogenated corticoid devoid of this activity is triamcinolone ($\triangle^1$-9α-fluoro-16-hydroxycortisol), a highly active glucocorticoid which possesses little or no mineralocorticoid potency. On the other hand, cortisone, a glucocorticoid with little mineralocorticoid activity is at least as effective in producing the ESCN as is DOC, although the latter is much more mineralocorticoid than is the former (690). It is especially noteworthy that, when given in combination with $NaH_2PO_4$, even cortisol, the principal natural glucocorticoid of man, can produce such cardiac changes in rats and other species, including the rhesus-monkey (691); the same is true of the natural corticoid mixture that is secreted by the adrenal of animals treated with large amounts of ACTH (619, 690).

All the steroid hormones that were found to be highly effective in producing the ESCN are potent corticoids. In experiments in which high doses of triamcinolone (a pure glucocorticoid) or DOC (a pure mineralocorticoid) produced no marked degree of cardiopathy in $NaH_2PO_4$-sensitized rats, combined treatment with small doses of both these steroids sufficed to induce pronounced and extensive cardiac necroses (618). It would appear, therefore, that the concurrent administration of mineralo- and glucocorticoids is most effective in conditioning the cardiac muscle to the necrotizing action of certain electrolytes. This finding seems to be especially interesting, because in so many other respects these two types of corticoids are antagonists.

In spite of this fundamental observation, very little is known as yet about interactions between steroids in the production of the ESCN. It will be noted that among the $6\alpha$-methyl-$\triangle^4$-pregnenes and their halogenated derivatives only $9\alpha$-fluoro-'Medrol' showed any cardiotoxicity, while most of the corresponding $2\alpha$-methylated-$\triangle^4$-pregnene compounds (such as Me-Cl-COL, Me-F-COL) were extremely active. On the other hand, all of the $C^{18}$, $C^{19}$ and $C^{21}$-(17-epi)-steroids (the groups to which the characteristic female and male sex hormones belong) are devoid of cardiotoxic activities (613).

Further experiments were needed, therefore, to establish whether the steroid hormones found to be inactive when given alone or supplemented by treatment with electrolytes would be activated by simultaneous administration of a pure mineralocorticoid with only a slight ESCN-producing ability. As it is well recognized that DOC has only a minimal cardiac-necrotizing property when it is administered with $NaH_2PO_4$, it was especially interesting to see whether this property would be aggravated or prevented by concurrent treatment with various steroids. We therefore administered, simultaneously with the DOC and $NaH_2PO_4$, the following steroids which are devoid of cardiotoxic effect:

1. $6\alpha$-methyl-$\triangle^4$-pregnenes;
2. $6\alpha$-methyl-$\triangle^{1,4}$-pregnadienes (their halogenated and their non-halogenated derivatives);
3. sex hormones: estradiol, methyltestosterone.

The necrotizing action of $9\alpha$-fluoro-$16\alpha$-hydroxy-$16\alpha$, $17\alpha$-acetonidecortisol, a recently synthetized steroid hormone and, for comparison with the results of the methylated $\triangle^{1,4}$-pregnadienes, of a corresponding non-methylated compound (triamcinolone) was studied.

## *Material and Techniques*

*General experimental design.* One hundred and twenty rats, with an average initial body weight of 100 g (range: 94–110 g), were subdivided into twelve equal groups. The animals in Group 1 served as controls to show the necrotizing activity of DOC when given with $NaH_2PO_4$ alone. In addition to DOC and to this sodium salt, Groups 2–12 received various other steroids simultaneously, as indicated in Table II.

*Treatment.* All the steroid hormones were injected in the form of a microcrystal suspension in 0.2 ml of water once daily, always subcutaneously. The daily dose of each hormone was 100 μg, with the exception of that of DOC which was 2.5 mg. The sources of the steroids used in this investigation are listed at the beginning of the monograph (see acknowledgements). As a sensitizing electrolyte, $NaH_2PO_4$ was administered at the dose of 300 mg in 2 ml of water, twice daily, by stomach tube.

*Evaluation of the experiment.* After 12 days of the hormone plus electrolyte treatment the experiment was terminated and the survivors of all groups were killed with chloroform. However, by that time, several of the experimental animals had died, exhibiting macroscopically visible, large patches of myocardial necroses, as well as intense renal calcification.

At autopsy, kidneys and hearts were carefully examined with the aid of a stereoscopic dissecting microscope. The calcium deposition in the renal tissue was clearly recognizable as a narrow band at the corticomedullary junction in every case; therefore, the kidneys were not examined histologically. Although, under these conditions, the necrotic lesions in the myocardium were also easily visible as yellowish or grayish patches between the darker healthy muscle tissue, we nevertheless verified the macroscopic findings with histologic evidence. Each heart was fixed with neutral formalin and stained by the fuchsin technique. It was found, however, that the lesions in the heart (just as those in the kidneys) can be graded at least as accurately by mere inspection of the whole heart as by the studies of a few histologic sections through each specimen.

## *Results and Discussion*

In evaluating the data, we must keep in mind that each steroid that was concurrently administered with DOC in this experiment was also assayed previously in rats with and without conditioning by $NaH_2PO_4$; but the results of these tests were uniformly negative. It may be said, therefore, that under the experimental conditions described here, none of the steroids used could be shown to produce cardiac necroses when given with $NaH_2PO_4$. On the other hand, treatment with $NaH_2PO_4$ alone also consistently failed to produce any cardiac changes.

It will be seen from the figures given in Table II that DOC when given without any other steroid exerted only negligible ESCN-producing activity in the $NaH_2PO_4$-sensitized rat (Group 1). Among the steroids tested in combination with DOC, all the 6α-methylated $\triangle^4$-pregnene and $\triangle^{1,4}$-pregnadiene compounds (Groups 2–7), as well as triamcinolone (Group 9) and 9α-fluoro-16α, 17α-acetonide-cortisol (Group 12 ) markedly increased the cardiotoxic effect of DOC, while estradiol (Group 10) and methyltestosterone (Group 11) proved to be inactive in this respect.

Since all the synthetic steroids that enhanced the ESCN-inducing activity of DOC have glucocorticoid properties, the present results confirm our previous statement: gluco- and mineralocorticoids, which, when given separately, are devoid of any cardiotoxic activity invariably elicit the ESCN in the $NaH_2PO_4$-conditioned rat when they are administered concurrently.

As regards any correlation between the actions and structures of the steroids, it is noteworthy that 6α-methyl-11α-hydroxyprogesterone (Group 2) was much more effective than was the corresponding keto-derivative (Group 3), in activating the ESCN-producing capacity of DOC. The results obtained with both methylated and halogenated $\triangle^{1,4}$-pregnadienes showed that an increase in the number of fluorine atoms enhanced the cardiotoxic properties of the compound (compare Group 3 with Group 4). It is more likely, however, that halogenation in the 9α-position is favorable in this respect, since the previously tested 2α-methylated, 9α-halogenated-compounds (such as Me-Cl-COL), as well as the 9α-fluoro-16α-hydroxy-16α, 17α-acetonide-cortisol investigated here (Group 12), were extremely cardiotoxic. But this assumption apparently contradicts the finding which indicated that 6α-methyl-9α-21-desoxycortisol (Group 7) was much less potentiated by DOC than was its non-hallogenated form (Group 6). The last observation may be due to the well established fact that, depending upon the structure of the corticoid, halogenation sometimes enhances the mineralocorticoid potencies, while in other cases (see for example, triamcinolone) it does not influence the maintenance of the gluco-

*Table II*

Interactions between Steroid Hormones in the Production of Experimental Myocardial Necrosis

| Group | Treatment* | Final body weight (g) | Cardiac necrosis | | Nephrocalcinosis | | Mortality | |
|---|---|---|---|---|---|---|---|---|
| | | | (Severity) | (Incidence) | (Severity) | (Incidence) | (%) | Survival time (days) |
| 1 | None | 110 ± 4.6 | 0.4 ± 0.27 | 20 | 3.0 ± 0 | 100 | 20 | 11.8 |
| 2 | 6α-methyl-11-β-hydroxyprogestrone | 99 ± 9.7 | 2.3 ± 0.30 | 90 | 2.8 ± 0.13 | 100 | 80 | 9.6 |
| 3 | 6α-methyl-11-ketoprogesterone | 116 ± 5.2 | 1.1 ± 0.46 | 40 | 2.9 ± 0.10 | 100 | 30 | 11.3 |
| 4 | 6α-methyl-21-fluoro-11-β, 17α-dihydroxy-$\Delta^{1,4}$-pregnadiene-3,20-dione | 123 ± 10.4 | 1.2 ± 0.44 | 50 | 2.8 ± 0.13 | 100 | 70 | 8.8 |
| 5 | 6α-methyl-9α,21-difluoro-11α,17α-dihydroxy-$\Delta^{1,4}$-pregnadiene-3,20-dione | 74 ± 2.3 | 2.7 ± 0.23 | 100 | 2.5 ± 0.17 | 100 | 100 | 6.0 |
| 6 | 6α-methyl-21-desoxy-cortisol | 124 ± 14.4 | 2.1 ± 0.32 | 90 | 3.0 ± 0 | 100 | 70 | 9.9 |
| 7 | 6α-methyl-9α,21-difluoro-21-desoxy-cortisol | 94 ± 6.6 | 1.3 ± 0.45 | 50 | 2.4 ± 0.27 | 100 | 70 | 9.1 |
| 8 | 6α-methyl-cortisol, 'Medrol' | 83 ± 11.5 | 2.5 ± 0.30 | 90 | 3.0 ± 0 | 100 | 90 | 8.0 |
| 9 | $\Delta^{1}$-fluoro-16-hydroxy-cortisol (Triamcinolone) | 100 ± 1.0 | 1.5 ± 0.45 | 60 | 2.8 ± 0.13 | 100 | 80 | 8.1 |
| 10 | Estradiol | 90 ± 3.8 | 0.3 ± 0.30 | 10 | 2.9 ± 0.10 | 100 | 10 | 11.6 |
| 11 | Methyltestosterone | 109 ± 6.0 | 0.3 ± 0.30 | 10 | 3.0 ± 0 | 100 | 10 | 11.6 |
| 12 | 9α-fluoro-16α-hydroxy-16α,17α-acetonide-cortisol | 97 ± 5.8 | 1.9 ± 0.45 | 80 | 2.8 ± 0.15 | 100 | 90 | 8.4 |

* All animals in Groups 1–12 were also treated with desoxycorticosterone acetate plus $NaH_2PO_4$ as described in the text.

corticoid character of the steroid hormone. Of course, a mainly mineralocorticoid-acting halogenated corticoid combined with another active mineralocorticoid cannot compete with the necrotizing ability of the nonhalogenated, i.e. gluco- plus mineralocorticoid, mixture.

On the other hand, these investigations clearly demonstrated that characteristic sex hormones, e.g., estradiol and methyltestosterone, do not affect the production of the ESCN in the DOC + $NaH_2PO_4$-conditioned rat. These results, however, do not give further information on the clinical observation that males have a significantly higher predisposition for cardiac infarcts than have females. In other words, we do not yet have any direct evidence to show that the production of an ESCN by one steroid could be prevented by another. Yet, the many antagonisms between steroids in other respects and the fact that pregnancy offers considerable protection against this type of cardiopathy (620) suggest that research along these lines may be profitable.

Nephrocalcinosis is also listed in Table II as resulting from the combined steroid-electrolyte treatment. It should be stated, however, that the calcium deposition in the renal tissue has no direct bearing upon the development of cardiac necroses. The development of nephrocalcinosis is due to the administration of $NaH_2PO_4$, since the ESCN can also be elicited in rats conditioned for the cardiotoxic activity of certain steroid hormones with $NaClO_4$ or $Na_2SO_4$ instead of phosphates. In these animals, renal damage never occurred (621, 622). Earlier experiments showed that under experimental conditions comparable to those used here, treatment with $NaH_2PO_4$ alone produced nephrocalcinosis of the grade $1.6 \pm 0.17$ in a group of 40 rats (613). It will be noted that DOC maximally aggravated the renal calcification produced by $NaH_2PO_4$ in the present investigation (cf. Table II, Group 1). If these two control values are kept in mind as standards for comparison, it may be concluded that no interaction between the steroids tested significantly decreased the development of nephrocalcinosis.

### *Summary*

After a brief review of previous investigations concerning the role of the steroid component in the production of the ESCN, a description is given of more recent experiments designed to study the interactions of steroid hormones in the pathogenesis of myocardial necroses. All the steroids tested here, in combination with DOC, had previously been found to be inactive in this respect when injected alone as well as after conditioning with $NaH_2PO_4$.

Results obtained in the DOC plus $NaH_2PO_4$-sensitized rats indicated:

1. DOC, a mainly mineralocorticoid compound, has only a minimal cardiotoxic property when given alone.
2. Of the steroids tested, those with glucocorticoid properties greatly aggravated the ESCN-producing activity of DOC.
3. It was concluded, therefore, that the concurrent actions of mineralo- and glucocorticoids are the most effective in eliciting cardiac necroses.
4. Estradiol and methyltestosterone were without influence on the slight necrotizing effect of DOC.
5. Some correlations between the cardiotoxic actions and structures of the steroids used are discussed.
6. As regards the extracardiac manifestations, it was demonstrated that DOC maximally enhances the development of nephrocalcinosis produced by $NaH_2PO_4$, but none of the steroids interacted beneficially in this respect.

### *c) Conditioning by Corticoids for the Production of Cardiac Lesions with Noradrenaline*

Several earlier investigators reported that heavy overdosage with adrenaline can produce myocardial lesions in various experimental animals (182,194, 489, 798). However, the changes so induced are inconstant, and consist only of minute, microscopic lesions that appear to have little in common with the massive, infarct-like necroses of the ESCN. In preliminary experiments we confirmed these findings with adrenaline, but found that noradrenaline is slightly more potent and constant in its ability to elicit such cardiac lesions in rats.

In view of what we have just said (see p. 135–141) about the role of corticoids in the production of the ESCN, it was interesting to determine whether the histologically different cardiopathy induced by noradrenaline also depends upon conditioning by corticoids.

*Materials and Techniques*

Ninety rats, with an average initial body weight of 100 g (range: 90–110 g) were subdivided into nine equal groups and treated as indicated in Table III.

Bilateral *adrenalectomies* were performed under ether anesthesia on the first day of the experiment. *Triamcinolone* ($\triangle^{1,4}$-pregnadiene-3,20-dione-9α-fluoro-11β,16α,17α-21-tetrol) at the daily dose of 500 μg and *DOC* at the daily dose of 3 mg were administered as microcrystal suspensions, in 0.2 ml of water, subcutaneously, throughout the experiment. *Noradrenaline* was given at the dose of 250 μg, in 0.2 ml of oil, subcutaneously, on the eighth and ninth days only, that is, one week after adrenalectomy and/or the initiation of pretreatment with the corticoids.

The experiment was terminated on the 11th day. The hearts were fixed in neutral formalin and stained with the acid fuchsin technique for the demonstration of early prenecrotic changes.

*Results and Discussion*

It will be noted that, under our experimental conditions, neither triamcinolone (Group 1) nor DOC (Group 2) produced any cardiac lesion when given alone. Noradrenaline alone (Group 3) induced only occasional foci in the myocardium of a few rats. On the other hand, combined treatment with noradrenaline and triamcinolone (Group 4) elicited widespread myocardial lesions in all experimental animals, and a mortality of 20%. The effect of this combined treatment was not prevented by adrenalectomy (Group 5). Both in the intact (Group 6) and in the adrenalectomized (Group 7) rats, DOC also increased the cardiotoxic effect of noradrenaline, but less markedly than did triamcinolone. Triamcinolone combined with DOC was not significantly more effective than was triamcinolone alone, either in intact (Group 8) or in adrenalectomized rats (Group 9).

It is especially noteworthy that the lesions produced with noradrenaline (alone or in combination with corticoids), unlike the large, yellow, macroscopically easily detectable lesions of the ESCN, were almost never detectable by simple inspection, or even with the aid of a hand-loupe. Histologic investigation showed that their inconspicuousness on fresh preparations is presumably due to the virtually complete absence of necrotic areas and of fibers that undergo fuchsinophilic denegeration. Even when the lesions were very pronounced and widespread (e.g., in Groups 4, 5, 8 and 9) the foci consisted almost exclusively of connective tissue with occasional histiocytes.

*Table III*

Conditioning by Corticoids for the Production of Cardiac Lesions with Noradrenaline

| Group | Treatment | Cardiac lesions | Mortality (%) |
|---|---|---|---|
| 1 | Triamcinolone | 0 | 0 |
| 2 | DOC | 0 | 0 |
| 3 | Noradrenaline | 0.4 ± 0.17 | 0 |
| 4 | Noradrenaline + Triamcinolone | 2.2 ± 0.15 | 20 |
| 5 | Noradrenaline + Triamcinolone + Adrenalectomy | 2.2 ± 0.15 | 10 |
| 6 | Noradrenaline + DOC | 1.2 ± 0.25 | 30 |
| 7 | Noradrenaline + DOC + Adrenalectomy | 0.8 ± 0.15 | 30 |
| 8 | Noradrenaline + Triamcinolone + DOC | 2.0 ± 0.20 | 10 |
| 9 | Noradrenaline + Triamcinolone + DOC + Adrenalectomy | 2.8 ± 0.15 | 0 |

Thus, the affected areas resembled the condition to which pathologists often refer as 'spotty myolysis' because it is characterized mainly by the disappearance of muscle fibers in certain areas. The remaining connective tissue is rather translucent on fresh preparations; hence, it does not differ in colour noticeably from the normal myocardium, although, histologically, the change is extremely pronounced.

Another reason why these lesions are so difficult to see with the naked eye is that their outlines are made extremely irregular by numerous fine processes which project into the essentially healthy adjacent areas (Fig. 1–4).

*Figs. 1–4 Characteristic aspects of the 'spotty myolysis' in the heart of a rat of Group 8 (Table III), treated with noradrenaline, triamcinolone and DOC.*

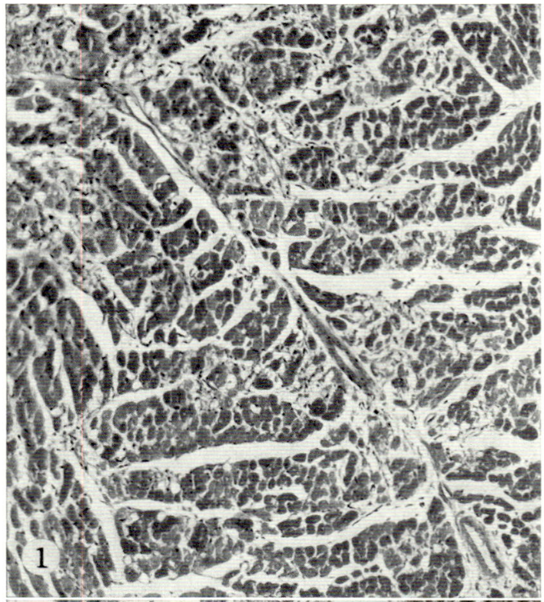

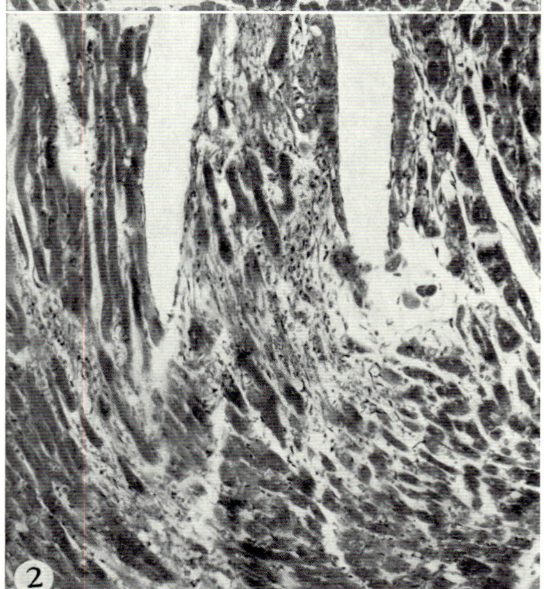

*Fig. 1* More or less diffuse disappearance of muscle fibers throughout the myocardium, and particularly, around the central small artery. Note the absence of necrotic muscle fibers (Fuchsin × 100).

*Fig. 2* Particularly severe lesions in the papillary muscles near the apex of the same heart (Fuchsin × 100).

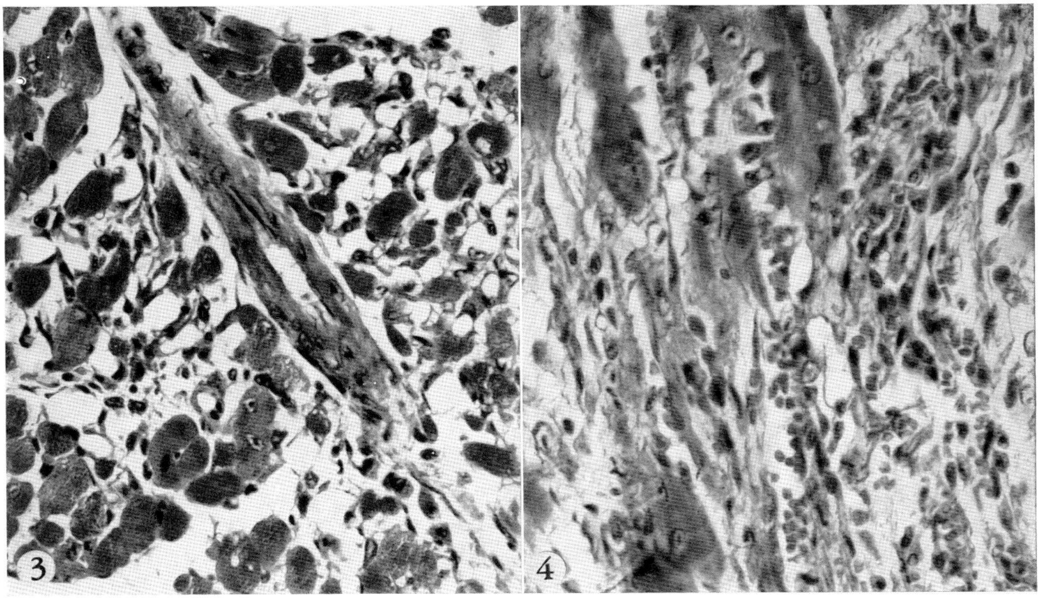

*Fig. 3* Higher magnification of a region in Fig. 1. Here the apparently empty spaces left by the disappearing muscle fibers are particularly obvious (Fuchsin × 250).

*Fig. 4* Higher magnification of a region in Fig. 2. Muscle-fiber dissolution proceeds without any evidence of necrosis (which would be manifested by nuclear disintegration) or fuchsinophilia (which, on histologic preparations, render the fibers red and, on a black-and-white photographs, black). (Fuchsin × 400).

It is evident, from these observations, that a virtually pure glucocorticoid, such as triamcinolone, is highly effective in conditioning the myocardium for the production of widespread lesions with noradrenaline. DOC, a mineralocorticoid, is distinctly less effective in this respect, particularly in adrenalectomized animals (cf. Groups 6 and 7), perhaps, because, in these, even endogenous glucocorticoids are missing. Since triamcinolone alone was already almost maximally effective in sensitizing the heart for this effect of noradrenaline, it cannot be concluded from our experiments that the additional administration of DOC does not aggravate this effect. Still, if there exists a synergism between triamcinolone and DOC, it is certainly not pronounced, because the difference in mortality rate was also essentially the same for Groups 4 and 5 as for Groups 8 and 9. In any event, it is clear that there does not exist any antagonism between gluco- and mineralocorticoids with respect to their sensitizing effect upon the cardiotoxic action of noradrenaline.

The synergism between the cardiotoxic effects of adrenergic and corticoid hormones is of interest to us, because both types of substances are produced in excess during stress. These findings show, furthermore, that corticoids can condition the heart for the production of lesions which differ histologically from the ESCN. Finally, our observations suggest caution in the use of a combined treatment with adrenergic and glucocorticoid compounds, such as has been recommended, for example, for asthmatic patients.

*Summary*

Experiments in albino rats indicate that a diffuse type of myocardial lesion reminiscent of the 'spotty myolysis' of the clinical pathologists—can be produced with great regularity, in both intact and adrenalectomized animals, by combined treatment with noradrenaline and corticoids.

*d) Sensitization by DHT for Induction of Cardiac Lesions by Various Agents*

Our previous experiments (pp. 125–146) showed that suitable conditioning with corticoids selectively enhances the susceptibility of the heart muscle to the cardiotoxic action of various agents. On the other hand, it was also observed by Selye *et al.* (689) that the production of an ESCN by combined treatment with certain corticoids plus $NaH_2PO_4$ is greatly enhanced by various stressors.

A histologically somewhat different type of cardiac lesion is produced by treatment with certain sterols of the vitamin D group, e.g., DHT, in combination with $NaH_2PO_4$. In itself, hypervitaminosis-D produces only calcification in the cardiac muscle fibers and the coronary arteries (578, 579), but when DHT is given in combination with $NaH_2PO_4$, the character of the cardiac lesions changes; calcification becomes less prominent, and an acute, suppurative myocarditis results (615).

In the following we shall report on experiments which indicate that intense acute overdosage with DHT alone, though not sufficient to produce cardiac necroses in itself, suffices to predispose the cardiac muscle to the production of necroses by various agents (e.g., cold, papain, plasmocid, noradrenaline, vasopressin) in doses, in themselves, virtually ineffective.

### *Materials and Techniques*

One hundred twenty rats, with an average initial body weight of 95 g (range 90–102 g), were subdivided into 12 equal groups and treated as indicated in Table IV.

DHT was administered by stomach tube in the form of a microcrystal suspension at the dose of 150 µg, in 0.5 ml of water, twice daily during the first two days and once on the third day.

Exposure to *cold* consisted in the immersion of the rats in icy water, for a period of 3.5 minutes, twice during the second day.

*Papain* was used as a filtered solution; 0.2 ml (10%) was injected into the jugular vein on the second day.

*Plasmocid* (8-[3-diethylaminopropylamino]-6-methoxyquinoline), 0.4 mg, in 0.2 ml of water, was injected intraperitoneally three times during the second day.

*Noradrenaline,* 300 µg, in 0.2 ml of oil, was administered subcutaneously twice on the second day.

*Vasopressin,* 10 I.U. in 1 ml of water, was injected subcutaneously twice on the second day.

At the end of the third day, all surviving rats were killed with chloroform. The hearts were fixed in neutral formalin for subsequent embedding in paraffin and histochemical determination of calcium with von Kóssa's technique.

### *Results and Discussion*

As shown by the data in Table IV, even at the high dose level at which it was given here, DHT did not produce any significant cardiac lesions during this acute three-day experiment (Group 2). Among the other agents that we employed, papain and plasmocid are known to produce widespread necroses in the myocardium, but only if they are given at higher dose levels. Cold, noradrenaline and vasopressin rarely induce any extensive myocardial necroses, however, except in animals that are specially conditioned (e.g., by corticoids). In any event, in this series, the comparatively mild and brief treatment with cold (Group 3), papain (Group 5), plasmocid (Group 7), noradrenaline (Group 9), or vasopressin (Group 11) caused little or no histologically detectable cardiac damage. On the other hand, these same agents produced pronounced and often fatal cardiac necroses when they were administered concurrently with doses of DHT in themselves ineffective (Groups 4, 6, 8, 10 and 12).

Histologic examination of the hearts revealed furthermore that, in the DHT-conditioned rat, the various additionally given agents produced histologic changes that simulated a much more severe DHT intoxication rather than the specific effects that would have been induced by higher doses of the eliciting agents themselves. For example, vasopressin, in itself, can produce minor cardiac lesions and, following corticoid conditioning, even extensive necroses, but it does not produce any lesions in the coronary arteries or calcification of the myocardium (613). Yet, in group 12, in which vasopressin was administered conjointly with DHT, the latter in doses themselves ineffective, the resulting picture was typical of a severe DHT intoxication. Throughout the myocardium, the muscle fibers as well as the stroma between them became impregnated with von Kóssa-tingible calcium deposits (Fig. 5). The coronary arteries exhibited the Mönckeberg-sclerosis type of calcification, as well as an often very pronounced perivascular edema.

Essentially similar changes were obtained in all the remaining groups in which DHT was administered in conjunction with another potentially cardiotoxic agent, yet the calcification was not always equally pronounced. Often, in the same heart, certain regions were calcified; in others, the structural alterations consisted primarily of interstitial edema and inflammation frequently accompanied by necrosis of muscle fibers.

### *Summary*

Rats were treated, during three days, with doses of DHT which, in themselves, caused no detectable cardiac lesions. In the hearts of these animals, necrosis, inflammation and coronary calcification could be produced by various agents (cold, papain, plasmocid, noradrenaline, vasopressin) which, in themselves, likewise produced no significant cardiac lesions under similar conditions of dosage.

*Table IV*

Effect of Dihydrotachysterol upon the Potential Cardiotoxic Action of Various Agents

| Group | Treatment | Cardiac necrosis | Mortality (%) |
|---|---|---|---|
| 1 | None | 0 | 0 |
| 2 | DHT | 0.1 ± 0.10 | 0 |
| 3 | Cold | 0 | 0 |
| 4 | Cold + DHT | 1.2 ± 0.28 | 10 |
| 5 | Papain | 0.2 ± 0.15 | 0 |
| 6 | Papain + DHT | 2.3 ± 0.37 | 10 |
| 7 | Plasmocid | 0.1 ± 0.10 | 0 |
| 8 | Plasmocid + DHT | 2.6 ± 0.23 | 30 |
| 9 | Noradrenaline | 0.5 ± 0.17 | 0 |
| 10 | Noradrenaline + DHT | 1.6 ± 0.23 | 0 |
| 11 | Vasopressin | 0 | 0 |
| 12 | Vasopressin + DHT | 1.1 ± 0.38 | 0 |

After brief sensitization with small doses of DHT, even agents which normally have no tendency to produce coronary lesions or calcification of the myocardium (e.g., vasopressin) elicit these changes which are usually induced by more prolonged and intense treatment with DHT alone. Apparently, the potentially cardiotoxic effect of mild DHT overdosage can be accentuated by a variety of nonspecific agents.

## B. Electrolytes and Electrolyte-Steroid Interactions

### *a) The Role of Sodium in Stress-Induced Cardiac Necrosis.*

Having established that both corticoids and steroids of the vitamin-D group (e.g., DHT) can sensitize the heart to the cardiotoxic actions of diverse agents, our next task was to study the role of electrolytes in the production of cardiac lesions by stress. However, in order to clarify the aim of our experiments we have to recall some basic

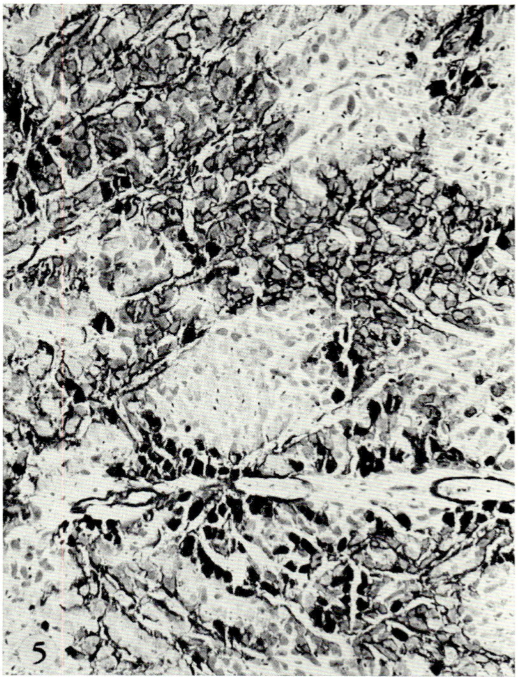

*Fig. 5* Intense calcification of the coronary arteries and the myocardium in a rat of Group 12 (Table IV) that was treated with vasopressin and DHT. In certain regions *(top)* calcification affects predominantly the stroma between the muscle fibers, while in other places *(bottom)* the entire muscle fibers are calcified (von Kóssa; × 100).

observations of Selye concerning the participation of electrolytes in the development of the ESCN (613, 615, 619, 621, 622, 626, 684).

As mentioned before, the ESCN was accidently discovered in rats injected with Me-Cl-COL and treated simultaneously with large amounts of $NaH_2PO_4$ by stomach tube. Soon after this observation, we learned that both $NaH_2PO_4$ and $Na_2HPO_4$ (as well as neutral mixtures of both these salts) are highly active in this respect. It was assumed, therefore, that this infarctoid cardiopathy is not due merely to changes in pH that might be induced either by the acid or by the basic phosphate. When $NaH_2PO_4$ and NaCl were given in equimolecular amounts to rats conditioned with Me-Cl-COL, only the former salt caused necroses in the myocardium. The inactivity of NaCl led us to conclude at the time that, for the production of the infarctoid cardiopathy, the phosphate ion is the essential part of $NaH_2PO_4$. This is the reason why, in the first reports, the ESCN was described as a 'phosphate-steroid-cardiopathy'. But it will be seen that the assumption that $PO_4$ is the active moiety in the sodium phosphate was not entirely correct, because Na is likewise indispensable.

Subsequently, it has also been possible to produce similar cardiac lesions by combined treatment with Me-Cl-COL and other inorganic phosphorus compounds, such as: $NaH_2PO_4$, $NaH_2PO_2$, $Na_4P_2O_7$ and $(NaPO_3)_6$. We then learned that not only phosphates and their immediate derivatives but many other Na-salts can produce cardiac necroses under these experimental conditions. Na-sulfates and sulfites, as well as $NaClO_4$, are approximately as active as the corresponding phosphorus compounds. As the chloride and several other organic and inorganic sodium salts were found to be ineffective, the question arose whether the cation plays any role in the production of the ESCN. $KH_2PO_4$ (unlike $NaH_2PO_4$) does not produce an ESCN in the Me-Cl-COL-conditioned rat. None of 18 non-sodium salts tested elicited the typical picture of the ESCN. This is all the more noteworthy because we purposely employed phosphates, sulfates and perchlorates, that is, salts of anions that are highly effective in activating the ESCN-producing effect of Na.

The general conclusions from all these observations can be summarized as follows: a) only Na-salts are active in producing an ESCN; b) not all Na-salts permit the production of an ESCN; c) both the cation and the anion play important roles in the production of the ESCN; d) Na occupies a central position and certain anions, especially $PO_4$, $SO_4$ and $ClO_4$, sensitize the heart for the cardiotoxic actions of this cation. After these facts were established, the question arose whether anions that do not sensitize (for example, Cl) are merely inert or whether they actively inhibit the efficacy of Na. Systemic studies were performed, therefore, on rats treated with a series of Na-salts in addition to Me-Cl-COL plus $Na_2HPO_4$. Among all the Na-salts tested, only NaCl exerted a statistically significant protective action. This inhibition by one Na-salt of cardiac necroses produced by other Na-salts offers the most convincing proof of the active role played by anions.

It was found, furthermore, that certain Na-salts (phosphates, sulfates, perchlorate) can, while others (chloride, acetate, citrate, lactate) cannot replace the stressors in precipitation of myocardial necroses after Me-Cl-COL-conditioning (613). No salts of cations other than Na were effective, but these observations again show that the anion also plays an important role in the pathogenesis of this type of myocardial necrosis.

We were particularly impressed by the fact that, although NaCl and the organic Na-salts were almost always totally ineffective after Me-Cl-COL pretreatment, they occasionally produced very pronounced cardiac necroses, in rats damaged through fortuitous circumstances. It was, therefore, postulated that, after suitable sensitization with corticoids, certain Na-salts (phosphates, sulfates, per-

*Table V*

Role of Sodium in Production of Myocardial Necroses by Stress

| Group | Treatment | Cardiac necrosis |
|---|---|---|
| 1 | None | 0 |
| 2 | NaCl | 0 |
| 3 | Na-Acetate | 0 |
| 4 | Na-Citrate | 0 |
| 5 | Na-Lactate | 0 |
| 6 | Me-Cl-COL | 0 |
| 7 | Me-Cl-COL + NaCl | 0 |
| 8 | Me-Cl-COL + Na-Acetate | 0.1 ± 0.10 |
| 9 | Me-Cl-COL + Na-Citrate | 0 |
| 10 | Me-Cl-COL + Na-Lactate | 0.2 ± 0.20 |
| 11 | Restraint | 0.1 ± 0.10 |
| 12 | Restraint + NaCl | 0.1 ± 0.10 |
| 13 | Restraint + Na-Acetate | 0.2 ± 0.20 |
| 14 | Restraint + Na-Citrate | 0.1 ± 0.10 |
| 15 | Restraint + Na-Lactate | 0.1 ± 0.10 |
| 16 | Restraint + Me-Cl-COL | 0.4 ± 0.18 |
| 17 | Restraint + Me-Cl-COL + NaCl | 1.9 ± 0.14 |
| 18 | Restraint + Me-Cl-COL + Na-Acetate | 2.6 ± 0.30 |
| 19 | Restraint + Me-Cl-COL + Na-Citrate | 2.1 ± 0.25 |
| 20 | Restraint + Me-Cl-COL + Na-Lactate | 3.0 ± 0 |

*Table VI*

Role of Sodium in Production of Myocardial Necrosis by Stress

| Group | Treatment | Cardiac necrosis | |
|---|---|---|---|
| | | (Severity) | (Incidence) |
| 1 | None | 0 | 0 |
| 2 | $NaHCO_3$ | 0 | 0 |
| 3 | Na-Butyrate | 0 | 0 |
| 4 | Na-Glutamate | 0 | 0 |
| 5 | Na-Glycerophosphate | 0 | 0 |
| 6 | Na-Formate | 0 | 0 |
| 7 | Na-Pyruvate | 0 | 0 |
| 8 | Na-Succinate | 0 | 0 |
| 9 | Na-Tartrate | 0 | 0 |
| 10 | Me-Cl-COL | 0 | 0 |
| 11 | Me-Cl-COL + $NaHCO_3$ | 0.1 ± 0.10 | 10 |
| 12 | Me-Cl-COL + Na-Butyrate | 0.1 ± 0.10 | 10 |
| 13 | Me-Cl-COL + Na-Glutamate | 0 | 10 |
| 14 | Me-Cl-COL + Na-Glycerophosphate | 0.2 ± 0.20 | 20 |
| 15 | Me-Cl-COL + Na-Formate | 0 | |
| 16 | Me-Cl-COL + Na-Pyruvate | 0 | |
| 17 | Me-Cl-COL + Na-Succinate | 0.3 ± 0.16 | 20 |
| 18 | Me-Cl-COL + Na-Tartrate | 0.1 ± 0.10 | 10 |
| 19 | Restraint | 0 | |
| 20 | Restraint + $NaHCO_3$ | 0.2 ± 0.20 | 10 |
| 21 | Restraint + Na-Butyrate | 0.3 ± 0.15 | 30 |
| 22 | Restraint + Na-Glutamate | 0 | |
| 23 | Restraint + Na-Glycerophosphate | 0.2 ± 0.18 | 20 |
| 24 | Restraint + Na-Formate | 0.4 ± 0.16 | 30 |
| 25 | Restraint + Na-Pyruvate | 0.7 ± 0.28 | 50 |
| 26 | Restraint + Na-Succinate | 0.4 ± 0.15 | 40 |
| 27 | Restraint + Na-Tartrate | 0.3 ± 0.17 | 30 |
| 28 | Restraint + Me-Cl-COL | 0.2 ± 0.25 | 20 |
| 29 | Restraint + Me-Cl-COL + $NaHCO_3$ | 2.4 ± 0.20 | 100 |
| 30 | Restraint + Me-Cl-COL + Na-Butyrate | 2.9 ± 0.10 | 100 |
| 31 | Restraint + Me-Cl-COL + Na-Glutamate | 2.7 ± 0.25 | 100 |
| 32 | Restraint + Me-Cl-COL + Na-Glycerophosphate | 2.6 ± 0.32 | 100 |
| 33 | Restraint + Me-Cl-COL + Na-Formate | 3.0 ± 0 | 100 |
| 34 | Restraint + Me-Cl-COL + Na-Pyruvate | 2.5 ± 0.22 | 100 |
| 35 | Restraint + Me-Cl-COL + Na-Succinate | 2.7 ± 0.18 | 100 |
| 36 | Restraint + Me-Cl-COL + Na-Tartrate | 3.0 ± 0 | 100 |

chlorate) produce cardiac necroses under ordinary conditions, while others (chloride and several organic salts) are inactive in themselves, but become highly effective during stress. We now wish to report upon experiments which substantiate this concept.

### *Materials and Techniques*

Two hundred rats, with a mean initial body weight of 100 g (range: 95–110 g) were subdivided into 20 equal groups, as indicated in Table V. *Me-Cl-COL* was administered subcutaneously, in the form of its acetate, as a microcrystal suspension of 100 µg in 0.2 ml of water, once daily. All the *Na-salts* were given by stomach tube, at the dose of 2 mM, in 2 ml of water twice daily. *Neuromuscular* stress was induced by maintaining the rats on a board with adhesive tape, for a period of 17 hours on the fifth day of the experiment. The animals of all groups were killed on the sixth day. The hearts were fixed in neutral formalin and embedded in paraffin for subsequent staining with the fuchsin technique.

### *Results and Discussion*

It is evident from our data that, in these rats, cardiac necroses do not occur spontaneously (Group 1), or after treatment with any of the Na-salts (Groups 2–5) or Me-Cl-COL alone (Group 6). Treatment with Me-Cl-COL + Na-salts (Groups 7–10), restraint alone (Group 11) or restraint + Na-salts (Groups 12–15) produced only minute necrotic foci in occasional animals. These lesions were never large enough to be detectable by the naked eye or the hand loupe. Combined treatment with restraint + Me-Cl-COL (Group 16) was somewhat more effective, but (owing to the low dosage of Me-Cl-COL) even here the lesions were very small and only occasionally visible under loupe magnification. By contrast, in the animals treated with restraint + Me-Cl-COL in combination with the otherwise ineffective Na-salts (Groups 17–20) pronounced cardiac necroses were invariably detectable by naked-eye inspection, because they affected large areas of the myocardium. Deaths occurred only among the rats treated with restraint + Me-Cl-COL combined with either Na-citrate (40% mortality, Group 19) and Na-lactate (10% mortality, Group 20).

The principal outcome of these experiments is that certain Na-salts (ineffective in themselves and during simultaneous treatment with either Me-Cl-COL or a stressor) become highly effective in producing massive myocardial necroses, when given in combination with Me-Cl-COL and a stressor, such as forced restraint. Further studies will be necessary to elucidate the mechanism through which otherwise ineffective Na-salts can produce acute myocardial necroses in Me-Cl-COL-conditioned rats during restraint. It is also still uncertain whether there exists any close pathogenetic relationship between the experimental cardiac necroses thus produced and the acute cardiac infarcts that occur in man. It is significant, however, that both these conditions can be elicited by an acute stress situation.

Finally we note that, under similar experimental conditions, several other Na-salts ($NaHCO_3$, Na-butyrate, -glutamate, -glycerophosphate, -formate, -pyruvate, -succinate, -tartrate) were also tested. These experiments were published in detail elsewhere (42) and Table VI serves merely to summarize the results obtained.

*Summary*

Certain Na-salts (chloride, acetate, citrate and lactate) are well tolerated even by rats simultaneously treated with Me-Cl-COL or a severe stressor, such as forced restraint. However, these same salts produce massive and sometimes fatal myocardial necroses, in rats exposed to the stress of forced restraint after conditioning with Me-Cl-COL. It appears that during stress the metabolism of certain otherwise innocuous Na-salts and/or steroids is so altered that they acquire severe cardiotoxic properties.

### *b) Sensitization by DHT and Calcium Acetate for the Induction of Cardiac Lesions by Various Agents.*

The results obtained in our previous experiments showed that corticoids (e.g., Me-Cl-COL) and sterols of the vitamin-D group (e.g., DHT) are both capable of conditioning the heart muscle to the cardiotoxic actions of different agents (see pp. 125–149). Consequently the question arose as to whether there are differences in the manner in which electrolytes affect the heart, following conditioning by corticoids on the one hand, and by sterols of the vitamin-D group on the other.

It was previously established that, in rats, the oral administration of $NaH_2PO_4$ qualitatively alters the cardiotoxic actions of DHT, so that an acute, purulent myocarditis results (615). It has been found, furthermore, that the production of an ESCN by combined treatment with certain corticoids and Na-salts is greatly enhanced in rats exposed to various stressor agents or given dietary supplements of fats or carbohydrates (613).

The experiments described here will show that in rats given calcium acetate instead of sodium phosphate, otherwise ineffective amounts of DHT also produce a suppurating myocarditis, although the pattern of the accompanying soft-tissue calcification is somewhat different. It will be seen, furthermore, that the cardiac damage caused by calcium acetate plus DHT—like that of the ESCN that is induced by corticoids plus Na-salts—can be precipitated by various stressors, and by oral administration of corn oil or glucose supplements.

### *Materials and Techniques*

One hundred sixty rats, with an average initial body weight of 100 g (range 94–109 g) were subdivided into 16 equal groups and treated as indicated in Table VII.

Calcium acetate (1 mM), DHT (25 µg) and glucose (600 mg) were all administered in 2 ml of water, by gavage, twice daily, throughout the experiment. The animals that were to be treated with calcium acetate plus DHT simultaneously received the above-mentioned doses of the two compounds mixed in 2 ml of water. Corn oil was administered by stomach tube, at the dose of 1 ml twice daily, throughout the experiment.

Treatment with the various potentially precipitating agents was initiated on the fifth day, since preliminary experiments had shown that, by that time, treatment with calcium acetate plus DHT alone produces only minimal cardiac lesions and no mortality. The cold baths consisted in immersing the rats in icy water for 5-minute periods, once on the fifth day and twice on the sixth day. Noradrenaline was given subcutaneously, at the dose of 300 µg in 0.2 ml of olive oil, once on the fifth day and twice on the sixth day. The restraint procedure consisted in immobilizing the rats for a period of 17 hours beginning on the morning of the fifth day. Motor denervation of all four extremities was performed, under surgical anesthesia, on the fifth day.

The experiment was terminated on the seventh day. Immediately after autopsy, the hearts were fixed in neutral formalin and stained by von Kóssa's technique for the histochemical demonstration of calcium on paraffin-embedded sections.

## *Results and Discussion*

Perusal of our data (Table VII) indicates that no cardiac lesions occurred either in the controls (Group 1) or in those subjected to motor denervation (Group 5), treatment with corn oil (Group 6), glucose

*Table VII*

Sensitization by DHT and Calcium Acetate for the Induction of Cardiac Lesions by Various Agents

| Group | Treatment | Cardiac lesions | Mortality (%) |
|---|---|---|---|
| 1 | None | 0 | 0 |
| 2 | Cold Baths | 0.1 ± 0.10 | 0 |
| 3 | Noradrenaline | 0.4 ± 0.30 | 0 |
| 4 | Restraint | 0.5 ± 0.25 | 0 |
| 5 | Motor denervation | 0 | 0 |
| 6 | Corn oil | 0 | 0 |
| 7 | Glucose | 0 | 0 |
| 8 | DHT | 0 | 0 |
| 9 | Calcium acetate | 0 | 0 |
| 10 | DHT + Calcium acetate | 0.8 ± 0.15 | 0 |
| 11 | DHT + Calcium acetate + Cold Baths | 2.5 ± 0.23 | 10 |
| 12 | DHT + Calcium acetate + Noradrenaline | 3.0 ± 0 | 20 |
| 13 | DHT + Calcium acetate + Restraint | 2.1 ± 0.28 | 50 |
| 14 | DHT + Calcium acetate + Motor denervation | 1.1 ± 0.17 | 30 |
| 15 | DHT + Calcium acetate + Glucose | 1.5 ± 0.27 | 80 |
| 16 | DHT + Calcium acetate + Corn Oil | 1.8 ± 0.32 | 80 |

(Group 7), DHT (Group 8), or calcium acetate (Group 9), alone. Cold baths (Group 2), noradrenaline (Group 3) and restraint (Group 4) induced only minimal lesions when given by themselves.

Treatment with DHT plus calcium acetate (Group 10) produced definite but mild cardiac lesions, consisting of calcification of the Mönckeberg-sclerosis type in the coronary arteries and calcium deposition within the cardiac muscle fibers or in their surrounding stroma. Previous experiments have shown that this type of lesion can be produced by various vitamin-D derivatives (including DHT) alone, although without supplements of sensitizing salts much larger doses of the sterols are required to obtain calcification of similar intensity (613, 578). In addition to tissue calcification, there were, in the myocardia of most of the animals treated with DHT plus calcium acetate, definite inflammatory, suppurating lesions, with extensive fiber necrosis and massive infiltration with polymorphonuclear leukocytes. These changes cannot be produced even with fatal doses of DHT alone.

The same type of cardiac and coronary lesions occurred, but with significantly greater intensity, in the rats which were treated with cold baths (Group 11), noradrenaline (Group 12), restraint (Group 13), motor denervation (Group 14), oil (Group 16) or glucose (Group 15), in addition to the DHT plus calcium acetate.

Neither DHT nor calcium acetate alone produced any appreciable degree of nephrocalcinosis, but the kidneys of the rats treated with DHT plus calcium acetate exhibited extensive calcification, mainly in the stroma of the cortical region. Calcium deposition within the tubules at the corticomedullary junction line—such as occurs in rats treated with DHT plus $NaH_2PO_4$ (613, 616)—was absent or negligible in the animals of the present experimental series. In this respect, therefore, calcium acetate cannot replace $NaH_2PO_4$. The intensity of the nephrocalcinosis produced by DHT plus calcium acetate (Group 10) was not significantly altered by any of the agents administered to the rats of Groups 11–16; hence, the corresponding figures are not listed in the table.

Deaths occurred only in the groups which, in addition to DHT plus calcium acetate, were treated with one of the agents capable of precipitating the development of cardiac lesions.

It is obvious from these observations that calcium acetate can replace sodium phosphate as a sensitizing agent for the production of myocardial and coronary calcification, as well as suppurating myocarditis, in the rat. Still, there is a difference between the two salts as regards their effect upon the course of DHT intoxication; calcium acetate produces a greater degree of soft-tissue calcification and an almost exclusively cortical nephrocalcinosis, owing to the deposition of insoluble calcium salts in the stroma of the renal cortex, while $NaH_2PO_4$ produces a more intense myocarditis and calcium deposition within the tubular lumina, particularly at the corticomedullary junction line. This difference is apparently due to the fact that although DHT sensitizes tissue for calcification under the influence of an excess of either calcium or phosphate, the two ions have different tissue affinities.

Evidently, after sensitization by DHT plus calcium acetate the most diverse agents can precipitate intense cardiac lesions and cause high mortality. Presumably, the eliciting or precipitating effect is rather nonspecific and largely due to stress. This explanation appears to be particularly probable as regards the precipitation of cardiac lesions by cold baths, restraint and motor denervation.

Adrenergic hormones are known to produce a Mönckeberg-type of arterial calcification in some species (e.g., the rabbit) but not in the rat. However, threshold doses of DHT plus calcium acetate can so sensitize the cardiovascular system of the rat that this normally insensitive species reacts to noradrenaline as does the naturally sensitive rabbit.

Nothing is known about the mechanism through which oral administration of fat and carbohydrate elicits cardiac lesions in rats conditioned with DHT plus calcium acetate. It is noteworthy, however, that these same dietary supplements are also highly effective in eliciting an ESCN in rats conditioned by otherwise ineffective amounts of corticoids plus sodium salts (613).

### *Summary*

Calcium acetate can replace sodium phosphate as a sensitizing agent that permits the production of severe cardiovascular and renal lesions with otherwise ineffective doses of DHT. Still, the effect of the two electrolytes is not the same. Under the influence of DHT, sodium phosphate induces comparatively little cardiac and vascular calcification, much suppurating myocarditis, and a type of nephrocalcinosis that is primarily characterized by the formation of calcium casts within the tubular lumina at the corticomedullary junction line. On the other hand, under the same conditions, calcium acetate induces only mild myocarditic changes, much calcium deposition in the cardiovascular system, and a type of nephrocalcinosis that is almost exclusively limited to the stroma of the renal cortex.

In rats simultaneously treated with comparatively small doses of DHT plus calcium acetate the resulting cardiovascular lesions can be considerably aggravated by a variety of stressor agents (cold baths, restraint, motor denervation). Furthermore, although noradrenaline does not normally produce any cardiovascular calcification in the rat, it is highly effective in this respect when the animal is pretreated with comparatively small doses of DHT plus calcium acetate.

Finally, the oral administration of corn oil or glucose likewise aggravates the cardiovascular effects of DHT plus calcium acetate intoxication; these dietary supplements also act upon the course of the DHT plus calcium acetate syndrome in the same manner as they were previously shown to act upon the cardiopathy induced by corticoids plus sodium salts.

### *c) Interactions between Electrolytes, Corticoids and DHT in the Production of Cardiovascular Disease and Nephrocalcinosis*

It will be recalled that our previous experimental series showed that in the production of a suppurating myocarditis with DHT, calcium acetate can replace sodium phosphate as a conditioning agent (see pp. 155–160). Thus, in this respect the DHT-cardiopathy differs fundamentally from the ESCN, since only Na-salts can produce such cardiac lesions when given in combination with corticoids.

In view of this latest finding, it seemed of interest to establish: 1. whether in animals sensitized with threshold doses of DHT, calcium acetate acquires the property of synergizing the cardiotoxic effect of corticoids, such as Me-Cl-COL; and 2. whether conversely, in the presence of subthreshold doses of Me-Cl-COL, all corticoid-sensitizing Na-salts enhance the toxicity of DHT.

Calcium salts and phosphates are closely implicated in the mechanism of vitamin D intoxication. Hence, their ability to aggravate the changes produced by DHT (alone or in combination with corticoids) would not be unexpected; our main problem was to determine whether such corticoid-sensitizers as $NaClO_4$ and $NaHSO_4$ could also be made effective in this respect.

*Materials and Techniques*

Three experiments were performed on 440 rats with a mean initial body weight of 100 g (range 93–110 g). The animals were subdivided into 44 equal groups and treated as indicated in the Tables VIII–X. Except for the sodium lactate (which was a partially purified product of Fisher Scientific Co.), all salts were of 'reagent' degree of purity. They were invariably administered by stomach tube, at the dose of 1 mM in 2 ml of water, twice daily. DHT was given—also twice daily, by stomach tube—in the first (Table VIII) and third (Table X) experiments, at the dose of 25 μg, and in the second experiment (Table IX) at the dose of 15 μg. Whenever DHT and an electrolyte were given simultaneously, the individual doses of the two compounds were administered together in a total of 2 ml of water. Me-Cl-COL was injected subcutaneously, once daily, in the form of a microcrystal suspension of its acetate, at the dose of 50 μg in 0.2 ml of water, in all 3 experiments.

The hearts and kidneys of all animals were fixed in neutral formalin, for the subsequent histochemical demonstration of calcium deposition with the von Kóssa technique.

*Results*

*First experiment.* In the first experiment the controls received only Me-Cl-COL — DHT, whereas each of the 23 experimental groups was given, in addition to these steroids, various electrolytes as indicated in the preceding section. The experiment was terminated after 6 days.

It is clear from the data in Table VIII that equimolecular amounts of sodium, administered in the form of 11 of its salts (Groups 2–12), exerted very different effects. The perchlorate (Group 3) produced by far the most severe cardiopathy. However, pronounced cardiac lesions also were produced by $Na_2HPO_4$ (Group 5), $NaHSO_4$ (Group 6), $CaH_4(PO_4)_2$ (Group 14), and calcium acetate (Group 23). $NaH_2PO_4$ (Group 4) and $K_2HPO_4$ (Group 16) produced moderate cardiac lesions, whereas all the other salts exhibited little or no such activity.

The most pronounced nephrocalcinosis was elicited by $Na_2HPO_4$ (Group 5), but severe renal calcification also was produced by all other phosphates (Group 4, 13–17), as well as by $NaClO_4$ (Group 3) and calcium acetate (Group 23).

The highest mortality occurred among the rats treated with $NaMnO_4$ (Group 8) due to the intense hemorrhagic gastritis produced by this oxidant; however, since all the rats so treated died during the first 3 days, the absence of cardiac and renal lesions in this group is uninformative. The next highest mortality was induced by $NaClO_4$

*Table VIII*

Effect of Various Electrolytes on the Toxicity of Me-Cl-COL + DHT (First Experiment)

| Group | Treatment* | Cardiac lesions | Nephrocalcinosis | Mortality (%) |
|---|---|---|---|---|
| 1 | None | 0.1 ± 0.10 | 0 | 0 |
| 2 | $NaCl$ | 0 | 0.3 ± 0.15 | 0 |
| 3 | $NaClO_4$ | 2.7 ± 0.30 | 1.9 ± 0.34 | 80 |
| 4 | $NaH_2PO_4$ | 0.5 ± 0.23 | 1.6 ± 0.17 | 0 |
| 5 | $Na_2HPO_4$ | 1.7 ± 0.33 | 3.0 ± 0 | 10 |
| 6 | $NaHSO_4$ | 1.7 ± 0.40 | 0.9 ± 0.17 | 0 |
| 7 | $Na_2SO_4$ | 0.2 ± 0.20 | 0.2 ± 0.15 | 0 |
| 8 | $NaMnO_4$ | 0 | 0 | 100 |
| 9 | $NaNO_3$ | 0.2 ± 0.15 | 0.1 ± 0.10 | 40 |
| 10 | $NaHCO_3$ | 0.2 ± 0.15 | 0 | 0 |
| 11 | Na-acetate | 0.1 ± 0.10 | 0 | 0 |
| 12 | Na-lactate | 0.1 ± 0.10 | 0.2 ± 0.15 | 0 |
| 13 | $MgH_4(PO_4)_2$ | 0.2 ± 0.15 | 1.7 ± 0.18 | 0 |
| 14 | $CaH_4(PO_4)_2$ | 1.0 ± 0.32 | 1.4 ± 0.30 | 50 |
| 15 | $KH_2PO_4$ | 0 | 1.7 ± 0.32 | 0 |
| 16 | $K_2HPO_4$ | 0.6 ± 0.30 | 2.2 ± 0.35 | 0 |
| 17 | $(NH_4)_2HPO_4$ | 0 | 1.0 ± 0.20 | 10 |
| 18 | $MgSO_4$ | 0 | 0.2 ± 0.20 | 10 |
| 19 | $KHSO_4$ | 0 | 0.2 ± 0.15 | 0 |
| 20 | $NH_4HSO_4$ | 0 | 0.1 ± 0.10 | 0 |
| 21 | $KClO_4$ | 0 | 0.3 ± 0.15 | 0 |
| 22 | $Mg(Cl_4)_2$ | 0 | 0 | 0 |
| 23 | Ca-acetate | 2.0 ± 0.32 | 1.8 ± 0.28 | 10 |
| 24 | K-acetate | 0 | 0.4 ± 0.25 | 0 |

* In addition to the treatments mentioned in this column, the rats of all groups were given Me-Cl-COL + DHT, as indicated in the text.

and—judged by their clinical symptoms (cyanosis, dyspnea)—these animals died as a direct result of the cardiac damage. The 4 animals that died after $NaNO_3$ administration appeared to have succumbed to methemoglobin formation (judged by the brownish color of their blood). In the other groups, the immediate cause of death could not be established, but here the mortality was due presumably to cardiac lesions and/or uremia subsequent to nephrocalcinosis.

Apparently, following conditioning with doses of Me-Cl-COL and DHT, in themselves inactive, severe cardiac lesions and nephrocalcinosis can be induced by many electrolytes, not only by the classical 'sensitizing Na-salts' that are effective in this respect even after sensitization with Me-Cl-COL alone. The cardiotoxic effect cannot be ascribed to sodium as such, since several Na-salts are inert in this respect, even after combined treatment with Me-Cl-COL + DHT. The efficacy of salts in which the cation is not sodium (e.g., calcium acetate and dibasic potassium phosphate) may be due in part to the well known sensitization to DHT by calcium or phosphate. Yet, even the activity of phosphate depends in part upon the cation, since ammonium phosphate and monobasic potassium phosphate were inert, while magnesium phosphate exhibited only a trace of activity.

As was to be expected, nephrocalcinosis has been produced under these experimental conditions by all phosphates and calcium salts. However, interestingly, several electrolytes not known to be related in any way to vitamin-D actions (e.g., $NaClO_4$ and $NaHSO_4$) also produced nephrocalcinosis after sensitization with DHT + Me-Cl-COL.

*Second experiment.* The second experiment was designed to determine the relative importance of DHT and Me-Cl-COL in this phenomenon of sensitization. For this purpose, one group of rats received Me-Cl-COL + DHT, whereas the others were given DHT, Me-Cl-COL, or Me-Cl-COL + DHT in combination with certain electrolytes. Among the last, calcium acetate, sodium perchlorate, acid sodium sulfate and acid sodium phosphate were selected because of their previously established intense sensitizing effect (see first experiment), whereas equimolecular amounts of sodium chloride were administered for control purposes. This experiment, terminated after 10 days, is summarized in Table IX.

It is evident that under the conditions prevailing in this second experiment, DHT produced only minimal cardiac lesions and no nephrocalcinosis, even when it was given in combination with

Me-Cl-COL (Group 2). Calcium acetate, given either with DHT (Group 1) or with Me-Cl-COL (Group 3), likewise exhibited little or no effect, but after sensitization with Me-Cl-COL + DHT it produced severe cardiac lesions and marked nephrocalcinosis (Group 4). Essentially similar results were obtained with $NaClO_4$ (Groups 5–7) and $NaH_2PO_4$ (Groups 11–13); these electrolytes also produced much less pronounced cardiac and renal lesions when administered with either DHT or Me-Cl-COL alone than when they were given with Me-Cl-COL + DHT. $NaHSO_4$ induced only negligible cardiac lesions in rats conditioned with DHT alone (Group 8), but in combination with Me-Cl-COL and with Me-Cl-COL + DHT (Groups 9 and 10), this electrolyte produced approximately equally severe cardiac lesions. In no instance did it induce any significant degree of nephrocalcinosis. NaCl proved to be totally inert under all experimental conditions used (Groups 14–16).

As mentioned in our introductory remarks, only certain sodium salts can sensitize the myocardium for the production of necrosis, inflammation, and calcification by such mineralocorticoids as Me-Cl-COL. We then learned that this effect of the 'sensitizing Na-salts' can be further increased by threshold doses of DHT. Calcium acetate does not sensitize for the production of an ESCN by Me-Cl-COL, but it greatly enhances the production of myocardial damage by DHT (as shown by the first experiment). Therefore, in the second experiment, we had to use a much smaller amount of DHT; otherwise maximal lesions would have been obtained in Group 1, and the possible sensitizing effect of Me-Cl-COL could not have been tested. Under the conditions of this second experiment, the possibility of such a sensitization by the corticoid has been demonstrated clearly. Apparently, in rats simultaneously treated with subthreshold amounts of Me-Cl-COL + DHT, salts that sensitize for either of these two sterols become extremely effective in producing cardiac lesions. Conversely, NaCl does not enhance the cardiotoxicity of either DHT or Me-Cl-COL, remains ineffective even when both these sterols are administered.

It is not yet clear why the effect of $NaHSO_4$ (a salt that is highly active in producing an ESCN in combination with Me-Cl-COL) is not further aggravated by the concurrent administration of DHT.

*Third experiment.* The third experiment was performed to verify whether the toxicity of $NaH_2PO_4$ in rats sensitized with Me-Cl-COL or Me-Cl-COL + $NaH_2PO_4$ could be diminished by $CaCl_2$, and the consequent precipitation of less soluble calcium phosphates in the gastrointestinal tract. This experiment was terminated after 12 days.

From Table X it is evident that the intensity of the cardiac lesions and nephrocalcinosis produced by $NaH_2PO_4$ in combination with either Me-Cl-COL or Me-Cl-COL + DHT is considerably reduced by the concurrent oral administration of $CaCl_2$.

Apparently, the sensitizing effect exerted by certain electrolytes in rats conditioned by sterols largely depends upon the absence of other electrolytes that could precipitate the potentially sensitizing salts. Yet, precipitation does not abolish this electrolyte effect completely, as shown by the nephrocalcinosis in Group 4 of Table X and the cardiac lesions and nephrocalcinosis in Group 14 of Table VIII. Presumably,

*Table IX*

Effect of Various 'Sensitizing Salts' upon the Toxicity of Me-Cl-COL + DHT (Second Experiment)

| Group | Treatment | Cardiac lesions | Nephrocalcinosis | Mortality (%) |
|---|---|---|---|---|
| 1 | DHT + Ca-acetate | 0.2 ± 0.5 | 0.2 ± 0.2 | 10 |
| 2 | Me-Cl-COL + DHT | 0.4 ± 0.17 | 0 | 10 |
| 3 | Me-Cl-COL + Ca-acetate | 0.1 ± 0.10 | 0 | 0 |
| 4 | Me-Cl-COL + DHT + Ca-acetate | 1.9 ± 0.32 | 1.2 ± 0.25 | 20 |
| 5 | DHT + $NaClO_4$ | 1.0 ± 0.33 | 0.1 ± 0.10 | 10 |
| 6 | Me-Cl-COL + $NaClO_4$ | 1.7 ± 0.55 | 0.3 ± 0.15 | 60 |
| 7 | Me-Cl-COL + DHT + $NaClO_4$ | 3.0 ± 0 | 1.1 ± 0.10 | 100 |
| 8 | DHT + $NaHSO_4$ | 0.1 ± 0.10 | 0.1 ± 0.10 | 0 |
| 9 | Me-Cl-COL + $NaHSO_4$ | 1.7 ± 0.44 | 0 | 10 |
| 10 | Me-Cl-COL + DHT + $NaHSO_4$ | 1.6 ± 0.64 | 0 | 30 |
| 11 | DHT + $NaH_2PO_4$ | 0.5 ± 0.30 | 2.0 ± 0.32 | 20 |
| 12 | Me-Cl-COL + $NaH_2PO_4$ | 1.6 ± 0.28 | 1.9 ± 0.28 | 40 |
| 13 | Me-Cl-COL + DHT + $NaH_2PO_4$ | 3.0 ± 0 | 2.8 ± 0.20 | 100 |
| 14 | DHT + NaCl | 0 | 0.1 ± 0.10 | 0 |
| 15 | Me-Cl-COL + NaCl | 0 | 0 | 0 |
| 16 | Me-Cl-COL + DHT + NaCl | 0 | 0.2 ± 0.20 | 0 |

*Table X*

Protection by $CaCl_2$ against Conditioning by $NaH_2PO_4$ (Third Experiment)

| Group | Treatment | Cardiac lesions | Nephrocalcinosis | Mortality (%) |
|---|---|---|---|---|
| 1 | Me-Cl-COL + $NaH_2PO_4$ | $1.0 \pm 0.20$ | $1.5 \pm 0.40$ | 40 |
| 2 | Me-Cl-COL + $NaH_2PO_4$ + $CaCl_2$ | $0.3 \pm 0.25$ | $0.1 \pm 0.10$ | 10 |
| 3 | Me-Cl-COL + DHT + $NaH_2PO_4$ | $2.0 \pm 0.32$ | $2.8 \pm 0.20$ | 60 |
| 4 | Me-Cl-COL + DHT + $NaH_2PO_4$ + $CaCl_2$ | 0<br>0 | $1.0 \pm 0.20$ | 0 |

in rats maximally sensitized with DHT + Me-Cl-COL, under the conditions prevailing in the gastrointestinal tract (pH, enzymes), a sufficient amount of calcium phosphate can be absorbed to produce at least some toxic manifestations.

## *Summary*

In rats sensitized with doses of DHT in themselves ineffective, calcium acetate greatly enhances the production of a necrotizing cardiopathy by Me-Cl-COL. This fact is important, because without DHT only certain Na-salts exhibit such a cardiotoxic effect in corticoid-conditioned animals. Conversely, in the presence of subthreshold amounts of Me-Cl-COL, a variety of otherwise inactive Na-salts can enhance the toxicity of simultaneously given, minute amounts of DHT.

Apparently, electrolytes sensitize the heart to the toxic effects of corticoids and of sterols of the vitamin-D group through some closely related mechanisms; consequently, these two types of steroids can potentiate each other's electrolyte-dependent actions. This interpretation has been substantiated further by observations showing essentially similar interactions between Me-Cl-COL and DHT as regards the production of nephrocalcinosis by various electrolytes.

The oral administration of $CaCl_2$ largely neutralizes the cardiotoxic and nephrocalcinotic actions of Me-Cl-COL + $NaH_2PO_4$ or Me-Cl-

COL + DHT + $NaH_2PO_4$. This antagonism is due presumably to the precipitation of comparatively insoluble calcium phosphates. Still, following suitable sensitization with Me-Cl-COL + DHT, even the oral administration of calcium phosphate suffices to produce some cardiac lesions and nephrocalcinosis.

These experiments furnish additional support for the concept that interactions between hormonal steroids, sterols of the vitamin-D group, and electrolytes can exert important pathogenic effects upon the cardiovascular system and the kidney.

## C. Dietary Deficiencies and Other Sensitizing Factors

### *a) Sensitization by K-deficiency for the Production of Myocardial Necrosis by Various Stressor Agents*

It has been shown by FOLLIS (203) that, in rats maintained on a K-deficient diet, forced exercise (swimming with a weight attached to the feet), increased the incidence of myocardial necrosis. On the other hand, it is also known that rats maintained on a diet deficient in K for a period of 3–5 weeks develop cardiac lesions spontaneously (Lit.: 613, 802).

In the following we report on experiments showing that the cardiac muscle is selectively sensitized to the induction of necrosis by various agents in rats maintained on a K-deficient diet for a brief period (for only one week). The diet duplicates 'selective conditioning' to the normally latent cardiotoxic effects of stressor agents. This has previously been found to occur after pretreatment with certain corticoids (e.g., Me-Cl-COL).

#### *Materials and Techniques*

Two hundred thirty rats, with an average initial body weight of 52 g (range: 50–56 g) were subdivided into 23 equal groups and treated as indicated in Table XI.

The *K-deficient diet* (for its composition see 'General Methodology', p. 119) was administered to all the odd-numbered groups listed in Table XI, during the 8 days of the experiment. The even-numbered groups were kept on Purina Fox Chow, but the amount of their food was so reduced as to keep the body weight approximately equal to that of the animals on the K-deficient diet. In this manner, it was hoped to eliminate any possible nonspecific effect of malnutrition which might have been related to the fact that K-deficient animals do not grow at the normal rate.

The potentially cardiotoxic agents used were the following:

*Noradrenaline,* 200 µg in 0.2 ml of oil, administered subcutaneously, twice on the sixth day.

*Vasopressin,* 10 I.U. in 0.5 ml of water, introduced subcutaneously, twice on the sixth day.

*Thyroxine,* 125 µg in 0.2 ml of water, given subcutaneously, daily, throughout the experiment.

*DHT,* 25 µg in 0.2 ml of water, administered by stomach tube, daily, throughout the experiment.

*Plasmocid.* 8-(3-3-diethylaminopropylamino)-6-methoxyquinoline; 0.4 mg in 0.2 ml of water, injected intraperitoneally, 3 times during the sixth day.

*Restraint.* The animals were immobilized for a period of 17 hours on the sixth day.

*Cold.* The rats were immersed in icy water for two periods of 3–5 minutes on the sixth day.

*Heat.* Immersion was carried out in water at 48 °C for two periods of 3–5 minutes on the sixth day.

*Vagotomy.* Bilateral transection of the vagus nerves was performed on the sixth day. As in all surgical procedures, this was carried out under ether anesthesia.

*Quadriplegia.* The motor nerves of all 4 extremities (sciatic, femoral and obturator nerves, brachial plexuses) were severed, thus depriving the rat of the use of its limbs.

*Trauma.* The stomach, ileum and cecum were crushed—3 times each—with a hemostat.

All the surviving rats were sacrificed on the eight day. In each instance, the heart was fixed in neutral formalin and embedded in paraffin. Calcium was demonstrated histologically by the von Kóssa method.

### *Results and Discussion*

It is evident from the data in Table XI that even the comparatively mild nutritional deficiency induced by the low K diet for one week greatly sensitized the heart to the necrosis-producing effects of various agents. This was true in the case of substances (e.g., noradrenaline, vasopressin, DHT and plasmocid) that, at higher dose levels, could produce cardiac lesions in animals on normal diets (613). It also occurred as the result of various forms of stress (e.g., restraint, cold, heat, vagotomy, quadriplegia or intestinal trauma) which normally exerted no specific cardiotoxic effects.

Histologically, the lesions were rather similar to those designated ESCN which were induced by combined treatment with certain electrolytes and steroids. Irrespective of the precipitating agent used, the cardiac lesions in the K-deficient rats consisted of more or less extensive patches of necrosis, distributed throughout the heart, but with particular frequency in the subendocardial layers, the papillary muscles, and the auricles. The necrotic muscle fibers were occasionally impregnated with calcium, but usually the debris derived from them was removed by histiocytes, and eventually they were replaced by scar tissue. Often, Anitschkow myocytes ('caterpillar cells') and multinucleated giant cells appeared in the affected regions. In extreme lesions, the contractile elements disappeared completely from large portions of the ventricular wall. In the auricles, in these instances, only occasional muscle fibers remained. As an incidental observation, it was noted that at the low dose level at which it was given, dihydrotachysterol failed to produce any renal calcification in the control rats. On the other hand, in the rats given the K-deficient diet, its administration resulted in intense nephrocalcinosis. Since the brief period of K-deficiency itself produced no such renal lesion, it was concluded that dietary potassium deprivation sensitized the kidney to the production of nephrocalcinosis by DHT.

In evaluating these data, it should be kept in mind that the 'low-K diet' prepared by the Nutritional Biochemicals Corporation, used in these investigations, is also comparatively poor in magnesium. It was found to contain 52 mg of magnesium per kg. This is close to the minimum amount necessary for growth, according to Tufts and Greenberg (753). Since both potassium and magnesium salts exert a protective effect against the ESCN phenomenon, it is possible that the relative poverty of magnesium also played a sensitizing role in the present experiments. In any event, it is clear that one week of the deficient diet sufficed to render rats unusually sensitive to the induction of massive myocardial necrosis by a great variety of agents. These agents apparently had as their only feature a capacity to produce stress.

A possible relationship between true cardiac infarcts in man and the ESCN phenomenon has been discussed elsewhere (613). It is re-emphasized here that the cardiac lesions elicited by various agents in rats on low-K diet in the present experiments resemble the ESCN in their histologic characteristics and their distribution within the heart. There is, moreover, no evidence of alteration in the coronary vessels. Nonspecific systemic stress can elicit such myocardial lesions after

*Table XI*

Effect of Potassium Deficiency upon the Potential Cardiotoxic Action of Various Agents

| Group | Treatment | Cardiac necrosis | Mortality (%) |
|---|---|---|---|
| 1 | K-Deficiency | 0 | 0 |
| 2 | Noradrenaline | 0.4 ± 0.23 | 0 |
| 3 | Noradrenaline + K-Deficiency | 1.6 ± 0.38 | 30 |
| 4 | Vasopressin | 0 | 0 |
| 5 | Vasopressin + K-Deficiency | 1.7 ± 0.30 | 20 |
| 6 | Thyroxine | 0 | 0 |
| 7 | Thyroxine + K-Deficiency | 0.3 ± 0.15 | 30 |
| 8 | DHT | 0 | 0 |
| 9 | DHT + K-Deficiency | 2.0 ± 0.44 | 10 |
| 10 | Plasmocid | 0.1 ± 0.10 | 0 |
| 11 | Plasmocid + K-Deficiency | 1.3 ± 0.20 | 100 |
| 12 | Restraint | 0 | 10 |
| 13 | Restraint + K-Deficiency | 2.4 ± 0.34 | 30 |
| 14 | Cold | 0 | 0 |
| 15 | Cold + K-Deficiency | 2.1 ± 0.30 | 60 |
| 16 | Heat | 0.1 ± 0.10 | 30 |
| 17 | Heat + K-Deficiency | 1.0 ± 0.20 | 10 |
| 18 | Vagotomy | 0.2 ± 0.17 | 80 |
| 19 | Vagotomy + K-Deficiency | 1.2 ± 0.39 | 0 |
| 20 | Quadriplegia | 0 | 0 |
| 21 | Quadriplegia + K-Deficiency | 1.0 ± 0.27 | 0 |
| 22 | Trauma | 0 | 0 |
| 23 | Trauma + K-Deficiency | 0.7 ± 0.20 | 10 |

conditioning with certain corticoids (635) and following maintenance during a brief period on a potassium deficient diet. It remains to be seen whether this type of cardiopathy has any equivalent in human disease. Our experiments merely indicate that, following suitable dietary conditioning, various stressors may precipitate myocardial necrosis in rats.

*Summary*

In rats maintained for one week on a K-deficient diet, the myocardium showed no detectable structural alterations. This diet also contained only minimum maintenance levels of magnesium. However, in similar animals, extensive myocardial necrosis was induced by a variety of factors which were ineffective in causing this lesion in animals on normal diet. The factors utilized were noradrenaline, vasopressin, thyroxine, DHT, plasmocid, forced restraint, cold or hot baths, vagotomy, quadriplegia and intestinal trauma. It is concluded that a brief period of nutritional deficiency can 'selectively condition' the myocardium to the cardiotoxic effect of various forms of stress.

### *b) Sensitization by K- or Mg-deficiency for the Production of Myocardial Necroses by Papain*

In the course of our studies concerning the sensitizing effects of dietary deficiencies the question arose whether the myocardial necroses normally produced by the intravenous injection of proteases would also be influenced by dietary means.

Experiments performed to check this possibility showed that:

1. dietary deficiency in K or Mg sensitizes the rat to the production of myocardial necroses by papain extracts;
2. the sensitizing effects of K-deficient ration can be abolished by $MgCl_2$-supplements, and those of an Mg-deficient diet by KCl-supplements.

*Materials and Techniques*

Eighty rats, with an initial body-weight of 50 g (range: 49–54 g), were subdivided into 8 equal groups and treated as indicated in Table XII.

The composition of the *K- and Mg-deficient diets* is specified on pp. 119–120 ('General Methodology'). Since the rats on the K-deficient or Mg-deficient diets did not gain weight normally, we added one group of 'weight controls' which received the normal Purina Fox Chow Diet (Ralston Purina Co. of Canada) in an amount so reduced as to keep the body-weight approximately equal to that of the animals on the K- or Mg-deficient diets. Another group, 'age controls', was fed on Purina Fox Chow ad libitum, but they were also of the same weight as those of the previously mentioned groups, because they were selected from a correspondingly younger age-group. By so doing, we felt that the effects of papain were sufficiently controlled, as regards the possible influence a decrease in body-weight might have on the effects of the enzyme preparation.

The *electrolyte* (KCl and $MgCl_2$) solutions were given by stomach tube twice daily throughout the experiment. The individual dose of each of these salts was 0.5 mM in 2 ml of water.

On the 7th day, 0.1 ml of a 5% *papain* solution (filtered) was injected into the jugular vein, under ether anesthesia to all rats.

All the surviving rats were killed on the 9th day of the experiment, that is 2 days after the papain injection. Complete post mortem examinations were made on all animals that were sacrificed and also on those that died soon after the papain injection. In each case, the heart was fixed in neutral formalin and embedded in paraffin, for staining with special fuchsin stain, which is especially suitable for the demonstration of the so-called 'fuchsinophilic degeneration' that characterizes early stages of cardiac necroses.

*Results and Discussion*

It is evident from the data in Table XII that even the comparatively mild nutritional deficiency, induced by keeping rats on K- or Mg-deficient diets for only one week, greatly sensitized the heart for the destructive effect on the proteolytic enzyme preparation.

This hypersensitivity cannot be ascribed merely to the smaller size of the deficient animals. The mean final body-weight of the rats in Group 2, 45 g (range 43–48 g), corresponds quite closely to that of the 'age controls', 47 g (range 45–50 g). On the other hand, the mean final body-weight in Group 5, 73 g (range 60–78 g), closely approximates that of the partially starved 'weight controls' in Groups 7, 62 g (range 59–67 g).

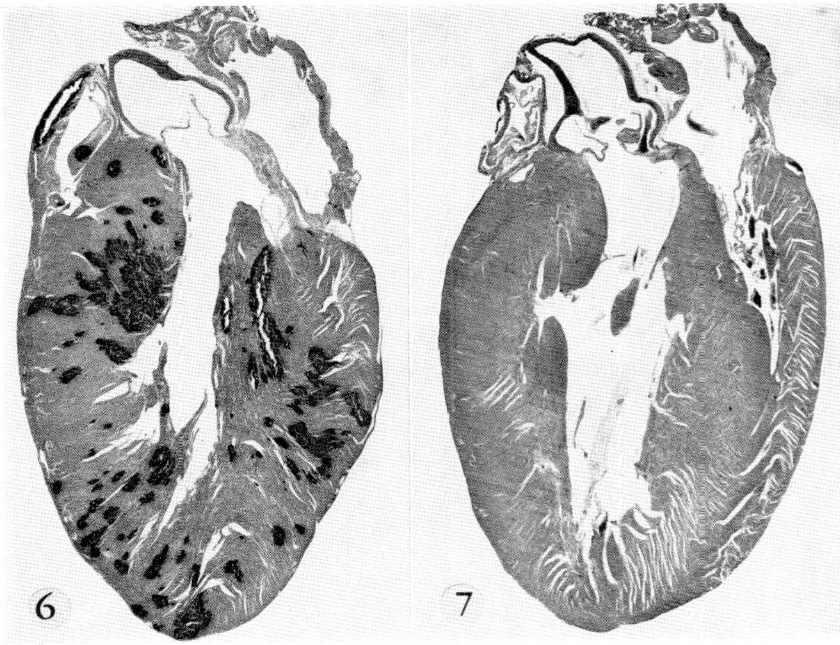

*Figs. 6–7* General view of the myocardial necroses produced by papain in a Mg-deficient rat (Fig. 6), in comparison with the heart of a similarly treated animal protected by a KCl-supplement (Fig. 7). (von Kóssa × 9).

It is particularly noteworthy that the sensitization to papain by the deficient diets failed to occur, not only in the rats kept on the normal Purina Fox Chow ration (Groups 7 and 8), but also in the K-deficient animals given $MgCl_2$-supplements (Group 3) and in the Mg-deficient rats (Group 6) that received additional KCl.

One histologic feature of the cardiac necroses produced by papain that deserves especial mention is the virtually complete absence of 'fuchsinophilic degeneration'. As it was pointed out elsewhere (613), the cardiac necrosis elicited by combined treatment with Me-Cl-COL and certain salts, or by mere exposure to stress, is always preceded by the appearance of fuchsinophilic material and even those parts of the myocardium that do not undergo necrosis tend to show widespread fuchsinophilic degeneration and interstitial edema. Although in the present experimental series necroses were often extremely widespread,

*Table XII*

Sensitization by K- or Mg-Deficiency for the Production of Myocardial Necrosis by Papain

| Group | Treatment | Cardiac necrosis | Mortality (%) |
|---|---|---|---|
| 1 | K-Deficiency | 0 | 0 |
| 2 | K-Deficiency + Papain | 2.1 ± 0.28 | 50 |
| 3 | K-Deficiency + Papain + $MgCl_2$ | 0.1 ± 0.10 | 20 |
| 4 | M-Deficiency | 0 | 0 |
| 5 | Mg-Deficiency + Papain | 2.6 ± 0.17 | 40 |
| 6 | Mg-Deficiency + Papain + KCl | 0.3 ± 0.15 | 10 |
| 7 | Weight controls (partially starved) + Papain | 0.3 ± 0.15 | 0 |
| 8 | Age controls (young) + Papain | 0.5 ± 0.17 | 10 |

papain appears to have affected certain muscle fibers quite selectively causing them to undergo immediate necroses and the fibers that did not succumb showed no detectable histologic evidence of damage. Apparently papain, unlike most other agents that can produce necroses in the heart, either kills the cardiac muscle fibers outright or leaves them structurally intact (Fig. 6).

In evaluating these data, it should be kept in mind that the 'K-deficient Diet' of the Nutritional Biochemical Corp.—that we, like so many other laboratories, have used—is also comparatively poor in Mg. We found it to contain 52 mg/kg of Mg, which is close to the minimal amount necessary for growth, according to Tufts and Greenberg (753). Hence, in Group 3, the $MgCl_2$ may have acted, in part, as a specific supplement for a relative Mg-deficiency that could have played a part in the sensitization to papain. On the other hand, the Mg-deficient diet contained ample amounts of KCl, yet, additional supplements of this salt were required in Group 6, to restore the heart's papain resistance towards normal. In view of these considerations, it is evident that the amounts of Mg and KCl required to maintain the structural integrity of cardiac muscle fibers under normal conditions do not provide optimal protection against papain; an excess of either KCl or $MgCl_2$ is necessary to accomplish this. These observations confirm and extend our earlier finding, according to which KCl and MgCl supplements augment the heart's resistance to the production of papain necroses in rats kept on the well-balanced Purina Fox Chow diet (633); it is particularly noteworthy, however, that in this respect, K and Mg can largely substitute for each other.

*Summary*

In rats kept either on an Mg- or on a K-deficient diet for one week, the production of myocardial necroses by the intravenous injection of papain extract is greatly aggravated. This sensitizing effect of the K-deficient diet can be abolished by supplements of $MgCl_2$, and that of the Mg-deficient diet by KCl.

### *c) Influence of Variations in Dietary Intake of Chlorides upon Diverse Necrotizing Cardiopathies*

Investigations by SELYE (613) showed that $MgCl_2$ and KCl are especially active in preventing the ESCN produced by the combined administration of corticoids and certain Na-salts. Additional experiments (some of which will be described on pp. 224–239) indicated that the chlorides of other cations (like NaCl, $NH_4Cl$, or $CaCl_2$), as well as a mixture of these electrolytes containing equivalent amounts of the anion, are to a certain extent all effective inhibitors of the ESCN and of the infarctoid cardiac changes normally elicited with $NaClO_4$ after sensitization by diets deficient in K or Mg (42, 626).

From these observations, it may be concluded that both the cations ($K^+$ and $Mg^{++}$) and the anion ($Cl^-$) play an important role in the yet unclarified biochemical processes that sensitize or desensitize the myocardium to the action of potentially cardiotoxic agents. It has also been showed that transient occlusion of the pylorus (accompanied by hypochloremia) regularly elicits acute, massive myocardial necrosis in suitably conditioned animals (624).

Consequently, it was interesting to examine the participation of the Cl-ion in the pathogenesis of necrotizing cardiopathies by varying the dietary intake of chlorides. Rats kept on a high- or low-chloride diet were subsequently treated with diverse cardiotoxic agents as described below.

*Materials and Techniques*

*Experiments with a low chloride diet.*—Two hundred and twenty rats, with an average initial body-weight of 50 g (range 45–56 g), were subdivided into 22 equal groups and treated as indicated in Table XIII.

The experimental animals (even-numbered groups) were kept on a low chloride diet, while the controls (odd-numbered groups) received a basic diet, throughout the period of observation. In this manner, we hoped to eliminate any possible nonspecific effect that might have been due to the pure synthetic diet. The rats on the low chloride diet received distilled water ad libitum to drink; those on the basic diet, tap water. The composition of the diets is given on pp. 121–122.

The total chloride content of the low chloride diet was 0.035%, while that of the basic diet, 0.935% (according to the data given by the General Biochemicals, Inc.). Reports in the literature show that diets deficient in chlorides retard somatic growth, in the rat (204). We therefore carried out preliminary studies designed to confirm this finding, using our low chloride diet. It was seen that the growth rate of rats on this diet was diminished as compared with that of controls on the basic diet; this difference was, however, significant only after the 20th day. To avoid any difficulties due to possible size differences between the groups, all the treatments were initiated, and the entire experiment was terminated, prior to the 20th day.

Preliminary experiments, on animals of similar body weight, showed that the doses of the various cardiotoxic agents used here produce only slight cardiac damage, if any. Hence, these doses were suitable for demonstrating possible sensitization by the low chloride diet. The potentially cardiotoxic agents used were the following:

*Noradrenaline* was given at the dose of 150 μg in 0.2 ml of oil, twice daily, subcutaneously, on the 17th and 18th days of the experiment. *Vasopressin* was injected twice daily on the 17th and the following day, at the dose of 10 I.U. in 1.0 ml of water, subcutaneously. *Plasmocid,* 6-methoxy-8-(3-diethylamino-propylamino)-quinoline dihydroiodide, was injected three times daily, at 4-hour intervals, on the 17th and 18th days, at the dose of 0.3 mg in 0.2 ml of water, intraperitoneally. *Papain* (5 percent—filtered solution) was injected once on the 17th day; 0.1 ml into the jugular vein. *DHT* was always given in the form of a microcrystal suspension, twice daily, by stomach tube. This treatment was administered from the 13th to the 18th day of the experiment. The rats in group 11 and group 12 received 70 μg of DHT daily, in two equal portions, always in 1.0 ml of water. In groups 13 and 14, 20 µg of DHT was administered mixed with Ca-acetate, in 1.0 ml of water, twice daily. *Calcium acetate* was given (together with DHT) in a concentration of 0.25 mM in 1.0 of water, twice daily, by stomach tube, between the 13th and the 18th day. *F-COL* was injected subcutaneously, as a microcrystal suspension, at the dose of 500 µg daily, in 0.2 ml of water, from the 13th to the 18th day. *$Na_2HPO_4$,* dibasic sodium phosphate was administered from the 13th to the 18th day, in a concentration of 0.25 mM in 1.0 ml of water, twice daily, by stomach tube. *Sodium acetate* was likewise given by stomach tube, twice daily, in a concentration of 0.25 mM in 1.0 ml of water from the 13th to the 18th day. *Restraint* was applied, on the 17th day, for 17 hours. *Quadriplegia,* through motor denervation of all four extremities, was performed on the 17th day.

The experiment was terminated on the 19th day by killing the surviving rats with chloroform. In all instances, the hearts were first inspected with the aid of a dissecting loupe, immediately after autopsy, and then fixed in absolute alcohol, containing 10% neutral formalin, for subsequent embedding in paraffin. The sections were stained with von Kóssa's technique for the histochemical demonstration of calcium (using hematoxylin-phloxine counterstain), as well as with the fuchsin method.

*Experiments with a high chloride diet.*—To observe the effect of a high chloride diet upon the development of necrotizing cardiopathies, two hundred female Sprague-Dawley rats, with a mean initial body weight of 51 g (range: 46–58 g), were subdivided into 20 equal groups and treated as indicated in Table XIV.

All the animals of the odd-numbered groups (listed in Table XIV) were maintained on a synthetic basic diet, while those of the even-numbered groups were kept on a high chloride diet. The total chloride content of the high chloride diet was 1.62% (determined by the General Biochemicals Inc.). The *basic diet* used here was identical in its composition with that used in the first experimental series. The composition of the high chloride diet is given in the chapter 'General Methodology', p. 122.

In order to establish the possible protective effect of the high chloride diet, the doses of the cardiotoxic agents (with the exception of noradrenaline, vasopressin and F-COL) were higher than in the previous experimental series, namely: plasmocid 0.5 mg; papain 0.15 ml (10%); DHT 100 µg to groups 11 and 12, 75 µg to groups 13 and 14,

Ca-acetate 0.5 mM; Na-acetate 1 mM and $Na_2HPO_4$ 0.5 mM. However, the date of initiation, duration of treatment, route of administration, and all other experimental conditions remained as previously.

Because of the high mortality rate, the surviving rats of groups 13 and 14 were killed on the 17th day; all animals in the remaining groups were sacrificed on the 19th day, the termination of the experiment. The results were evaluated histologically, as previously described, and are summarized in Table XIV.

### *Results*

*Effect of low chloride diet.*—As will be seen from the data in Table XIII, chloride deficiency markedly enhanced the cardiotoxic effect of most of the agents used. Only the necrotizing actions of noradrenaline and vasopressin were not effected.

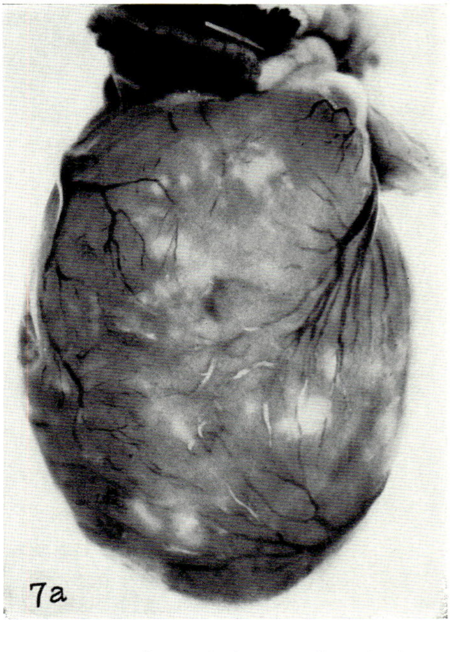


*Fig. 7a* Macroscopic appearance of the calcifying cardiopathy in a rat treated with DHT plus Ca-acetate while kept on the low chloride diet.

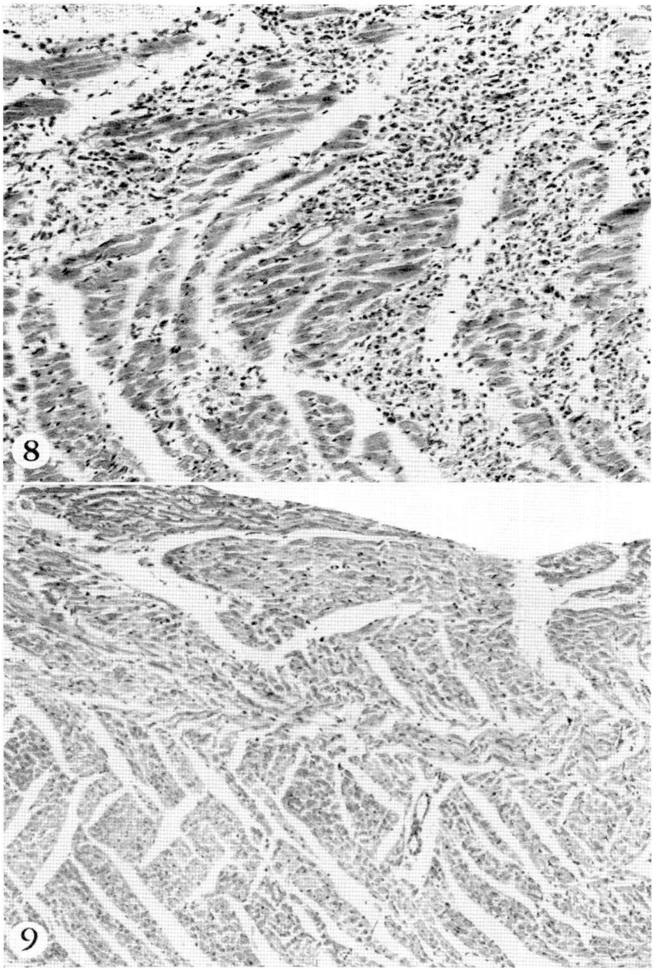


*Figs. 8–9 Sensitization by low chloride intake to necrotizing effect of papain.* Fig. 8: Extensive necroses throughout the wall of the right ventricle, in a papain treated rat kept on a chloride-deficient diet. Fig. 9: Absence of cardiac lesions in a similarly papain-treated control rat allowed a normal intake of chlorides (von Kóssa × 120).

The body weights of the animals maintained on the experimental and on the basic diets were essentially the same at the time when treatment with the various cardiotoxic agents began, yet the low chloride diet markedly aggravated the severity and incidence of the cardiac lesions normally produced by plasmocid (Groups 7 and 8), papain (Groups 9 and 10), DHT (Groups 11 and 12) DHT + Ca-acetate (Groups 13 and 14); F-COL + $Na_2HPO_4$ (Groups 15 and 16), F-COL + Na-acetate (Groups 17 and 18), as well as those elicited by restraint (Groups 19 and 20) and quadriplegia (Groups 21 and 22), after conditioning with F-COL.

*Table XIII*

Effect of Low Chloride Diet upon Cardiac Lesions Produced by Small Doses of Various Agents

| Group | Treatment* | Cardiac lesions | | Mortality (%) |
|---|---|---|---|---|
| | | (Severity) | (Incidence) | |
| 1 | None (Basic Diet) | 0 | 0 | 0 |
| 2 | None (Low Chloride Diet) | 0 | 0 | 0 |
| 3 | Noradrenaline + Basic Diet | 1.1 ± 0.27 | 60 | 0 |
| 4 | Noradrenaline + Low Chloride Diet | 1.0 ± 0.20 | 60 | 0 |
| 5 | Vasopressin + Basic Diet | 1.3 ± 0.31 | 60 | 0 |
| 6 | Vasopressin + Low Chloride Diet | 1.5 ± 0.23 | 70 | 0 |
| 7 | Plasmocid + Basic Diet | 0.3 ± 0.18 | 20 | 0 |
| 8 | Plasmocid + Low Chloride Diet | 2.7 ± 0.13 | 90 | 40 |
| 9 | Papain + Basic Diet | 0.4 ± 0.17 | 30 | 0 |
| 10 | Papain + Low Chloride Diet | 2.8 ± 0.20 | 100 | 50 |
| 11 | DHT + Basic Diet | 0.2 ± 0.20 | 20 | 0 |
| 12 | DHT + Low Chloride Diet | 3.0 ± 0 | 100 | 60 |
| 13 | DHT + Ca-Acetate + Basic Diet | 0.5 ± 0.25 | 30 | 0 |
| 14 | DHT + Ca-Acetate + Low Chloride Diet | 3.0 ± 0 | 100 | 40 |
| 15 | F-COL + $Na_2HPO_4$ + Basic Diet | 0.3 ± 0.18 | 20 | 0 |
| 16 | F-COL + $Na_2HPO_4$ + Low Chloride Diet | 2.7 ± 0.21 | 100 | 100 |
| 17 | F-COL + Na-Acetate + Basic Diet | 0 | 0 | 0 |
| 18 | F-COL + Na-Acetate + Low Chloride Diet | 2.2 ± 0.13 | 90 | 70 |
| 19 | F-COL + Restraint + Basic Diet | 0.8 ± 0.25 | 50 | 0 |
| 20 | F-COL + Restraint + Low Chloride Diet | 2.6 ± 0.15 | 100 | 20 |
| 21 | F-COL + Quadriplegia + Basic Diet | 0.2 ± 0.20 | 10 | 0 |
| 22 | F-COL + Quadriplegia + Low Chloride Diet | 1.9 ± 0.26 | 80 | 10 |

* All the odd-numbered groups were kept on a synthetic (basic) diet, as described in the text.

The comparatively small doses of *plasmocid,* which produced only occasional, mild lesions in the control rats, regularly caused large, patchy myocardial necroses and myocarditic lesions in the chloride-deficient animals. It will be recalled that the plasmocid lesions differ from most of the other experimental cardiopathies that we studied in that the former cannot be greatly influenced by treatment with electrolytes or corticoids. Nevertheless, as in many other cardiopathies, Na-deficiency offers protection against plasmocid also (644). The miliary, disseminated cardiac necroses normally caused by the intravenous injection of *papain* were much more severe in the rats kept on a chloride-deficient diet; this sensitization also manifests itself in the mortality rate (Table XIII). Chloride deficiency not only aggravated the calcification and necrosis of the cardiac muscle normally produced by DHT, but intensive calcification also occurred in the skeletal muscles, gastrointestinal tract, and renal cortex. The calcification of the tissues was even more marked in the chloride-deficient rats treated with DHT + Ca-acetate; in these animals, muscular paralysis developed in addition to acute, suppurative myocarditis. The combination of *$Na_2HPO_4$ + F-COL* in the amounts used was not sufficient to induce ESCN in the control rats, whereas 100% of the chloride-deficient animals died, exhibiting the typical picture of this infarctoid cardiopathy. It is especially interesting, furthermore, that in the animals kept on the low chloride diet, otherwise completely ineffective treatment with *F-COL + Na-acetate* elicited macroscopically visible, large patches of cardiac necroses resembling the typical ESCN. Nephrocalcinosis developed in many, but not in all, of these rats. The *stressor effect* of neuromuscular effort (induced by forced restraint) or quadriplegia only occasionally produced the usual small necrotic foci ('micronecroses') in the control animals conditioned with F-COL; but there again, dietary chloride deficiency sensitized the heart muscle so that, as a result of stress, large macroscopically visible necroses developed.

On the other hand, the spotty, myolytic type of cardiac damage elicited with *noradrenaline* (Groups 3 and 4) and with *vasopressin* (Groups 5 and 6) was not altered by a lowered dietary intake of chlorides.

*Effect of high chloride diet.*—As shown in Table XIV an increase in the dietary intake of chlorides from a basic 0.953 to 1.62% protects the myocardium against the necrotizing actions of many unrelated agents. Here again, however, the cardiotoxicity of noradrenaline and of vasopressin was not significantly influenced.

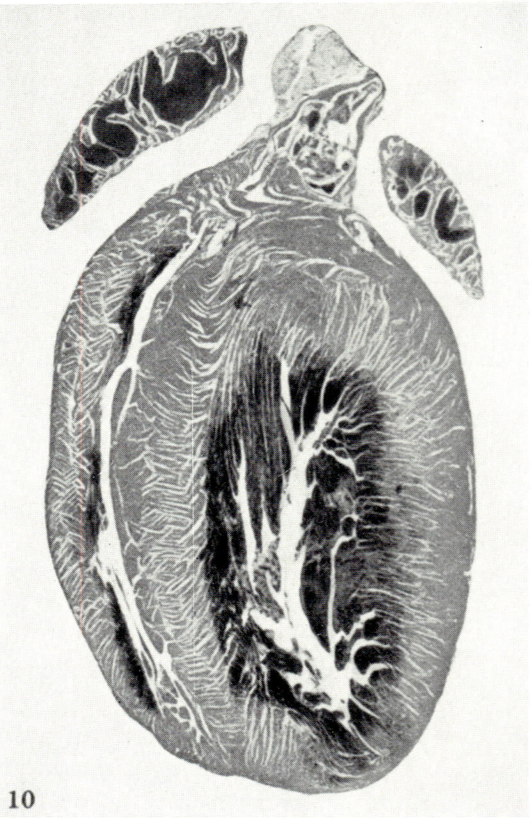

*Fig. 10* Sensitization by chloride deficiency to the necrotizing action of F-COL + Na-acetate. The general view of the myocardial necrosis and calcification *(black area)* in a rat given F-COL + Na-acetate while on a low chloride diet. On a normal diet this treatment is consistently ineffective in producing any cardiac lesion without subsequent exposure to stressor agents (von KÓSSA × 9).

The mean body weight of the rats kept on the basic and high-chloride diets was essentially the same at the initiation of the cardiac-damaging treatments. Yet, the dietary excess of chlorides significantly protected the animals against the cardiac lesions normally produced by plasmocid (Groups 7 and 8), papain (Groups 9 and 10), DHT (Groups 11 and 12), and DHT + Ca-acetate (Groups 13 and 14). Not only the decrease in the severity and incidence of the cardiac lesions, but also the lowered mortality rate, illustrates the desensitizing action of a high

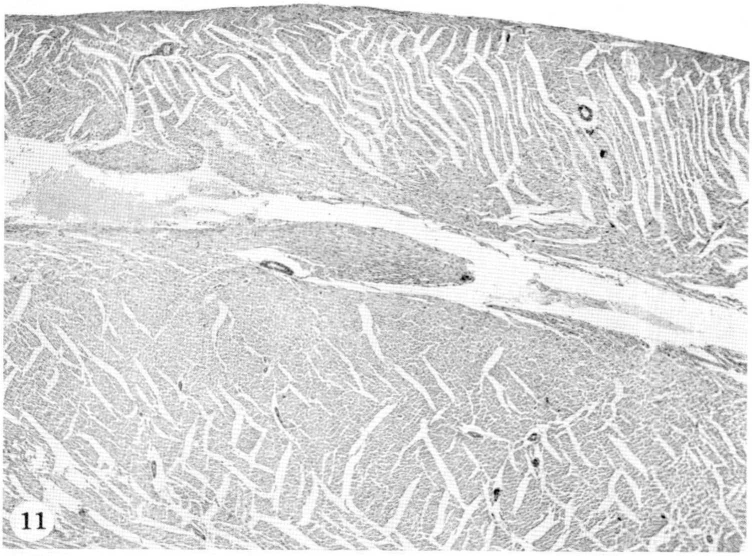


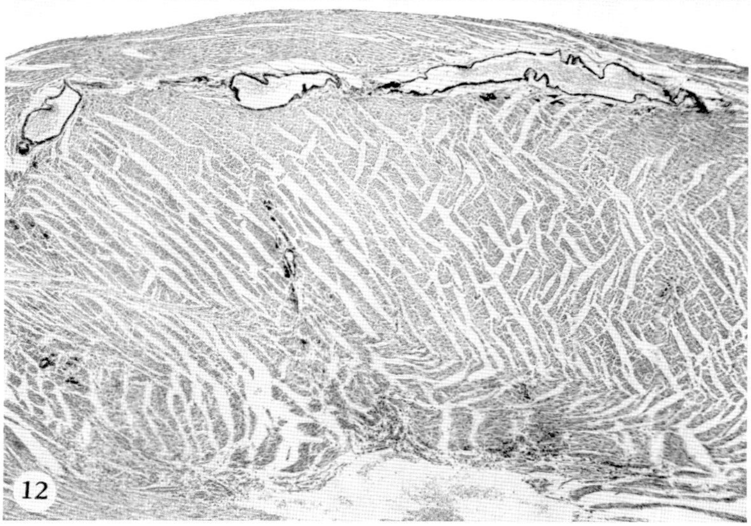


*Figs. 11–12 Prevention by high chloride diet of cardiac calcification after DHT treatment.* Fig. 11: Absence of calcification and necrosis in heart of a rat kept on high chloride diet and given a large amount of DHT. Fig. 12: Severe calcifying lesions produced by same doses of DHT on the basic diet (von Kóssa × 30).

intake of chlorides in all four cardiopathies. It is especially noteworthy that a dietary excess of chloride abolished the cardiotoxic action of DHT and that of DHT + Ca-acetate; in an earlier experiment, Na-deficiency similarly inhibited the calcifying and slight necrotizing action of DHT, but not the more severe myocarditic lesions resulting from DHT + Ca-acetate (644). Interestingly, in the animals treated

*Table XIV*

Effect of High Chloride Diet upon Cardiac Lesions Produced by Large Doses of Various Agents

| Group | Treatment* | Cardiac lesions (Severity) | Cardiac lesions (Incidence) | Mortality (%) |
|---|---|---|---|---|
| 1 | None (Basic Diet) | 0 | 0 | 0 |
| 2 | None (High Chloride Diet) | 0 | 0 | 0 |
| 3 | Noradrenaline + Basic Diet | 0.4 ± 0.28 | 30 | 0 |
| 4 | Noradrenaline + High Chloride Diet | 0.5 ± 0.25 | 40 | 0 |
| 5 | Vasopressin + Basic Diet | 0.8 ± 0.37 | 50 | 0 |
| 6 | Vasopressin + High Chloride Diet | 1.1 ± 0.21 | 70 | 0 |
| 7 | Plasmocid + Basic Diet | 2.9 ± 0.12 | 100 | 80 |
| 8 | Plasmocid + High Chloride Diet | 0.4 ± 0.16 | 20 | 0 |
| 9 | Papain + Basic Diet | 3.0 ± 0 | 100 | 90 |
| 10 | Papain + High Chloride Diet | 0.5 ± 0.23 | 30 | 10 |
| 11 | DHT + Basic Diet | 2.6 ± 0.34 | 100 | 20 |
| 12 | DHT + High Chloride Diet | 0.2 ± 0.20 | 10 | 10 |
| 13 | DHT + Ca-Acetate + Basic Diet | 3.0 ± 0 | 100 | 70 |
| 14 | DHT + Ca-Acetate + High Chloride Diet | 0.6 ± 0.27 | 40 | 0 |
| 15 | F-COL + $Na_2HPO_4$ + Basic Diet | 2.1 ± 0.18 | 90 | 50 |
| 16 | F-COL + $Na_2HPO_4$ + High Chloride Diet | 0 | 0 | 100 |
| 17 | F-COL + Na-Acetate + Restraint + Basic Diet | 2.8 ± 0.16 | 100 | 70 |
| 18 | F-COL + Na-Acetate + Restraint + High Chloride Diet | 0.2 ± 0.17 | 10 | 70 |
| 19 | F-COL + Restraint + Basic Diet | 1.0 ± 0.39 | 60 | 40 |
| 20 | F-COL + Restraint + High Chloride Diet | 0.1 ± 0.10 | 10 | 30 |

* All the odd-numbered groups were kept on a synthetic (basic) diet, as described in the text.

with DHT, as well as in those treated with DHT + Ca-acetate, the high chloride diet suppressed the exclusively cortical nephrocalcinosis normally induced by overdosage with this vitamin-D derivative.

Many of the animals that were fed the high chloride diet died after the first injection of fluorocortisol, with rather persistent, tonic extensor cramps. The mortality rate was the highest in the rats receiving a dietary excess of chlorides and treated with F-COL + $Na_2HPO_4$; here, the clinical picture of acute phosphate intoxication was the dominant feature and resulted in 100% fatality within a few hours. Since, these animals did not show any histologically detectable cardiac changes, this part of the experiment is rather inconclusive (Groups 15 and 16). The results obtained in the rats pretreated with F-COL + Na-acetate (Groups 17 and 18) and especially in those conditioned with F-COL alone (Groups 19 and 20) and then exposed to the stressor effect of forced restraint are more instructive, since there the unexpected side action of F-COL resulted in only 40 and 20% mortality, respectively, among the rats with a high chloride intake. None of the survivors showed marked myocardial damage, whereas in the control animals the lesions were constant and pronounced.

On the other hand, a dietary excess of chlorides did not prevent the occurrence of spotty myolysis in the rats treated with noradrenaline (Groups 3 and 4) and in those treated with vasopressin (Groups 5 and 6). The lesions (more or less complete disappearance of individual muscle fibers) induced with these agents were mild in the control animals, but, as a result of a high intake of chlorides, their incidence seemed to be slightly increased, although this apparent sensitization was not statistically significant.

### *Discussion*

It is obvious from the results described in the foregoing that dietary chloride deficiency sensitizes the heart to various potentially cardiotoxic agents, whereas dietary chloride excess exerts an opposite action. Nothing is known as yet about the mechanism through which variations in the dietary intake of chlorides so uniformly influence (aggravate or prevent) the various types of necrotizing cardiopathies that formed the subject of our investigations.

Although the diets used in the present experimental series were identical as regards the ratios and amounts of cations, the variations in their chloride content naturally necessitated changes in other anions.

The chloride-deficient diet differed from the basic diet in that in the former the chloride was replaced by equivalent quantities of corresponding bicarbonates. Therefore, since the bicarbonate is generally considered innocuous (745, 764) the noxious effect of this diet may be attributed to its deficiency in chlorides. On the other hand, the great increase in the intake of chlorides with no change in the ratio of cations resulted in a high chloride diet relatively deficient in bicar bonate and inorganic sulfate. However, the uniform and dramatic preventive effect of this high chloride diet as compared with the marked opposite effect of chloride deficiency suggests that the variations in this anion may be the most important factor responsible for the results observed. This assumption is further supported by earlier findings in which, among the various electrolytes administered, no salts of anions other than chlorides offered significant protective action in the ESCN or in other experimental cardiopathies (613).

All these observations suggest that chlorides play an important role in the pathogenesis of many types of experimental cardiopathies produced by biochemical means. It remains to be established whether variations in the intake of chlorides similarly influence the occurrence of spontaneous necrotizing cardiopathies in man, especially those unaccompanied by acute obstruction of the coronary vessels.

The pathogenesis of the necrotizing cardiopathy normally produced with noradrenaline and vasopressin (changes to which we usually refer as 'spotty myolysis') seems to be basically different from all other types of cardiac necroses studied, since only the latter were significantly influenced by the administration of electrolytes, by dietary Na-deficiency (42, 644) or by variations in dietary intake of chlorides. It is interesting in this connection that Raab (503) concluded from his experiments that a sudden liberation of catecholamines within the heart muscle fibers could be responsible for the development of the ESCN. By depleting the catecholamines with reserpine, he succeeded in protecting the myocardium against this type of necrosis. Perhaps noradrenaline and vasopressin act at the final stage of the biochemical chain-reaction that results in necroses, whereas all other agents (steroids and electrolytes) exert their influence at intermediate points. Yet it would be difficult to explain on this basis why pretreatment with KCl and $MgCl_2$ offers considerable protection against the myocardial necroses normally produced by intravenous administration of proteases (633, 640, 649) and even against the acute infarcts that follow surgical occlusion of coronary vessels (47).

*Summary*

Experiments on rats were performed to examine the effect of variations in dietary intake of chlorides upon diverse experimental cardiac lesions, which differ widely from each other in both their causative agents and their histologic characteristics.

It was found that chloride deficiency significantly enhances the susceptibility of the heart to the production of necrosis, inflammation, and/or calcification by plasmocid, papain, DHT, Ca-acetate + DHT, $Na_2HPO_4$ + F-COL, Na-acetate + F-COL, as well as by the stressor effect of forced restraint or quadriplegia after conditioning with F-COL. On the other hand, a dietary excess of chlorides proved to be effective in protecting the myocardium against all the cardiotoxic agents enumerated above.

The observation that a number of diverse cardiopathies are uniformly aggravated by a low chloride diet, and prevented by a dietary excess of chlorides, suggests that chlorides may play an important role in the pathogenesis of various necrotizing cardiopathies.

The spotty myolysis normally due to the administration of nor-adrenaline or vasopressin remained uninfluenced by variations in the dietary intake of chlorides; hence, it was concluded that this type of cardiac lesion differs basically in its mechanism from all the other forms studied.

### *d) Sensitization by Chloride Deficiency to Corticoid-induced Cardiac Necroses.*

Our previous experimental series suggested that not only the variations in dietary intake of certain cations (such as K and Mg) but also of the anions (i.e., Cl) play an important role in the pathogenesis of various necrotizing cardiopathies (see p. 175). On the other hand, it was also observed that after suitable sensitization with corticoids, certain Na-salts (phosphates, sulfates and perchlorate) produce cardiac necrosis under ordinary conditions, while others (chloride, carbonate, and several organic salts) are inactive in themselves but become highly effective during stress (see p. 149). Thus, it appears that during stress the metabolism of certain otherwise innocuous Na-salts and/or steroids is so altered that the combination of these agents acquires severe cardiotoxic properties.

In the following we wish to report upon experiments showing that a similar activation of an electrolyte-steroid interaction occurs even without exposure to stressors when rats are kept on a diet low in chloride.

### *Materials and Techniques*

One hundred and fifty rats, with a mean initial body weight of 49 g (range 42–56 g), were subdivided into 15 equal groups and treated as indicated in Table XV. The rats were kept on either a synthetic basic diet or on a chloride deficient ration, 7 days prior to, as well as during, the treatment with Na-salts and/or F-COL. They were allowed to drink distilled water ad libitum. The composition of the basic diet and that of the chloride-deficient ration is detailed on pp. 121–122.

The *Na-salts* were administered by stomach tube, in a concentration of 0.5 ml in 2 mM of water, twice daily. F-COL was injected subcutaneously as a microcrystal suspension, at the dose of 500 μg daily, in 0.2 ml of water. The F-COL and the electrolytes were administered from the 8th day until the termination of the experiment. The survivors of all groups were killed with chloroform on the fifteenth day. At autopsy, the hearts were fixed in neutral formalin and embedded in paraffin for subsequent staining with haemotoxylin-phloxine. The kidneys were studied for calcium using von Kóssa's silver nitrate technique.

### *Results and Discussion*

It is evident from the data (see Table XV) that cardiac necroses do not occur spontaneously (Group 1) or after combined treatment with F-COL plus Na-salts in rats on the basic diet (Groups 2–5). Similarly, the chloride-deficient diet (Group 6), with or without administration of either the Na-salts (groups 7–10) or F-COL (Group 11), produced no histologically detectable cardiac abnormality. However, in the animals fed the chloride-deficient diet and given F-COL plus the Na-salts, acute and sometimes fatal cardiac necroses developed (Groups 12–15). These cardiac lesions were invariably detectable with the naked eye, because they affected large areas of the myocardium; they were distributed throughout the heart, but with particular frequency in the

*Table XV*

Electrolyte-Steroid Cardiotoxicity Activated by Chloride Deficiency

| Group | Treatment | Cardiac necrosis | | Mortality (%) |
|---|---|---|---|---|
| | | (Severity) | (Incidence) | |
| 1 | Basic Diet | 0 | 0 | 0 |
| 2 | Basic Diet + F-COL + $NaHCO_3$ | 0 | 0 | 0 |
| 3 | Basic Diet + F-COL + Na-Citrate | 0 | 0 | 0 |
| 4 | Basic Diet + F-COL + Na-Glutamate | 0 | 0 | 0 |
| 5 | Basic Diet + F-COL + Na-Succinate | 0 | 0 | 0 |
| 6 | Cl-Deficient Diet | 0 | 0 | 0 |
| 7 | Cl-Deficient Diet + $NaHCO_3$ | 0 | 0 | 0 |
| 8 | Cl-Deficient Diet + Na-Citrate | 0 | 0 | 0 |
| 9 | Cl-Deficient Diet + Na-Glutamate | 0 | 0 | 10 |
| 10 | Cl-Deficient Diet + Na-Succinate | 0 | 0 | 10 |
| 11 | Cl-Deficient Diet + F-COL | 0 | 0 | 0 |
| 12 | Cl-Deficient + F-COL + $NaHCO_3$ | 2.3 ± 0.25 | 100 | 100 |
| 13 | Cl-Deficient Diet + F-COL + Na-Citrate | 2.4 ± 0.18 | 100 | 90 |
| 14 | Cl-Deficient Diet + F-COL + Na-Glutamate | 1.9 ± 0.31 | 80 | 70 |
| 15 | Cl-Deficient Diet + F-COL Na-Succinate | 2.2 ± 0.27 | 90 | 90 |

subendocardial layers and papillary muscles. The yellowish patches consisted of necrotic and disintegrated muscle fibers partly infiltrated by polymorphonuclear leukocytes and monocytes. In about 10% of these rats (Groups 12–15) a slight degree of nephrocalcinosis at the cortico-medullary junction was detected. No such renal lesion was observed in any of the remaining groups. With the exception of two deaths in Groups 9 and 10 that were probably caused by technical errors (e.g., inspiration of the electrolyte solution), mortality occurred only in the rats with cardiac necroses; in other words, in those animals fed the chloride-deficient diet and given both the F-COL and Na-salts.

The principal outcome of these experiments is that the combined administration of F-COL and certain Na-salts (ineffective under ordinary conditions) becomes highly effective in eliciting acute cardiac necrosis when the chloride content of the diet is lowered from a basic 0.935% to 0.035%. It should be recalled in this connection that the chloride-deficient diet differed from the basic diet in that, in the former, the chlorides were replaced by corresponding bicarbonates. Since the bicarbonate is generally considered innocuous (745, 764), the toxic effect observed may be attributed to the deficiency in chloride. Further studies will be necessary to elucidate the mechanism through which chloride deficiency activates the cardiotoxicity of F-COL and/or certain Na-salts. It is significant, however, that the same electrolyte-steroid combination is similarly activated, even in the animals fed the normal laboratory ration (e.g., 'Purina Fox Chow' or a synthetic diet with an adequate chloride content) during exposure to stressful stimuli (42, 638).

*Summary*

The effects of variations in dietary chloride intake upon the cardiotoxic effect of F-COL and/or certain Na-salts were studied. It was observed that overdosage with fluorocortisol, $NaHCO_3$, Na-citrate, Na-glutamate or Na-succinate is well tolerated by rats kept on synthetic diets. However, combined administration of F-COL and the same Na-salts produces massive and sometimes fatal myocardial necroses when the chloride content of the diet is lowered from a basic 0.953% to 0.035%. It appears that chloride deficiency selectively sensitizes the heart muscle to this potentially cardiotoxic electrolyte-steroid interaction.

### e) *The Age Factor in the Production of Various Experimental Cardiopathies*

In the course of our studies on experimental cardiac necroses, incidentally, we noted that the production of such lesions is much easier in old than in young animals. Since, in man, the incidence of cardiac lesions is likewise greatly increased with the progress of age, we decided to examine the role of the age factor in the production of various experimental cardiopathies.

*Materials and Techniques*

Two hundred and forty rats were subdivided into 24 groups of ten. The approximate age of the animals was as follows: 4 weeks (50 g),

45 days (100 g), and 10 months (300 g). Each of the 8 potentially cardiotoxic agents used in this study was tested under otherwise identical conditions.

*Papain* (5%, filtered solution) was injected into the jugular vein, in the amount of 0.2 ml/100 g of body weight, once on the 1st day. All the surviving rats were killed 48 hours following the papain injection. *Plasmocid,* 8(3-diethylaminopropylamino)-6-methoxyquinoline, was given at the dose of 0.4 mg/100 g body weight, always in 0.2 ml of water, intraperitoneally, three times on the first day. The experiment was terminated 48 hours following the last injection. *Noradrenaline* was given twice daily, at the dose of 250 μg/100 g body weight, in 0.2 ml of oil, subcutaneously, during the first two days. *Vasopressin* was injected during the first and second days, at the dose of 10 I.U./ 100 g body weight, in 1 ml of water, twice daily, subcutaneously. The animals were killed 48 hours following the last noradrenaline and vasopressin injection. *Restraint* was applied for 17 hours, on the first day of the experiment. The animals were killed 48 hours after the initiation of the restraint. *Quadriplegia* was performed on the first day and this experiment was terminated on the second day following the operation. *DHT* was given in the form of a microcrystal suspension, at the daily dose of 300 μg/100 g body weight, in 0.5 ml of water, by stomach tube, during 5 days. The rats were then killed on the sixth day. *Me-Cl-COL* was injected subcutaneously, in the form of microcrystals of its acetate, at the daily dose of 100 μg/100 g body weight, during 5 days. *$Na_2HPO_4$* was administered at the dose of 1 mM/100 g body weight, twice daily, in 2 ml (the amount of 3 mM however, in 4 ml) of water by stomach tube, during 5 days. The experiment was terminated on the sixth day.

In all instances, the hearts were first inspected with the aid of a dissecting loupe, immediately after autopsy, and then fixed in neutral formalin for subsequent embedding in paraffin. The sections were stained with von Kóssa's technique for the histochemical demonstration of calcium (using a hematoxylin-phloxine counterstain), because several of the cardiotoxic agents produce calcium depositions in the heart.

*Results and Discussion*

It is evident, from the data in Table XVI, that, with increasing age (and size), the cardiotoxic effect of several among the agents used becomes more severe. These agents are: papain (Groups 1–3), noradrenaline (Groups 7–9), vasopressin (Groups 10–12), DHT (Groups 19–21), and combined treatment with the ESCN-producing combination of Me-Cl-COL + $Na_2HPO_4$ (Groups 22–24). On the other hand, the age factor does not appear to play any important role in the production of myocardial lesions by plasmocid (Groups 4–6) restraint (Groups 13–15), or quadriplegia (Groups 16–18).

Histologic study of the hearts essentially confirmed earlier data concerning the types of cardiac lesions produced by the agents that we employed.

In the case of stimuli with age-dependent cardiotoxic activity, the quality of the structural alterations was not especially dependent upon age; the lesions were merely more intense in the older animals and occasionally absent in the young ones.

It is not yet clear why the cardiotoxic effect of some agents is, while that of others is not, dependent upon age. As mentioned in our introduction, the myocardial lesions produced by the means we employed differ widely in their structural characteristics. For example, papain produced predominantly acute, disseminated necroses, DHT calcification in the heart and its arteries, while noradrenaline and vasopressin induced 'spotty myolysis'. However, the histologic lesions elicited by restraint or quadriplegia were rather similar to those evoked by noradrenaline or vasopressin, and yet the action of the latter hormones was evidently dependent upon age, while that of restraint and quadriplegia was not.

Of course, the dose of the hormones (as well as that of all other drugs) was adjusted in proportion to the body weight; hence, the older rats, with a mean body weight of 300 g, received 6 times as much as the young animals, which weighed only 50 g; no such adjustment was possible (or seemed necessary) in the event of restraint or quadriplegia.

It is also possible that the cardiotoxicity of restraint and quadriplegia was too mild to serve as a test object for this type of study. Nonspecific stressors, such as these, notoriously produce massive, infarct-like myocardial necroses only following 'conditioning' with steroids or, better, with steroids and Na-salts (613).

However, neither of these explanations is applicable to the results obtained by plasmocid. This drug produced a very definite cardiac lesion at the smallest dose level in the young rats that weighed 50 g but a 6 times higher dose was no more effective in the old animals whose body weight was 300 g. Essentially the same may be said about the mortality rates. The lethal effect of plasmocid seemed to be independent of the absolute dosage employed, while the other cardiotoxic agents that produced any mortality caused the greatest number of deaths among the oldest rats. In connection with the exceptional

*Table XVI*

The Age Factor in the Production of Various Experimental Cardiopathies

| Group | Treatment | Body weight (g) | Cardiac lesions | Mortality (%) |
|---|---|---|---|---|
| 1 | Papain | 50 | 0.2 ± 0.17 | 10 |
| 2 | Papain | 100 | 0.9 ± 0.27 | 0 |
| 3 | Papain | 300 | 2.6 ± 0.23 | 90 |
| 4 | Plasmocid | 50 | 1.2 ± 0.49 | 40 |
| 5 | Plasmocid | 100 | 1.8 ± 0.25 | 80 |
| 6 | Plasmocid | 300 | 1.4 ± 0.38 | 40 |
| 7 | Noradrenaline | 50 | 0.2 ± 0.15 | 0 |
| 8 | Noradrenaline | 100 | 0.7 ± 0.15 | 0 |
| 9 | Noradrenaline | 300 | 1.6 ± 0.23 | 0 |
| 10 | Vasopressin | 50 | 0 | 0 |
| 11 | Vasopressin | 100 | 0.4 ± 0.17 | 0 |
| 12 | Vasopressin | 300 | 1.3 ± 0.20 | 0 |
| 13 | Restraint | 50 | 0 | 0 |
| 14 | Restraint | 100 | 0.5 ± 0.28 | 0 |
| 15 | Restraint | 300 | 0.3 ± 0.17 | 0 |
| 16 | Quadriplegia | 50 | 0.2 ± 0.20 | 0 |
| 17 | Quadriplegia | 100 | 0.2 ± 0.17 | 0 |
| 18 | Quadriplegia | 300 | 0.2 ± 0.15 | 0 |
| 19 | DHT | 50 | 0.3 ± 0.15 | 10 |
| 20 | DHT | 100 | 1.8 ± 0.32 | 10 |
| 21 | DHT | 300 | 2.0 ± 0.27 | 10 |
| 22 | Me-Cl-COL + $Na_2HPO_4$ | 50 | 0 | 0 |
| 23 | Me-Cl-COL + $Na_2HPO_4$ | 100 | 0.6 ± 0.23 | 0 |
| 24 | Me-Cl-COL + $Na_2HPO_4$ | 300 | 1.6 ± 0.30 | 70 |

behavior of plasmocid it may be mentioned that, unlike most other agents that produce extensive myocardial necroses and myocarditis, treatment with plasmocid is also singularly irresponsive to aggravation by corticoids and Na-salts, or to prophylaxis by KCl and $MgCl_2$.

With our present-day methods, it may be difficult to verify the cause of these apparent discrepancies and to identify the specific mechanisms through which age influences the susceptibility of the myocardium to the production of morphologic lesions. Five of the 6 chemical agents that we used to produce myocardial lesions were significantly more effective in large than in small rats. Yet we have no proof that this difference is due to age rather than size. On the other hand, restraint and quadriplegia—which naturally could not be

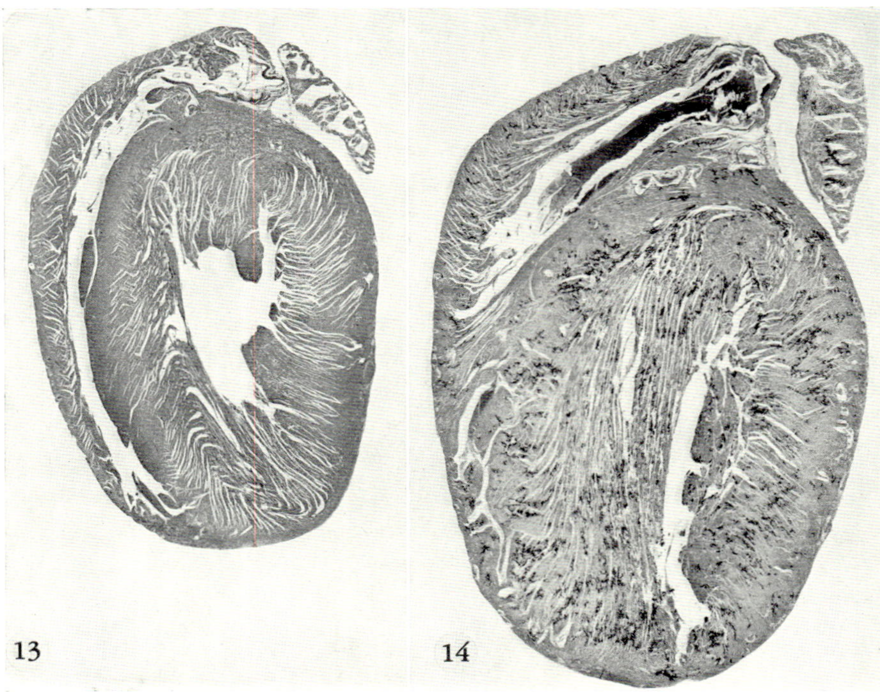


*Figs. 13–14* Cross-section through the whole heart of a 50 g (Fig. 13), a 300 g (Fig. 14) rat of Groups 19 and 21, respectively (and see Table XVI). Note complete absence of calcium deposition in the heart of the young animal, while that of the old rat is studded with calcified (here black) tissue lesions (von Kóssa × 11).

adjusted to body weight—were about equally effective in young and in old rats. Still, in view of the enormous importance of cardiovascular disease in gerontology, it is of interest that a variety of experimental cardiac lesions depends so largely upon the age factor.

Finally, in connection with the studies just described, it is interesting to recall that most of our previous experiments concerning cardiac necroses were performed on healthy young animals, while spontaneous infarcts tend to occur with the greatest frequency in middle-aged or older men, in whom even a moderate degree of coronary sclerosis may act as a predisposing factor for cardiac necrosis. We thought that in order to elucidate this problem, it would be useful, first, to produce a moderate degree of coronary sclerosis and hardening (for instance, by pretreatment with DHT) and then, to determine whether such an 'artificial aging' of the arterial system can sensitize the heart to the necrotizing effect of subsequent treatment with various agents. Consequently, if our hypothesis were correct, it would be expected that after DHT-pretreatment, the administration of various potentially cardiotoxic agents would affect the myocardium more markedly.

To verify this hypothesis, rats were pretreated with DHT during 10 days. This pretreatment in itself causes no significant changes in the myocardium, but induces a slight arteriosclerosis of the Mönckeberg-type. If, following such pretreatment, the rats are exposed to otherwise ineffective or only slightly effective treatment with vasopressin, noradrenaline, cold or papain, then severe myocardial necroses ensue. On the other hand, it was also shown that the necroses that are thus normally elicited in the arteriosclerotic heart can be prevented by KCl, $MgCl_2$ or hemorrhage. These experiments have been described in detail elsewhere (649), and Table XVII serves, here, to summarize the results.

*Summary*

Experiments on 240 female rats, 4 weeks to 10 months of age, were performed to examine the importance of the age factor in the production of various experimental cardiac lesions, which differ widely from each other, both as regards their causative agents and their histologic characteristics.

It was found that papain, noradrenaline, vasopressin, DHT and combined treatment with Me-Cl-COL + $Na_2HPO_4$ induce much more

*Table XVII*

Influence of Mönckeberg-Sclerosis upon the Induction of Cardiac Lesions by Various Agents

| Group | Treatment | Cardiac lesions | Mortality (%) |
|---|---|---|---|
| 1 | None | 0 | 0 |
| 2 | DHT | 0 | 0 |
| 3 | Hemorrhage | 0 | 0 |
| 4 | Vasopressin | 0.1 ± 0.10 | 0 |
| 5 | Noradrenaline | 0.6 ± 0.20 | 0 |
| 6 | Cold | 0.1 ± 0.10 | 0 |
| 7 | Papain | 0.8 ± 0.25 | 0 |
| 8 | DHT + Vasopressin | 0.8 ± 0.15 | 0 |
| 9 | DHT + Noradrenaline | 1.5 ± 0.33 | 10 |
| 10 | DHT + Cold | 1.3 ± 0.27 | 0 |
| 11 | DHT + Papain | 2.9 ± 0.10 | 90 |
| 12 | DHT + KCl | 0 | 0 |
| 13 | DHT + KCl + Vasopressin | 0 | 0 |
| 14 | DHT + KCl + Noradrenaline | 0.4 ± 0.17 | 0 |
| 15 | DHT + KCl + Cold | 0 | 0 |
| 16 | DHT + KCl + Papain | 0.2 ± 0.15 | 0 |
| 17 | DHT + $MgCl_2$ | 0 | 0 |
| 18 | DHT + $MgCl_2$ + Vasopressin | 0 | 10 |
| 19 | DHT + $MgCl_2$ + Noradrenaline | 0.5 ± 0.17 | 0 |
| 20 | DHT + $MgCl_2$ + Cold | 0 | 0 |
| 21 | DHT + $MgCl_2$ + Papain | 0 | 0 |
| 22 | DHT + Hemorrhage | 0 | 0 |
| 23 | DHT + Hemorrhage + Vasopressin | 0 | 0 |
| 24 | DHT + Hemorrhage + Noradrenaline | 0.4 ± 0.23 | 0 |
| 25 | DHT + Hemorrhage + Cold | 0 | 0 |
| 26 | DHT + Hemorrhage + Papain | 0.6 ± 0.27 | 10 |

pronounced cardiac lesions in old than in young rats, when the dose of these substances is adjusted to the body weight. On the other hand, under the same circumstances, plasmocid is essentially equally effective in producing cardiac lesions in young and old animals.

Two highly stressful procedures, which did not depend upon the injection of exogenous drugs or hormones (forced restraint and motor denervation of all 4 extremities) produced only mild and inconstant cardiac lesions, irrespective of the age of the experimental animals.

The role of the age factor in the pathogenesis of spontaneous and experimental cardiovascular disease is briefly discussed on the basis of these observations.

Finally, experiments are described to show that a slight degree of Mönckeberg-sclerosis (produced by pretreatment with DHT) greatly sensitizes the myocardium to the potential cardiotoxic actions of vasopressin, noradrenaline, cold baths, or papain. Thus, an 'artificial aging' of the coronary vessels may act as a predisposing factor for the induction of cardiac necroses.

## III. Desensitization of the Heart Muscle: Negative Conditioning Actions

### A. Stress, Hemodynamic Changes, and Stimuli Influencing Stress-Induced Cross-Resistance

#### *a) Adaptation to the Cardiac Necrosis-eliciting Effect of Stress.*

During the typical triphasic evolution of the General Adaptation Syndrome, resistance to diverse potentially pathogenic stimuli undergoes considerable and largely predictable variations. In this connection it is customary to distinguish: 1. specific resistance, that is, increased tolerance to only the particular kind of stimulus to which the body has been previously exposed, and 2. nonspecific- or cross-resistance, that is, increased tolerance to a stressor qualitatively different from that to which the body has been adapted. Depending primarily upon the intensity and the duration of the pretreatment, both these kinds of resistance can be either increased or decreased as a consequence of previous exposure to stress (597).

The possibility of raising or diminishing specific resistance, respectively, by moderate or excessive exposure to certain stimuli (e.g., cold, muscular exercise, solar irradiation) has long been recognized and need not detain us here. It is more pertinent to the subject of this paper that exposure to various stressors can also induce cross-resistance to agents that normally elicit highly selective organ lesions. For example, in the rat, stress can protect against the appendicitis-like changes normally induced by intravenous injection of histamine (584), the production of lung edema by adrenaline (587) or the anaphylactoid inflammation caused by parenteral administration of egg-white (585). Although many additional examples of such cross-resistance have been described (Lit.: 597, 629, 802), nothing was known about the underlying mechanism until quite recently when it became evident that, in most cases, these protective actions of stress are due to increased glucocorticoid activity (597).

However, some types of nonspecific resistance cannot be readily explained on the basis of a stress-induced hypercorticoidism. For example, in rats pretreated with methylchlorocortisol plus sodium acetate, sudden exposure to stressors (e.g., noradrenaline, intense muscular exercise, forced restraint or trauma) elicits large, infarct-like patches of necrosis in the heart, while no such cardiac lesions are elicited under similar conditions if the animals are gradually adapted to any one of these stressors before being exposed to the full, normally pathogenic, dose of the same stressor agents (626). Here, it is disease susceptibility that depends upon hypercorticoidism (Me-Cl-COL administration); hence, this type of nonspecific resistance cannot be due to stress-induced hypercorticoidism.

In the present report, we shall describe, first, an improved procedure for the demonstration of adaptation to the cardiac necrosis eliciting effect of single stressors and, second, induction of cross-resistance to this effect of one stressor by pretreatment with another stressor agent.

### *Materials and Techniques*

In the *first experiment,* fifty female rats (Quebec Breeding Farm), with a mean initial body weight of 104 g (range: 90–111 g) were subdivided into five equal groups and treated as indicated in Table XVIII. Since Me-Cl-COL is not readily available, F-COL was used in combination with Na-acetate to sensitize the animals to the cardiac necrosis eliciting effect of stress. This combined steroid-electrolyte treatment was given to all groups from the 6th day until the 15th day. F-COL was injected as a microcrystal suspension, 500 µg daily in 0.2 ml of water, subcutaneously. *Na-acetate* was administered by stomach tube, in a concentration of 1 mM in 2 ml of water, twice daily. Group 1 served as controls to confirm that this sensitizing electrolyte-steroid treatment alone does not produce cardiac necrosis. Two of the remaining groups (Group 3, 5) were gradually adapted to forced muscular exercise or restraint, respectively, while the others (Groups 2, 4) were exposed suddenly (that is without previous adaptation) to the stressor effects of one or the other stimulus.

Muscular exercise was performed in revolving cages 30 cm in diameter and turning at a speed of 18 revolutions per minute. *Repeated exercise* (gradually conducive to adaptation) consisted in running once daily during the first 14 days of the experiment; the animals exercised for 180 minutes on the first day, and this time was increased every third day by 30 minutes (Group 3). *Sudden exercise* (conducive to acute stress) consisted in running continuously from the 15th day until death ensued (Groups 2, 3).

*Restraint* was applied by strapping the rats with adhesive tape to a board, in the prone position. *Repeated* restraint consisted in exposure to this neuromuscular strain for 7 hours every second day from the beginning of the experiment until the 14th day (Group 5). *Sudden* restraint consisted in exposure to this stress from the 15th day until the animals died (Group 4).

In the *second experiment,* one hundred female rats (Quebec Breeding Farm), with a mean initial body weight of 100 g (range: 91–112 g) were subdivided into ten equal groups and treated as indicated in Table XVIIIa. All animals received the combined F-COL + Na-acetate treatment, under conditions identical with those of the previous experiment. Here—in an attempt to establish cross-resistance—the rats were adapted to one stressor agent and then exposed (together with the corresponding unadapted controls) to the cardiac necrosis eliciting effect of another stressor.

The *repeatedly* given stressors used for adaptation were cold baths, which consisted in immersing the rats in water at 6 °C for 1 minute, twice on the first day and gradually increasing this time until a maximum of 5 minutes twice daily was reached (Group 2); repeated muscular exercise once daily, as described above (Groups 4, 10); repeated restraint for 7 hours every second day (Group 6); noradrenaline injected subcutaneously in 0.2 ml of oil, twice daily throughout the experiment—the initial concentration of 50 μg per rat was increased by a further 50 μg on every third day (Group 8).

To elicit cardiac lesions, the following *suddenly* applied stressors were given without previous adaptation on the 15th and 16th day; muscular exercise until death (Groups 1, 2); cold baths in water at 0°C, three times daily for 5 minutes (Groups 3, 4); noradrenaline, 300 μg in 0.2 ml of oil per rat, was injected twice daily subcutaneously (Groups 5, 6); restraint for 48 hours (Groups 7, 8); multiple bone fractures of all four extremities (Groups 9, 10). On the 17th day, the experiment was terminated by killing the survivors with chloroform. At autopsy, the hearts were inspected with a binocular loupe and then fixed in neutral formalin for subsequent staining with hematoxylin-phloxine.

### *Results and Discussion*

The figures in Table XVIII show that combined administration of F-COL + Na-acetate did not result in any histologically detectable cardiac lesion (Group 1). However, large patches of infarct-like cardiac necroses were elicited in almost all of the electrolyte + steroid-pretreated rats suddenly exposed to intensive muscular exercise (Group 2) or forced restraint (Group 4). The myocardial lesions so induced were invariably detectable by naked-eye inspection, because they affected large areas of the heart muscle. Histologic sections showed necrotic foci that were distributed throughout the heart but with particular frequency in the subendocardial layers and papillary muscles. Around disintegrated muscle fibers, secondary inflammatory phenomena were often seen.

On the other hand, it is also clear that a gradual adaptation to the stressor agents was very effective in protecting the rats against the development of cardiac necroses (Groups 3, 5). In this regard, it is important to note that at the end of the experiment both the adapted and unadapted animals were exposed to stressors until they died. This procedure was necessary because adapted animals need much more severe and prolonged stress before exhibiting any signs of damage. The rats adapted to muscular exercise were actually able to run for 6 hours more on the 15th day before succumbing than were the unadapted; the latter all died within 12 hours of continuous exercise. Similarly, the adapted animals survived the same type of restraint about 6–8 hours longer than those unadapted; in the latter group, the mortality was already 100% at the end of the first 52 hours. Thus, the rats all died during exposure to stressors, but, of the adapted animals, only three developed a slight degree of cardiac damage and the remainder were all completely protected against this specific effect of stress (Groups 3, 5).

While in the first experiment the stimuli used for adaptation and eliciting were identical, in the second experimental series the rats were first adapted to one stressor and then exposed to another.

As shown by Table XVIIIa, in the F-COL + Na-acetate-sensitised rats, a great many noxious agents—muscular exercise (Group 1), cold baths (Group 3), noradrenaline (Group 5), restraint (Group 7), and bone fractures (Group 9)—all induce extensive and sometimes fatal cardiac necroses; this indicates the nonspecific character of this eliciting mechanism.

On the other hand, it is also obvious that adaptation to various stimuli protects the rats even against the cardiac necrosis eliciting effect of other stressors that are fundamentally different in nature. Thus, animals gradually adapted to cold baths did not develop cardiac necroses from sudden exposure to severe muscular exercise, although

*Table XVIII*

Adaptation to the Cardiac Necrosis-Eliciting Effect of Stressors

| Group | Treatment* | | Cardiac necrosis (Severity) | Cardiac necrosis (Incidence) |
|---|---|---|---|---|
| 1 | None | | 0 | 0 |
| 2 | Muscular exercise | Sudden | 2.1 ± 0.23 | 90 |
| 3 | Muscular exercise | Repeated | 0.2 ± 0.15 | 10 |
| 4 | Restraint | Sudden | 2.8 ± 0.13 | 100 |
| 5 | Restraint | Repeated | 0.3 ± 0.17 | 20 |

* In addition the rats in all groups were treated with F-COL and Na-acetate as described in the text.

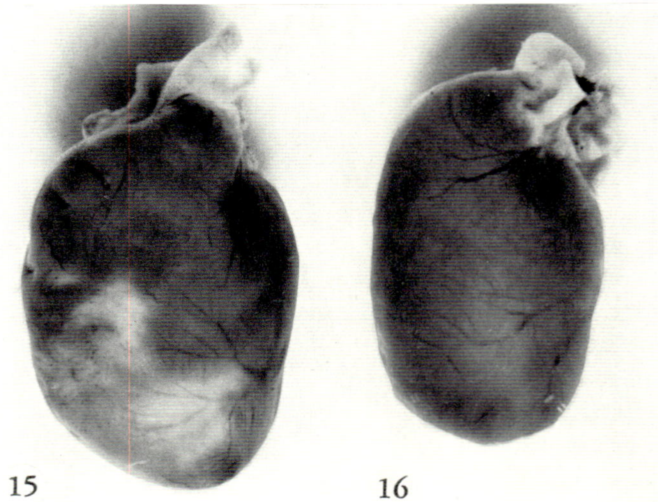

*Figs. 15–16 Production of cross-resistance of the heart by exposure to stressor agents.*—Fig. 15: Massive myocardial necrosis (white patch) resulting from noradrenaline overdosage, in a rat pretreated with F-COL plus Na-acetate. Fig. 16: Complete prevention of the necrosis by previous repeated exposure to forced restraint.

in 90% of the unadapted controls, severe cardiac lesions developed as a result of such forced neuromuscular work (cf., Groups 1, 2). Similar cross-resistance was observed when adaptation to muscular exercise (Groups 4, 10), restraint (Group 6), or noradrenaline (Group 8) was followed by sudden exposure to the eliciting effect of various other stressors.

The first experimental series confirms that, in rats sensitized with Na-acetate and certain corticoids (in this case F-COL), sudden exposure to unaccustomed muscular exercise or forced restraint induces severe cardiac necroses, while, after gradual adaptation, these same stressors largely lose their cardiotoxic effect. It would be tempting to ascribe this protection by gradual inurement to the fact that a given period of exercise or restraint is less damaging to the adapted than to the unadapted rat. Our adapted animals did, in fact, survive longer than the unadapted, yet the former showed little or no cardiac lesion, even though the stress period was prolonged until death. In other words, the unadapted controls were exposed to a shorter period of stress, and, still, only they exhibited severe cardiac necroses. It seems, therefore, that the cardiac muscle itself rather selectively acquires a high degree of topical resistance, which remains effective even when systemic resistance to the fatal effects of stress breaks down under the influence of excessive exposure.

The second experimental series revealed that a true cross-resistance to the cardiac necrosis eliciting effect of stress can be acquired: exposure to one stressor protects against the cardiotoxic effect of another stressor. This kind of resistance cannot result from any specific metabolic adjustment that adapts the body to cold, muscular exercise, forced restraint, noradrenaline or bone fracture, in particular,

*Table XVIIIa*

Cross-Resistance to the Cardiac Necrosis-Eliciting Effect of Stressors

| Group | Treatment* | | Cardiac necrosis | | Mortality (%) |
|---|---|---|---|---|---|
| | Repeated for Adaptation | Sudden for Eliciting | (Severity) | (Incidence) | |
| 1 | None | Muscular exercise | 1.8 ± 0.26 | 90 | 100 |
| 2 | Cold bath | | 0 | 0 | 100 |
| 3 | None | Cold bath | 1.7 ± 0.23 | 70 | 70 |
| 4 | Muscular exercise | | 0.2 ± 0.15 | 10 | 0 |
| 5 | None | Noradrenaline | 3.0 ± 0 | 100 | 70 |
| 6 | Restraint | | 0 | 0 | 0 |
| 7 | None | Restraint | 2.5 ± 0.18 | 90 | 90 |
| 8 | Noradrenaline | | 0 | 0 | 0 |
| 9 | None | Bone fracture | 1.5 ± 0.21 | 70 | 30 |
| 10 | Muscular exercise | | 0 | 0 | 0 |

* In addition to the treatments listed above, the rats in all groups received F-COL and Na-Acetate as described in the text.

since the specific effects of all these agents are fundamentally different. Of course, all stressors increase corticoid secretion, but such an adaptive response could hardly explain this kind of cross-resistance. Under no circumstance would the adrenal be likely to secrete corticoids in amounts that could significantly influence the severe hypercorticoidism that we induced by F-COL. Besides, the extreme compensatory adrenal atrophy that resulted from the F-COL treatment may be assumed to have greatly inhibited the endogenous secretion of corticoids that usually takes place under stress.

Our observations do not permit us to draw any conclusions concerning the mechanism that might be involved in this type of adaptation to stress. It is evident, however, that under our experimental conditions, pretreatment with one stressor protects against the production of cardiac necrosis resulting from subsequent exposure to either the same or another stressor agent.

*Summary*

In rats sensitized with F-COL + Na-acetate, sudden exposure to the stress of intense muscular exercise or forced restraint produces rapidly fatal, severe myocardial necroses. In rats gradually pretreated by short periods of muscular exercise or restraint, even fatal exposure to the same agent produces little or no cardiac necrosis and survival is greatly prolonged.

True cross-resistance to the cardiotoxic action of various stressors can be demonstrated under these circumstances, in rats sensitized by F-COL and Na-acetate; the cardiac necrosis-producing effect of muscular exercise could be prevented by pretreatment with cold, that of cold by muscular exercise, that of noradrenaline by restraint, that of restraint by noradrenaline, and that of bone fractures by muscular exercise.

### *b) Induction of Cross-resistance to Cardiotoxic Agents*

As already mentioned (see p. 198) the phenomenon of cross-resistance was first studied mainly in connection with the suppression of inflammatory lesions by nonspecific stress and it was concluded that, in most cases, the protective action of stress is due to increased anti-inflammatory corticoid production.

However, some of the more recently discovered instances of cross-resistance do not seem to be due to a stress-induced suppression of inflammation. For example, our experiments just described (p. 197) showed that in rats pretreated with F-COL plus Na-acetate, sudden exposure to stressor agents (e.g., muscular exercise, restraint, noradrenaline) elicits large, infarct-like patches of myocardial necroses. This change is not due to inflammation, yet, it is suppressed if, under otherwise similar conditions, the animals are gradually adapted to any one of these agents; they resist subsequent exposure to the full, normally pathogenic dose of the same stressor, or even different from that with which the subject has been pretreated.

Subsequent experiments showed that such cross-resistance of the heart can be obtained also against other types of experimental cardiopathies. For example, in rats sensitized with DHT plus $NaH_2PO_4$, sudden exposure to the stress of forced restraint or bone fracture produces a rapidly fatal syndrome, characterized by severe myocardial necroses and nephrocalcinosis. These cardio- and nephrotoxic effects of restraint can both be prevented by pretreatment with restraint or noradrenaline, and those of bone fractures by cold baths (46). Indeed, even the cardiopathy produced by DHT overdosage alone (680) as well as that induced by intravenous injection of proteolytic enzymes, such as papain, and the cardiac necroses resulting from plasmocid administration, can be prevented by adaptation to stressor agents (48, 659).

In rats sensitized with corticoids or DHT plus Na-salts, myocardial necroses can also be precipitated by the oral administration of various fats, for example, corn oil. As judged by the absence of any obvious adrenocortical stimulation, thymus atrophy, or loss of body weight, the feeding of the required amount of fat is not particularly stressful for the rat. Hence, it was concluded that the induction of necroses by a high fat intake is due to specific metabolic changes and depends upon a mechanism different from that operating in the case of exposure to stressors (667).

In the following experiment, we compared the protection afforded by pretreatment with stressors on the one hand, and dietary fat supplements on the other, as regards the induction of cardiac necroses.

*Materials and Techniques*

One hundred and ninety rats, with a mean initial body weight of 98 g (range: 83–108 g), were subdivided into 19 equal groups and treated as indicated in Table XIX. F-COL was used in combination with Na-acetate to sensitize the animals to the cardiac necrosis-eliciting effect of stress as well as to that of corn oil. This combined steroid-electrolyte treatment was given to all groups from the 4th day until the termination of the experiment. *F-COL* was injected as a microcrystal suspension, at the dose of 500 µg daily in 0.2 ml of water, subcutaneously. *Na-acetate* was administered by stomach tube, at the dose of 1 mM in 2 ml of water, twice daily. Group 1 served as controls to confirm that, under our experimental conditions. F-COL plus Na-acetate treatment alone does not produce cardiac necrosis. Some of the remaining groups were gradually adapted to various stressor agents (Groups 3–6, 15–18) or to forced oil-feeding (Groups 7, 9, 11, 13, 19), then, together with the unadapted controls (Groups 2, 8, 10, 12, 14) they were exposed suddenly to the potentially cardiac-necrosis-eliciting effect of various other stimuli.

The *repeatedly applied stressors* used for adaptation were: restraint, every second day from the 1st until the 11th day of the experiment—the animals were exposed to this neuromuscular strain during 3 hours on the 1st day, the duration being gradually increased to 7 hours (Groups 3, 15); muscular exercise consisted in running once daily during the first 11 days—the animals exercised for 60 minutes on the 1st day, and this time was gradually increased to 360 minutes per day (Groups 4, 16); cold baths, for 0.5 minutes twice on the first day, and for increasing periods up to a maximum of 4 minutes, twice daily, on the 11th day (Groups 5, 17); noradrenaline injected subcutaneously in 0.2 ml of corn oil, twice daily throughout the experiment—the initial concentration of 50 µg per rat was increased by a further 50 µg every third day (Groups 6, 18). The rats in Groups 7, 9, 11, 13 and 19 were adapted to corn oil instead of stressor agents. 0.2 ml of corn oil was administered twice daily by stomach tube on the 1st day, this amount being gradually increased to 1 ml twice daily by the 11th day.

To elicit cardiac lesions, the following *suddenly applied stressors* were given: restraint, for 17 hours, once on the 12th day (Groups 2–7); muscular exercise (conducive to acute stress) consisted in running continuously during 5 hours, once on the 12th and 13th days (Groups 8, 9); cold baths, twice for 4 minutes on the 12th day and three times on the 13th day (Groups 10, 11); noradrenaline, 300 µg in 0.2 ml of oil per rat, was injected twice daily, subcutaneously, on the 12th and 13th days (Groups 1, 13). As previously stated, corn oil need not be given in doses causing obvious manifestations of stress; it apparently elicits cardiac necroses owing to more specific metabolic effects. Hence, only 2 ml of corn oil were given by stomach tube, twice daily on the 12th and 13th days (Groups 14–19).

The experiment was terminated on the 14th day. At autopsy, the adrenals were dissected, fixed in Susa solution saturated with picric acid and weighed on an analytical balance. The hearts were studied in histologic sections stained with PAS.

*Results and Discussion*

Table XIX shows that combined administration of F-COL plus Na-acetate did not result in any detectable cardiac lesion (Group 1). However, large patches of infarct-like cardiac necroses were elicited in almost all of the electrolyte plus steroid-pretreated rats suddenly exposed to any of the stressors used, namely: restraint (Group 2), muscular exercise (Group 8), cold baths (Group 10) and overdosage with noradrenaline (Group 12), as well as in those given corn oil (Group 14). The myocardial lesions so induced were invariably detectable by macroscopic inspection, because they affected large areas of the heart muscle. Histologic sections showed necrotic foci that were distributed throughout the heart but with particular frequency in the subendocardial layers and papillary muscles. Around disintegrated muscle fibers, secondary inflammatory phenomena were often seen.

On the other hand, it is also obvious that adaptation to various stressors protects the rat against the cardiotoxic effect not only of the agent with which it had been pretreated ('specific resistance'), but also to that of other fundamentally different stressors ('cross-resistance'). Thus, Group 3 represents an example of induced 'specific resistance', in that adaptation to repeated restraint abolished the pathogenic (eliciting) effect of the same stressor. On the other hand, Groups 4–6 are clearcut examples of 'cross-resistance': animals gradually adapted to muscular exercise (Group 4), cold (Group 5), noradrenaline (Group 6) were protected against the induction of cardiac lesions by sudden exposure to severe restraint. However, when the rats were adapted to corn oil, they developed specific resistance to the same agent (Group 19), but no cross-resistance to the cardiac necrosis-eliciting effect of restraint (Group 7), muscular exercise (Group 9), cold baths (Group 11), or noradrenaline (Group 13).

Furthermore, the large doses of corn oil elicited severe, and often fatal, cardiac necroses in the otherwise not-pretreated, F-COL plus Na-acetate-sensitized animals (Group 14), but adaptation to various stressor agents gave complete cross-resistance against the actions of the fat (Groups 15–18).

Interestingly, in all groups that developed severe cardiac necroses, the F-COL-induced adrenal atrophy was just as, or even more severe than in the controls (cf. Group 1 with Groups 2, 7, 8, 9, 10 ,11 and 14). On the other hand, there was significant adrenal enlargement in those rats in which gradual adaptation to stressors protected against other stressors (Groups 3–6) or against corn oil (Groups 15–18). However, no such adrenal hypertrophy occurred in the rats in which adaptation to oil protected against the pathogenic actions of the same agent (Group 19).

There is no obvious correlation between the final body weight and the adrenal changes or the development of cardiac necroses. Even in the rats which exhibited the greatest weight loss (and therefore received comparatively more F-COL per body weight), there was adrenal enlargement (Groups 3, 15) and the most pronounced adrenal atrophy was found in heavier rats, which exhibited severe cardiac necroses (Group 14).

It is evident that the cardiac necroses produced under our experimental conditions, by sudden exposure to the severe stress of restraint, can be prevented by pretreatment, not only with restraint, but also with other stressors.

We have seen, furthermore, that, in the F-COL plus Na-acetate-sensitized rats, oral administration of corn oil is highly active as an elicitor of cardiac necroses; yet pretreatment with this fat protects only against the cardiotoxic action of subsequent treatment with the same substance and not against that produced by other agents. This fact suggests a difference in the mechanism responsible for the notions of stressors and fats. On the other hand, pretreatment not only with oil itself, but also with any of the stressors used in this study proved to be highly effective in preventing the subsequent induction of cardiac necroses by oil-feeding. Evidently, stressors can induce cross-resistance against the subsequent action of oil. It is highly unlikely

*Table XIX*

Cross-Resistance to Cardiotoxic Agents

| Group | Treatment* | | Final body weight (g) | Adrenal weight (mg) | Cardiac necrosis | | Mortality (%) |
|---|---|---|---|---|---|---|---|
| | Repeated for Adaptation | Sudden for Eliciting | | | (Severity) | (Incidence) | |
| 1 | None | None | 106 ± 2.4 | 21 ± 0.36 | 0 | 0 | 0 |
| 2 | None | Restraint | 101 ± 2.6 | 20 ± 0.41 | 3.0 ± 0 | 100 | 80 |
| 3 | Restraint | Restraint | 92 ± 1.2 | 31 ± 0.53 | 0 | 0 | 0 |
| 4 | Muscular exercise | Restraint | 101 ± 3.2 | 31 ± 0.70 | 0 | 0 | 0 |
| 5 | Cold bath | Restraint | 106 ± 4.1 | 32 ± 0.66 | 0 | 0 | 0 |
| 6 | Noradrenaline | Restraint | 102 ± 2.6 | 30 ± 0.41 | 0.7 ± 0.30 | 10 | 0 |
| 7 | Oil | Restraint | 101 ± 2.5 | 19 ± 0.27 | 2.8 ± 0.17 | 100 | 70 |
| 8 | None | Muscular exercise | 98 ± 1.6 | 18 ± 0.36 | 2.4 ± 0.23 | 100 | 70 |
| 9 | Oil | Muscular exercise | 102 ± 3.2 | 19 ± 0.40 | 2.1 ± 0.25 | 90 | 50 |
| 10 | None | Cold bath | 101 ± 3.4 | 20 ± 0.51 | 1.4 ± 0.18 | 70 | 20 |
| 11 | Oil | Cold bath | 104 ± 1.8 | 18 ± 0.46 | 1.2 ± 0.21 | 80 | 20 |
| 12 | None | Noradrenaline | 105 ± 2.4 | ** | 2.9 ± 0.10 | 100 | 100 |
| 13 | Oil | Noradrenaline | 99 ± 1.4 | ** | 2.5 ± 0.16 | 100 | 100 |
| 14 | None | Oil | 108 ± 2.8 | 15 ± 0.39 | 2.9 ± 0.30 | 100 | 80 |
| 15 | Restraint | Oil | 97 ± 2.3 | 31 ± 0.50 | 0 | 0 | 0 |
| 16 | Muscular exercise | Oil | 111 ± 1.7 | 29 ± 0.63 | 0 | 0 | 0 |
| 17 | Cold bath | Oil | 115 ± 4.2 | 27 ± 0.44 | 0 | 0 | 0 |
| 18 | Noradrenaline | Oil | 106 ± 2.7 | 28 ± 0.58 | 0 | 0 | 0 |
| 19 | Oil | Oil | 116 ± 2.5 | 21 ± 0.43 | 0.1 ± 0.10 | 10 | 0 |

* In addition to the treatments mentioned in this column, the animals of all groups were conditioned for the production of cardiac necroses by F-COL + Na-acetate, as indicated in the text.

** Since the animals in these two groups died earlier than the others, their adrenal weights are not included.

that oil acted as a stressor here, because pretreatment with oil failed to produce any adrenal enlargement. On the other hand, effective pretreatment with any of the stressors used resulted in an increase in adrenal weight, which suggests the possibility of some adrenal participation in the mechanism of this type of cross-resistance. Even though pretreatment with oil failed to cause such adrenal enlargment, it still offered effective protection against the eliciting action of oil. Yet, there seems to be some relationship between the actions of stressors and oil, since pretreatment with various stressors did protect the heart against the eliciting of necroses by oil.

*Summary*

Experiments on rats indicated that, following pretreatment with F-COL plus Na acetate, various stressors (restraint, muscular exercise, cold baths, noradrenaline) produce infarctoid cardiac necroses and high mortality. Gradual adaptation by pretreatment with restraint, muscular exercise, cold baths, or noradrenaline protects against this cardiac necrosis-eliciting effect of subsequent restraint. This is considered to be an additional example of 'cross-resistance' to a stress-induced lesions and illustrates the non-specificity of the stress mechanism.

In similarly conditioned rats, oral administration of oil likewise elicits cardiac necroses, but this effect appears to be due to some specific metabolic action, because as used here, the oil elicits no obvious manifestations of stress, and pretreatment with oil protects only against the cardiac necrosis-eliciting effect of oil itself and not against that of various stressors.

### *c) Influence of Blood Pressure upon the Production of Myocardial Necroses by Various Agents*

It has been shown that various electrolytes influence the pressor activity of corticoids. On the other hand, the desoxycorticosterone-hypertension, as well as the associated ESCN (with periarteritis and nephrocalcinosis) is aggravated by Na-salts (673). It was, therefore, necessary to establish the relationships between ESCN and blood pressure. In rats treated with $NaH_2PO_4$ plus Me-Cl-COL, there was a slight initial hypertension not significantly greater than that induced by Me-Cl-COL alone. $NaH_2PO_4$, in itself, did not alter the blood pressure in these experiments. However, in the animals that received the combined electrolyte-steroid treatment, the blood pressure fell below normal several days before death from myocardial necroses. Here, the antemortem hypotension was presumably due to heart failure induced by myocardial necroses. There is no evidence that the ESCN is preceded by any pronounced hypertensive episodes (22). It had been found, however, that both the massive, infarct-like ESCN and the more discrete 'spotty myolysis' produced by noradrenaline can be prevented by repeated blood-letting (631).

As a working hypothesis, we assumed that the prophylactic effect of hemorrhage is due to the decrease in the cardiac work which it induces by diminishing aortic pressure and blood viscosity. This interpretation—though still unproven—is compatible with the apparently paradoxical finding that, in corticoid-conditioned rats, cardiac necroses can be more readily induced by comparatively mild than by very severe stressors. Thus, transection of the spinal cord, at the level of the seventh cervical vertebra (an operation which produces pronounced hypotension) causes no detectable histologic lesion in the heart, while a similar intervention, performed at the height of the first lumbar vertebra (conducive to little or no drop of blood pressure), elicits multiple myocardial necroses in the corticoid-conditioned rat (631, 802).

The experiments to be described here were designed to determine whether necrotizing lesions of the myocardium, induced by various other means, are likewise largely dependent upon the blood-pressure level.

## *Materials and Techniques*

Two experimental series were performed on rats with an average initial body weight of 96 g (range: 90–112 g). The animals were subdivided into equal groups of ten each, and treated with agents known to produce various types of cardiac lesions, as indicated in Tables XX and XXI.

In the *first experiment,* the hemorrhage consisted in the removal of 2.5 ml of blood from the jugular vein, on the first day, under light ether anesthesia. A preliminary experiment on 10 rats showed that this induces a drop of the mean blood-pressure (tail-cuff method) from 98 ± 1.9 to 89 ± 2.0 mmHg. *Noradrenaline* was given twice, during the first day, at the dose of 300 μg in 0.2 ml of oil subcutaneously. A preliminary experiment on 10 rats showed that this treatment rapidly raises the blood-pressure from an initial value of 100 ± 2.1 to 117 ± 2.2 mmHg. *Papain* (5%, filtered solution) was injected into the jugular vein; 0.2 ml, once on the first day. *Plasmocid,* 8-(3-diethylaminopropylamino)-6-methoxyquinoline, was given at the dose of 0.5 mg in 0.2 ml of water, intraperitoneally, three times on the first day. *Cold baths* were applied for a period of 5 minutes, three times during the first day (11 AM., 3 PM. and 6 PM.).

The animals were killed 48 hours following the initiation of the experiment. The hearts were fixed in neutral formalin and stained with the fuchsin technique.

The *second experiment* was performed in order to establish the possible effect of hemorrhage upon the diffuse, purulent myocarditis that can be produced by combined treatment with derivatives of the vitamin-D group plus sodium phosphates. For this purpose, two groups of rats were given a mixture of 50 μg of *DHT* plus 1 mM of $NaH_2PO_4$ in 2 ml of water, twice daily, by stomach tube, during 4 days. The *hemorrhage* consisted in the removal of 2 ml of blood from the jugular vein on the first and third days of the experiment.

The animals were killed on the 5th day and their hearts prepared for histologic examination as in the first experiment. Since DHT-plus-phosphate treatment also produces nephrocalcinosis, specimens of the kidneys were stained with von Kóssa's technique, for the histochemical demonstration of calcium. At autopsy, it was noted that several of the animals subjected to hemorrhage had hepatic lesions; these were subsequently identified as focal necroses, on formalin-fixed specimens stained with hematoxylin-phloxine. The results of this second experiment are summarized in Table XXI.

### *Results and Discussion*

Perusal of Table XX indicates that, at the dose employed here, noradrenaline produced only minor cardiac lesions in a few animals (Group 2), and hemorrhage elicited no detectable morphologic change (Group 3).

The lesions produced by papain (Group 4) were almost completely prevented by hemorrhage (Group 5) and very significantly ($P < 0.01$)

aggravated by noradrenaline (Group 6). It is noteworthy that, under these conditions, the intense changes induced by combined treatment with the two agents exhibited the morphologic characteristics of typical papain-necroses and, hence, differed qualitatively from the changes caused by noradrenaline.

Only the necroses produced by plasmocid (Group 7) could not be prevented by hemorrhage (Group 8). This further substantiates our previously expressed view that plasmocid acts through some mechanism essentially distinct from that of most of the other experimental interventions that cause morphologic changes in the heart. It will be recalled that the plasmocid-lesions also differ from the many other experimental cardiopathies that we studied, in that only the former cannot be prevented by KCl or $MgCl_2$ and are not greatly aggravated by pretreatment with corticoids or sensitizing Na-salts (802). Curiously, noradrenaline appears to have aggravated the plasmocid effect (Group 9) just as it accentuated the actions of the other cardiotoxic agents. As regards cardiac lesions themselves, this aggravation was on the borderline of statistical significance ($P < 0.05$), but since neither noradrenaline nor plasmocid alone produced any mortality, it is significantly that combined treatment with the two drugs killed 90% of the rats.

It is not very remarkable that the relatively mild lesions produced by cold baths alone (Group 10) were completely prevented by hemorrhage (Group 11), but noradrenaline induced an impressive and highly significant ($P < 0.01$) aggravation of the cardiotoxic action of this stressor (Group 12).

The *second experiment* was of somewhat longer duration and, therefore, is not directly comparable to the first.

As Table XXI indicates, combined treatment with DHT and $NaH_2PO_4$ produced intense cardiac lesions (Group 1 of Table XXI). As expected on the basis of our earlier work (664), there developed a suppurating myocarditis with numerous macroscopically visible, small yellowish foci that were irregularly distributed throughout the myocardium. Histologically, the lesions were characterized by the presence of necrotic muscle fibers, numerous polymorphonuclear leukocytes and occasional calcium deposits in the blood vessels and in the affected muscle fibers. There was also pronounced nephrocalcinosis but no hepatic necrosis.

Hemorrhage completely prevented the cardiac lesions, but had no effect upon the nephrocalcinosis, and induced hepatic necroses in 4 out of 10 animals. The mortality rate was only slightly diminished (Group 2 of Table XXI). In all these respects, the effect of hemorrhage is the same here as it was in our earlier work on the influence of bloodletting upon the massive infarct-like lesions of the ESCN, produced by corticoids plus Na-phosphate. In the latter experimental arrangement, hemorrhage likewise protected against the cardiac lesions, but at the same time predisposed for hepatic necroses; this is presumably why it only slightly diminished the mortality rate (631).

Hemorrhage exerted a pronounced prophylactic effect against the production of various types of myocardial lesions by such diverse agents as papain, cold baths, and combined treatment with DHT plus $NaH_2PO_4$. Only the plasmocid-lesions could not be prevented in this manner. Noradrenaline aggravated the myocardial changes produced by all these agents, including those induced by plasmocid.

In none of these instances did combined treatment with cardiotoxic agents plus noradrenaline result in myocardial changes of the type produced by noradrenaline alone ('spotty myolysis'); the lesions

*Table XX*

Influence of Noradrenaline and Hemorrhage upon the Production of Myocardial Necrosis by Various Agents

| Group | Treatment | Cardiac lesions | Mortality (%) |
|---|---|---|---|
| 1 | None | 0 | 0 |
| 2 | Noradrenaline | 0.2 ± 0.15 | 0 |
| 3 | Hemorrhage | 0 | 0 |
| 4 | Papain | 1.4 ± 0.40 | 0 |
| 5 | Papain + Hemorrhage | 0.1 ± 0.10 | 0 |
| 6 | Papain + Noradrenaline | 2.6 ± 0.17 | 60 |
| 7 | Plasmocid | 1.6 ± 0.30 | 0 |
| 8 | Plasmocid + Hemorrhage | 1.8 ± 0.28 | 0 |
| 9 | Plasmocid + Noradrenaline | 2.4 ± 0.27 | 90 |
| 10 | Cold Baths | 0.3 ± 0.15 | 0 |
| 11 | Cold Baths + Hemorrhage | 0 | 0 |
| 12 | Cold Baths + Noradrenaline | 1.3 ± 0.30 | 0 |

always exhibited the morphologic features characteristic of the cardiotoxic agent that was given in combination with the adrenergic hormone. In other words, hemorrhage prevented, and noradrenaline aggravated, a variety of histologically quite distinct types of myocardial lesions.

It is not yet proven—but we believe it highly probable—that the effect of hemorrhage is due to a decrease, and that of noradrenaline to an increase, in cardiac work. The possibility should also be considered that hemorrhage acts merely through its nonspecific stressor effect, but some of our observations do not support this view. For example, the cardiac necrosis normally produced by plasmocid is prevented by pretreatment with various stressors (i.e., restraint, noradrenaline, muscular exercise, reserpine), but not by hemorrhage (659). On the other hand, the 'spotty myolysis' resulting from noradrenaline-overdosage cannot be prevented with previous exposure to restraint or to other stressors (660), but it is easily prevented by hemorrhage (631). These observations suggest that hemorrhage acts through some specific mechanism and not merely as a stressor agent.

### *Summary*

Various histologic types of cardiac lesions (necrosis, inflammation, fuchsinophilic degeneration, calcification) were produced in rats by papain, plasmocid, the stress of ice-cold baths or simultaneous treatment with DHT plus $NaH_2PO_4$. Irrespective of the morphologic

*Table XXI*

Influence of Hemorrhage upon the Syndrome Normally Produced by Combined Treatment with DHT plus $NaH_2PO_4$

| Group | Treatment | Cardiac lesions | Nephrocalcinosis | Hepatic necrosis | Mortality (%) |
|---|---|---|---|---|---|
| 1 | DHT + $NaH_2PO_4$ | 2.5 ± 0.2 | 2.7 ± 0.15 | 0 | 80 |
| 2 | DHT + $NaH_2PO_4$ + Hemorrhage | 0 | 2.1 ± 0.28 | 0.4 ± 0.1 | 60 |

appearance of the lesions thus induced, hemorrhage exerted a pronounced prophylactic effect against all these agents except plasmocid, while noradrenaline aggravated the changes thus induced by all agents including plasmocid.

The severe lesions produced by noradrenaline given in combination with the various agents just mentioned do not exhibit the histologic characteristics of noradrenaline-overdosage ('spotty myolysis') but they always retain the specific histologic features characteristic of the agent given in combination with the adrenergic hormone.

As a working hypothesis, it is postulated—though not yet proven—that hemorrhage acts by decreasing, and noradrenaline by increasing, cardiac work. Finally, some observations are reviewed to indicate that hemorrhage may act through a specific mechanism and not merely as a stressor agent.

### *d) Prevention of Cross-resistance to Cardiotoxic Agents by Low Chloride Intake*

Our previous experiments showed that by pretreatment with various stressors cross-resistance of the heart can be obtained against various types of experimental cardiopathies (see pp. 197–210). Since we extensively studied the effect of dietary electrolyte deficiencies upon the development of cardiac lesions, it was interesting to see whether the induction of cross-resistance can also be influenced by dietary means.

The experiments to be described in the following will show that an adequate intake of certain electrolytes is, in fact, necessary for the successful development of cross-resistance. More particularly, it will be seen that the acquisition of this type of insensitivity can be completely abolished by lowering the dietary chloride intake. A Mg-deficient diet is also known to sensitize the myocardium to stress (448), but does not abolish this form of cross-resistance: it may be concluded therefore that, in this regard, the metabolic action of Cl-deficiency is rather specific.

#### *Materials and Techniques*

Two hundred forty rats, with an average initial body weight of 96 g (range: 87–103 g) were used in three experimental series. Each group consisted of ten animals. Some of the groups were kept on a low chloride diet, throughout the period of observation. (For the composition of the diets used see 'General Methodology', p. 121). In this manner, we hoped to eliminate any possible nonspecific effect that might have been due to the pure synthetic diets. Distilled water was given ad libitum. During sensitization with these diets, the animals were treated with various cardiotoxic agents, as indicated in Tables XXII, XXIII and XXIV. Several stressor agents were used to induce cross-resistance in the heart: the manner of their application will be described later.

The *first experiment* (Table XXII) deals with the influence of low chloride intake upon the development of cross-resistance to the cardio- and nephrotoxic actions of DHT plus $NaH_2PO_4$ administration, as well as the cardiac-necrosis eliciting effect of stress. In order to induce increased resistance of the heart, some of the animals were repeatedly pretreated with restraint (Groups 2, 4, 6, 8), while the remainder served as controls (Groups 1, 3, 5, 7). Restraint was applied every second day, starting with 4 hours on the second day and then gradually increasing this time up to 7 hours. Treatment with various potentially cardiotoxic agents was initiated on the fourth day and continued until the termination of the experiment. 20 μg DHT was administered in the form of a microcrystal suspension together with 0.5 mM of $NaH_2PO_4$ in 2 ml of water, twice daily, through a stomach tube (Groups 1, 2, 5, 6). F-COL was injected as a microcrystal suspension, 500 μg daily in 0.2 ml of water, subcutaneously (Groups 3, 4, 7, 8). Na-acetate was administered by stomach tube, in a concentration of 1 mM in 2 ml of water, twice daily (Groups 3, 4, 7, 8). Since the combined administration of F-COL plus Na-acetate does not produce cardiac necroses alone, on a normal diet, the rats kept on our basic ration were exposed to the stress of bone fractures in order to elicit cardiac lesions. Multiple bone fracture of all four extremities was performed under light ether anesthesia, on the 10th day (Groups 3, 4). This experimental series was terminated on the 12th day by killing the survivors with chloroform.

The *second experiment* (Table XXIII) deals with the development of cross-resistance to the cardiotoxic actions of papain and of plasmocid, as influenced by a lowered chloride intake. In order to activate stress-defense two stressor agents were applied on the 14th day (i.e., after 13 days' sensitization with the basic or chloride-deficient rations): restraint for a period of 17 hours (Groups 2, 5, 8, 11) and cold baths.

The latter consisted in immersing the rats in ice-water, three times at four hour intervals, for 4 minute periods (Groups 3, 6, 9, 12). Groups 1, 4, 7 and 10 served as controls to show the intensity of the cardiotoxic effects of papain and plasmocid on the basic and chloride-deficient diets, respectively, without previous exposure to stressors. Papain (5%, unfiltered preparation) was injected on the 15th day to all animals of Groups 1–3 and 7–9; 0.2 ml was slowly administered via the jugular vein. Plasmocid, 6-methoxy-8-(diethyl-amino-propylamino)-quinoline-dihydroiodide, was injected in Groups 4–6 and 10–12, three times daily, at 4 hour intervals, on the 15th and 16th days, at the dose of 0.3 mg in 0.2 ml of water, intraperitoneally. This experiment was terminated on the 17th and 18th days, respectively, 48 hours after the papain or the last plasmocid injection.

The *third experiment* (Table XXIV) deals with the effect of Mg-deficiency upon stress-induced cross-resistance, under experimental conditions comparable with those of the second experiment. Some of the animals on the Mg-deficient ration were exposed to restraint (Groups 2, 4) and then treated with papain or plasmocid, together with the unpretreated controls (Groups 1, 3). The duration and intensity of the exposure to restraint, as well as the doses of papain and plasmocid, were the same as in the second experiment. The survivors were killed on the 17th (Groups 1, 2) and 18th (Groups 3, 4) days, respectively.

At autopsy, the hearts were inspected with the aid of a dissecting loupe; they were then fixed in Susa solution saturated with picric acid, for subsequent staining with PAS (or hematoxylin-phloxine), and in alcohol-formol, for the histochemical detection of calcium with von Kóssa's silver nitrate technique. When autopsy findings were positive, the kidney sections were also studied for calcium.

### *Results*

Table XXII shows that all unpretreated control rats, whether kept on the basic diet (Group 1) or on the chloride-deficient ration (Group 5), exhibited severe cardiac lesions and intense nephrocalcinosis, as a consequence of DHT + $NaH_2PO_4$ administration. Histologically, the cardiac muscle of these rats showed suppurating, inflammatory lesions, with extensive fiber necrosis. In addition, there was calcification of the Mönckeberg-sclerosis type in the coronary arteries. Calcium deposition within the cardiac muscle fibers or in their surrounding stroma was

*Table XXII*

Influence of Low-Chloride Intake upon the Development of Cross-Resistance to Cardiotoxic Agents

| Group | Treatment: To induce cross-resistance | Treatment: To elicit cardiac lesions | Cardiac necrosis (Severity) | Cardiac necrosis (Incidence) | Nephrocalcinosis (Severity) | Nephrocalcinosis (Incidence) | Mortality (%) |
|---|---|---|---|---|---|---|---|
| | | **On Basic Diet** | | | | | |
| 1 | None | DHT + $NaH_2PO_4$ | 2.6 ± 0.23 | 100 | 2.5 ± 0.23 | 100 | 70 |
| 2 | Restraint | DHT + $NaH_2PO_4$ | 0 | 0 | 0 | 0 | 0 |
| 3 | None | F-COL + Na-acetate + Bone fracture | 1.2 ± 0.42 | 50 | 0.2 ± 0.20 | 10 | 80 |
| 4 | Restraint | F-COL + Na-acetate + Bone fracture | 0 | 0 | 0 | 0 | 10 |
| | | **On Chloride-Deficient Diet** | | | | | |
| 5 | None | DHT + $NaH_2PO_4$ | 3.0 ± 0.00 | 100 | 1.9 ± 0.10 | 100 | 100 |
| 6 | Restraint | DHT + $NaH_2PO_4$ | 2.1 ± 0.40 | 80 | 1.7 ± 0.30 | 90 | 90 |
| 7 | None | F-COL + Na-acetate | 1.9 ± 0.43 | 78 | 0.5 ± 0.17 | 50 | 90 |
| 8 | Restraint | F-COL + Na-acetate | 1.7 ± 0.40 | 80 | 1.2 ± 0.42 | 60 | 90 |

especially marked in the subendocardial layers of both ventricles. It is evident, furthermore, that while in rats kept on our basic diet adaptation to restraint completely protected against the acute DHT + $NaH_2PO_4$-intoxication (Group 2), a similar pretreatment with stress was ineffective in the animals on a low-chloride intake (Group 6).

It will be recalled that combined administration of F-COL + Na-acetate does not, in itself, usually (e.g., in animals on normal laboratory diets) produce any histologically detectable cardiac damage, but merely predisposes the heart to the necrosis-eliciting effect of subsequent exposure to stressors. However, chloride deficiency selectively sensitizes the myocardium to this potentially cardiotoxic steroid-electrolyte interaction, so that massive and sometimes fatal cardiac necroses develop (see p. 187). Thus, in this regard, chloride deficiency replaces the effect of an acute stressor.

In accordance with these observations, bone fractures elicited severe cardiac lesions in 50% of the F-COL + Na-acetate-conditioned rats on a basic diet (Group 3). On the other hand, this steroid-electrolyte combination in itself produced cardiac necroses in the chloride-deficient animals (Group 7). Here again, pretreatment with restraint protected only the rats fed the basic diet (Group 4); nearly all the animals on the chloride-deficient ration died, presumably as a consequence of the cardiac lesions (Group 8).

It should be noted that this so-called ESCN differs basically in its histologic characteristics from the myocarditic lesions normally produced with DHT + $NaH_2PO_4$ administration. The former consist of massive, necrotic patches in which the muscle fibers are gradually resorbed and replaced, first by histiocytes and polymorphonuclear cells, later by connective tissue. The slight degree of nephrocalcinosis produced by F-COL + Na-acetate in the animals maintained on a chloride-deficient diet was aggravated by pretreatment with restraint (cf. Groups 7 and 8). In addition, in fifty per cent of the restrained-chloride-deficient animals (Group 8), severe, centrolobular hepatic necroses occurred, which were not present in the chloride-deficient not restrained controls (Group 7).

Table XXIII shows that, in rats kept on our basic diet, the intensive disseminated cardiac fiber necrosis following papain injection (Group 1) as well as the large patchy cardiac necrosis (usually associated with diffuse myocarditis) that normally results from plasmocid administration (Group 4) are both prevented by a previous period of restraint (Groups 2, 5), or by cold baths (Groups 3, 6). This protective

*Table XXIII*

Stress-induced Resistance of the Heart to the Cardiotoxic Actions of Papain or Plasmocid and the Abolishing Effect of Chloride Deficiency

| Group | Treatment* | | Cardiac necrosis | | Mortality (%) |
|---|---|---|---|---|---|
| | To induce cross-resistance | To elicit cardiac lesions | (Severity) | (Incidence) | |
| | | On Basic Diet | | | |
| 1 | None | Papain | 1.5 ± 0.30 | 90 | 60 |
| 2 | Restraint | Papain | 0 | 0 | 0 |
| 3 | Cold bath | Papain | 0 | 0 | 0 |
| 4 | None | Plasmocid | 1.6 ± 0.33 | 80 | 90 |
| 5 | Restraint | Plasmocid | 0 | 0 | 0 |
| 6 | Cold bath | Plasmocid | 0 | 0 | 0 |
| | | On Chloride-Deficient Diet | | | |
| 7 | None | Papain | 2.1 ± 0.27 | 100 | 50 |
| 8 | Restraint | Papain | 0.6 ± 0.27 | 40 | 10 |
| 9 | Cold bath | Papain | 1.6 ± 0.40 | 70 | 10 |
| 10 | None | Plasmocid | 1.1 ± 0.28 | 70 | 90 |
| 11 | Restraint | Plasmocid | 1.5 ± 0.23 | 90 | 90 |
| 12 | Cold bath | Plasmocid | 2.2 ± 0.42 | 80 | 90 |

action of stressors is also evident from the reduced mortality rates. However, in the rats kept on the chloride-deficient ration, only restraint offered significant protection against the development of papain-necroses (cf. Groups 7 and 8). In some cases, stress not only failed to prevent but seemed to actually aggravate the lesions normally induced by such treatment (cf. Group 10 with Groups 11 and 12).

Table XXIV shows that maintenance on a Mg-deficient diet does not interfere with the protective effect of stress (Groups 2, 4) against the cardiac lesions normally induced by papain or by plasmocid.

### *Discussion*

It is evident from these experiments that when rats are kept on a basic diet (containing all the necessary electrolytes) various types of cardiac lesions—e.g., the DHT + $NaH_2PO_4$ myocarditis, the infarctoid cardiopathy produced by stress after sensitization with F-COL + Na-acetate, the cardiac necroses caused by papain or plasmocid—can be prevented by pretreatment with stressors. Previous studies showed that this protective effect is shared by many diverse (659) agents, e.g.: forced restraint, cold baths, electric shocks, adrenaline, noradrenaline, or reserpine. Hence, this protection cannot be ascribed to any specific action of the prophylactic agents; it presumably reflects a rather non-specific generalized defensive phenomenon. This view received further support from the present experiments.

We learned, however, that adaptation to stressors no longer increases resistance of cardiac and renal tissues when the dietary chloride intake is lowered from a basic 0.953% to 0.035%. Nothing is known as yet about the mechanism through which a short period of chloride deficiency can thus block cross-resistance phenomena. Earlier investigations suggested that variations in dietary intake, not only of certain cations (such as K and Mg), but also of the anions (e.g., Cl), play an important role in the pathogenesis of some necrotizing cardiopathies. In particular, chloride deficiency was found to enhance the

*Table XXIV*

The Inability of Mg-Deficient Diet to Influence the Development of Cross-Resistance

| Group | Treatment* | | Cardiac necrosis | | Mortality (%) |
|---|---|---|---|---|---|
| | To induce cross-resistance | To elicit cardiac lesions | (Severity) | (Incidence) | |
| 1 | None | Papain | 2.3 ± 0.30 | 90 | 0 |
| 2 | Restraint | Papain | 0 | 0 | 0 |
| 3 | None | Plasmocid | 1.2 ± 0.42 | 60 | 10 |
| 4 | Restraint | Plasmocid | 0 | 0 | 0 |

* In addition to the treatments listed here, all rats were kept on a Mg-deficient diet throughout the experiment, as described in the text.

susceptibility of the myocardium to the production of various lesions (necrosis, inflammation and/or calcification) by a number of cardiotoxic agents, while dietary chloride excess proved to exert an opposite protective effect (p. 181). It is difficult to decide, therefore, on the basis of the present experiments, whether here chloride deficiency specifically blocked the normal development of cross-resistance or whether it merely so raised the sensitivity of the heart that the defensive stress-reactions were no longer effective. The first hypothesis appears to receive some support from the observation that the Mg-deficient ration—well-known to enhance disease susceptibility of the heart muscle—did not affect the normal development of cross-resistance.

Finally, it should be noted that the chloride-deficient diet differed from the basic diet in that in the former the chloride was replaced on a molar basis by corresponding bicarbonates. However, since bicarbonate is generally considered to be innocuous (745, 764), the detrimental effect of this diet may reasonably be attributed to its deficiency in chloride. At any rate, it is significant that the effectiveness of defensive stress-reactions, as well as the disease susceptibility of the heart muscle, are so basically altered by changes in the dietary intake of certain anions.

*Summary*

Experiments on rats indicate that acute overdosage with DHT plus $NaH_2PO_4$ produces rapidly fatal myocarditis and nephrocalcinosis, while exposure to restraint elicits an infarctoid cardiopathy and high mortality, following sensitization with F-COL plus Na-acetate. Yet, both types of lesions, like the cardiac necroses normally induced by papain or plasmocid, are equally prevented by previous exposure to a stressor agent. These are additional examples of nonspecific cross-resistance, showing that increased resistance of the myocardium can be obtained against the most diverse cardiotoxic agents through pretreatment with the same stressor (e.g., restraint).

Stress fails to exert this protective effect upon the myocardium if the dietary chloride intake is markedly lowered. On the other hand, sensitization with a Mg-deficient ration—also known to enhance the disease-susceptibility of the heart muscle—does not influence the normal development of cross-resistance.

Apparently, the reactivity of the myocardium, as regards defensive reactions, largely depends upon the dietary intake of certain anions.

## B. Electrolytes

### *a) Prevention of Stress-induced Cardiac Necrosis by Oral Administration of Electrolytes*

It has been already briefly mentioned that according to earlier observations (622) various chlorides inhibit the morbid changes that can be produced in Me-Cl-COL conditioned rats by simultaneous treatment with certain Na-salts (particularly the phosphates, sulfates and perchlorate). However, in this respect, under standard experimental conditions, equivalent amounts of $MgCl_2$ or KCl are far more effective than is NaCl (618, 619, 688). Comparative experiments with other electrolytes clearly showed that the cation is likewise of importance since certain chlorides proved to be far more effective than others in preventing the ESCN. In particular, $MgCl_2$ and KCl were most active, $NH_4Cl$ and $CaCl_2$ exhibited a moderate anti-ESCN activity, while NaCl was least effective. The nature of this desensitizing action is still obscure, but since even the forced oral administration of water gave some protection against the ESCN the possibility had to be considered that both water and the chlorides might act merely by increasing the urinary excretion of toxic electrolytes (684). It has also been definitely proven that the phenomenon of desensitization does not depend upon interference with any specific effect of the phosphate-ion since the protective effect of $MgCl_2$ or KCl is also manifest in Me-Cl-COL-conditioned rats in which an ESCN is produced by $Na_2SO_4$ or $NaClO_4$ instead of by $Na_2HPO_4$ (621, 622). To further study the important phenomenon of protection, a great number of electrolytes were tested, in various combinations (613).

All these investigations suggested the following general conclusions: a) The production of an ESCN by sensitizing Na-salts can be prevented by a variety of chlorides; b) KCl and $MgCl_2$ are the most active among the relatively non-toxic chlorides that we have tested; c) a number of K-salts other than the chlorides likewise exhibit considerable anti-ESCN activity, while the corresponding Mg-salts are less active or actually inert; d) the anti-ESCN action of various K-salts, other than the chloride, is greater than that of Mg, but KCl and $MgCl_2$ are about equally active; e) both the cation and anion play important roles in the prevention of the ESCN; f) there exists a strictly quantitative relationship between sensitizing and desensitizing electrolytes in that ¼ to ½ mM of KCl or $MgCl_2$ is the threshold amount necessary to produce a just significant inhibition of an ESCN induced by 1 mM of $Na_2HPO_4$. The possibility had to be considered that sensitizing and desensitizing electrolytes might inactivate each other, owing to chemical reactions that take place immediately after these salts are introduced into the gastro-intestinal tract. It has been found, however, that the oral administration of desensitizing salts counteracts the effects of sensitizing electrolytes, even if the latter are injected parenterally.

However, KCl and $MgCl_2$ prevent the occurrence of not only the typical ESCN induced by corticoids and Na-salts, but also the suppurative myocarditis that is normally elicited by combined treatment with DHT plus $NaH_2PO_4$ (664). It is important to note that in all of these previous experiments Na-salts were also given and consequently the prophylactic effect of K- and Mg-salts could be simply due to the well-known antagonism between these anions. Therefore, it was important to determine whether KCl and $MgCl_2$ offer protection against stress-induced cardiac lesions, also.

*Materials and Techniques*

In the *first experiment,* one hundred and forty rats, with a mean initial body weight of 100 g (range 94–104 g) were subdivided into 7 equal groups of 20 each. The order of treatment is indicated in Table XXV.

Me-Cl-COL was administered in the form of a microcrystal suspension, 500 µg in 0.2 ml of water, daily, subcutaneously, throughout the experiment. Some groups received the electrolyte solutions daily throughout the entire experiment (Groups 4, 6), while others only on the day of the exposure to restraint (Groups 5, 7). More precisely, KCl and $MgCl_2$ were administered to Groups 4 and 6 respectively, twice daily, in a concentration of 0.5 mM in 2 ml of water from the 1st until the 10th day. On the 11th day, all rats in Groups 4–7 received 2 mM of electrolyte (KCl or $MgCl_2$ respectively); at every 6th hour one dose of 0.5 mM, always by a stomach tube. Restraint was applied on the 11th day, for 17 hours. The experiment was terminated on the 12th day and the hearts were studied following staining with the fuchsin technique.

In the *second experiment,* thirty rats, with a mean initial body weight of 95 g (range: 90–100 g), were subdivided in 3 equal groups and

*Table XXV*

Prevention by Electrolytes of Cardiac Necrosis Produced by Stress after Sensitization with Me-Cl-COL

| Group | Treatment | Final body weight (g) | Cardiac necrosis (Severity) | Cardiac necrosis (Incidence) | Mortality (%) |
|---|---|---|---|---|---|
| 1 | Me-Cl-COL | 83 ± 2.4 | 0 | 0 | 0 |
| 2 | Restraint | 113 ± 2.3 | 1.0 ± 0 | 100 | 0 |
| 3 | Me-Cl-COL + Restraint | 77 ± 1.8 | 2.5 ± 0.10 | 100 | 30 |
| 4 | Me-Cl-COL + Restraint + KCl (11 days) | 82 ± 2.0 | 1.1 ± 0.17 | 60 | 0 |
| 5 | Me-Cl-COL + Restraint + KCl (1 day) | 80 ± 1.7 | 0.8 ± 0.15 | 40 | 20 |
| 6 | Me-Cl-COL + Restraint + $MgCl_2$ (11 days) | 81 ± 1.9 | 0.5 ± 0.20 | 20 | 10 |
| 7 | Me-Cl-COL + Restraint + $MgCl_2$ (1 day) | 79 ± 2.1 | 0.6 ± 0.16 | 30 | 20 |

treated as indicated in Table XXVI. Restraint was applied on the 1st day of the experiment for a period of 17 hours. On the same day, 2 mM of KCl (Group 2), or $MgCl_2$ (Group 3) were administered through a stomach tube in four equal doses: 0.5 mM electrolyte in 2 ml of water, once at every 6th hour. The control Group 1 received the corresponding amount of water by the same route. The experiment was terminated on the 2nd day, and the hearts studied similarly to the first experiment.

### *Results and Discussion*

It is evident from the date summarized in Table XXV that cardiac necroses do not occur spontaneously in the Me-Cl-COL sensitized rats (Group 1). On the other hand, however, exposure to restraint elicited cardiac lesions in 100% of the animals (Group 2). It is also clear from the figures given in this table that pretreatment with Me-Cl-COL greatly aggravated the intensity of the cardiac lesions (Group 3), while the administration of KCl and $MgCl_2$ significantly diminished both the incidence and severity of the lesions normally produced by restraint in the Me-Cl-COL-conditioned animals (Groups 4–7). Interestingly, the protective action of KCl and $MgCl_2$ was independent of the duration of the pretreatment with these electrolytes (cf. Groups 4 and 6 with Groups 5 and 7).

Table XXVI shows, furthermore, that the simple stress-cardiopathy produced by exposure to forced immobilization (Group 1; Table XXVI) can also be prevented by KCl (Group 2) and $MgCl_2$ (Group 3).

We note that the cardiac lesions produced by simple exposure to stress in the absence of any specific conditioning factors are not visible on naked-eye inspection. Even in rats sensitized with Me-Cl-COL and then exposed to restraint, the lesions are rarely observable with dissecting loupe. They manifest themselves histologically as scattered 'micro'-necroses of individual muscle fibers or small fiber groups. These foci become secondarily infiltrated, first by inflammatory cells and later by connective tissue, but the individual lesions are so small that they do not tend to terminate in permanent scar formation. Myocardial calcification or hyalinization likewise fails to occur and the coronary vessels are never affected. Fuchsinophilic degeneration of individual muscle fibers is, however, common in the myocardium of such stressed rats. Yet, it is remarkable that these minute miliary myocardial necroses produced by restraint are diminished or even abolished by KCl or $MgCl_2$. This 'anti-stress' effect of KCl and $MgCl_2$ may be of special importance, because—as it was demonstrated by many experiments in this monograph—acute stress situations can precipitate necrotizing cardiopathies in suitably conditioned animals, a situation probably comparable to the stress-induced cardiac infarcts in predisposed human beings.

Finally, as an additional finding it may be mentioned our observation that the administration of KCl and $MgCl_2$ protects the animals against an otherwise 100% lethal dose of diphtherotoxin (661). Not only were the intensive hemorrhagic necroses of the adrenal (characteristic of the acute, vasotoxic and stressor actions of this bacterial toxin) absent in the chloride-treated guinea-pigs, but the adrenals did not show any histologic signs of cortical hyperactivity. Unfortunately we could not produce any cardiac lesion with diphtherotoxin in these experiments.

*Table XXVI*

Effect of KCl and $MgCl_2$ upon the Cardiac Lesions Induced by Restraint

| Group | Treatment | Final body weight (g) | Cardiac necrosis (Severity) | Cardiac necrosis (Incidence) | Mortality (%) |
|---|---|---|---|---|---|
| 1 | Restraint | 86 ± 1.7 | 1.2 ± 0.20 | 100 | 0 |
| 2 | Restraint + KCl | 84 ± 1.9 | 0.4 ± 0.25 | 30 | 0 |
| 3 | Restraint + $MgCl_2$ | 86 ± 1.9 | 0 | 0 | 0 |

*Summary*

Experiments in the rat showed that the minute myocardial necroses normally produced by restraint alone, or with exposure to this neuromuscular stressor after conditioning by Me-Cl-COL, are diminished or abolished by KCl or $MgCl_2$. Apparently, these salts do not act merely by interfering with the exogenous conditioning corticoids (e.g., Me-Cl-COL) usually employed to sensitize animals for the cardiac necrosis-eliciting effect of stress.

### *b) Prevention by $MgCl_2$ and KCl of the Myocardial Necroses Normally Produced by Proteolytic Enzymes*

The previously cited, earlier investigations (see p. 224) have shown that Mg- and K-salts protect the heart from intoxication with $NaH_2PO_4$ and adrenocortical steroids (e.g., Me- Cl-COL, cortisol, cortisone) or sterols of the vitamin-D group (e.g., DHT); however, these might well have been isolated specific instances of protection, since both the corticoids and the compounds of the vitamin-D group are known to exert their effect largely as a result of specific influences upon inorganic salt metabolism. On the other hand, it is also known that stress may basically alter the electrolyte-balance of the organism (see pp. 86–91). Consequently the question arose whether the cardiac necroses normally produced by proteolytic enzymes would also be influenced by electrolytes.

The experiments described below will show that the cardiac lesions normally produced by the intravenous injection of papain extract are inhibited by $MgCl_2$ and KCl, and aggravated by $Na_2HPO_4$. These findings are more unexpected and perhaps of greater general significance as regards the pathologic physiology of heart muscle, because they suggest that the effect of various sensitizing and desensitizing salts is rather nonspecific.

### *Materials and Techniques*

Eighty rats, with an average initial body weight of 98 g (range: 93–110 g), were subdivided into eight equal groups and treated as indicated in Table XXVII.

*Me-Cl-COL* was given in the form of microcrystal suspension, at the dose of 100 µg, in 0.2 ml of water, subcutaneously, once daily, throughout the experiment. The individual dose of *KCl*, *$MgCl_2$* and *$Na_2HPO_4$* was 1 mM. This amount of one or two salts was dissolved in 2 ml of water and was given by stomach tube, twice daily throughout the experiment to the groups indicated in Table XXVII. On the 4th day, the rats of all eight groups received 0.3 ml of freshly prepared papain (5%, filtered) solution, via the jugular vein. The experiment was terminated on the 5th day. In each case, the heart and kidney were fixed in neutral formalin and stained with the von Kóssa technique (for demonstration of calcium) and lightly counterstained with hematoxylin-phloxine (to appraise general histologic structure).

The study of the kidneys was only incidental in this investigation, but since the nephrocalcinosis caused by an excess of $Na_2HPO_4$ is aggravated by certain corticoids (613), we wanted to verify whether, under our experimental conditions, the calcium deposition in the kidney would parallel the cardiac changes.

### *Results and Discussion*

The most obvious, macroscopically visible lesions elicited by the papain extract were multiple, band-like, yellow streaks of *necrosis in the myocardium*. The diffuse distribution of these miliary lesions was strikingly different from the infarct-like, massive patches of necrosis that are normally produced by more chronic treatment with Me-Cl-

COL plus $Na_2HPO_4$ (613). Histologic examination showed that these lesions are rather diffusely distributed throughout the walls of both ventricles and auricles, although the subendocardial regions appeared to be sites of predilection.

It is evident, from the summary of our findings (seen in Table XXVII) that both Me-Cl-COL (Group 2) and $Na_2HPO_4$ (Group 3) aggravated the cardiotoxic effect of papain alone (Group 1); however, the rats sensitized by combined treatment with Me-Cl-COL plus $Na_2HPO_4$ (Group 6) were by far most severely affected. It should be emphasized that such short treatment with Me-Cl-COL plus $Na_2HPO_4$, as was given in this series, rarely, if ever, produced any noteworthy cardiac damage in our earlier experiments in which papain was not administered; besides—as just stated—the type and distribution of the lesions caused by the steroid-electrolyte treatment alone are wholly different from those seen in the present experiment. It may be concluded, therefore, that both Me-Cl-COL and $Na_2HPO_4$, but particularly the combination of these agents, greatly sensitize or 'condition' the myocardium for the production of necroses by a subsequent injection of papain extract.

On the other hand, treatment with $MgCl_2$ (Group 4) or KCl (Group 5) greatly increased the resistance of the myocardium to the necrotizing effect of the papain extract. This protective effect, though less pronounced, was also manifest in the rats in which a particularly severe cardiopathy was induced by combined treatment with Me-Cl-COL plus $Na_2HPO_4$ (compare Group 6 with Groups 7 and 8). It is significant that 80% of the rats in Group 6 succumbed, while all the animals in Groups 7 and 8 survived the papain injection (although, here, the myocardial damage caused by the steroid-electrolyte treatment was so severe that $MgCl_2$ and KCl could not prevent it completely). Furthermore, histologic study of the hearts revealed that, in Group 6, large areas of necrotic muscle fibers were still present at the time of autopsy (two days after the papain injection), while in Groups 7 and 8 most of the necrotic fibers were already absorbed and replaced by histiocytes and young connective-tissue cells, indicative of active repair and early scar formation.

*Nephrocalcinosis* was present, but only moderately intense in the rats treated with $Na_2HPO_4$ alone (Group 3); it was extremely severe in those animals which received Me-Cl-COL in addition to the $Na_2HPO_4$ (Group 6). This merely confirms earlier findings that active mineralocorticoids greatly enhance susceptibility to the production of the

*Table XXVII*

Influence of Me-Cl-COL and Various Electrolytes upon the Cardiac and Renal Lesions Produced by an Intravenous Injection of Papain Extract

| Group | Treatment* | Cardiac necrosis | | Nephrocalcinosis | | Mortality (%) |
|---|---|---|---|---|---|---|
| | | (Severity) | (Incidence) | (Severity) | (Incidence) | |
| 1 | None | 1.6 ± 0.18 | 90 | 0 | 0 | 0 |
| 2 | Me-Cl-COL | 2.3 ± 0.18 | 100 | 0 | 0 | 0 |
| 3 | $Na_2HPO_4$ | 2.1 ± 0.19 | 100 | 0.8 ± 0.15 | 80 | 0 |
| 4 | $MgCl_2$ | 0.4 ± 0.16 | 20 | 0 | 0 | 0 |
| 5 | KCl | 0.7 ± 0.20 | 40 | 0 | 0 | 0 |
| 6 | Me-Cl-COL + $Na_2HPO_4$ | 2.9 ± 0.10 | 100 | 2.5 ± 0.18 | 100 | 80 |
| 7 | Me-Cl-COL + $Na_2HPO_4$ + $MgCl_2$ | 2.4 ± 0.15 | 100 | 0 | 0 | 0 |
| 8 | Me-Cl-COL + $Na_2HPO_4$ + KCl | 2.1 ± 0.16 | 100 | 0 | 0 | 0 |

* In addition to the treatments listed in this column, the rats of all groups were given a single i.v. injection of papain extract, as indicated in the text.

phosphate-nephropathy (613). It is interesting however, that even this intense nephrocalcinosis could be completely prevented, both by $MgCl_2$ (Group 7) and by KCl (Group 8).

Judged by macroscopic inspection, the incidence and severity of the *hepatic necroses* that normally occur after intravenous treatment with papain extract ran approximately parallel with the cardiac necroses. However, the hepatic changes are not listed in the Table, since these observations were incidental to the main subject of this investigation. Besides, we have controlled our autopsy findings by microscopic study of specimens taken from only a few rats of each group, so that an exact grading of the lesions was not possible.

It is generally assumed—though perhaps not definitely proven—that papain attacks the cardiac muscle directly, as a result of its proteolytic effect (347, 485). If this assumption is correct, our findings would appear to indicate that magnesium and potassium salts can protect the cardiac muscle against the immediate toxic effects of an active proteolytic enzyme preparation, while $Na_2HPO_4$ and Me-Cl-COL exert an opposite effect. Finally we note that the cardiotoxic action of other proteolytic enzymes (e.g., ficin) is similarly influenced by electrolytes and corticoids (640).

*Summary*

Experiments on rats indicate that the myocardial necroses normally induced by an intravenous injection of a papain extract are aggravated by pretreatment with Me-Cl-COL or $Na_2HPO_4$ and, particularly, by combined treatment with both these agents. On the other hand, $MgCl_2$ and KCl protect the cardiac muscle against the necrotizing action of papain extract.

The nephrocalcinosis, normally elicited by large amounts of $Na_2HPO_4$ in the rat, is greatly aggravated by Me-Cl-COL, but even the unusually intense nephrocalcinotic effect of this combined treatment can be abolished by the concurrent administration of $MgCl_2$ or KCl.

### *c) Effect of Various Chlorides upon the Development of $NaClO_4$-induced Cardiac Lesions*

In view of our findings concerning the interactions of anions and cations in the production of experimental cardiopathies, and particularly to further investigate the protective effect of chlorides, we wished to determine 1. whether the degree of cardiac necroses elicited with certain Na-salts (for example $NaClO_4$) is independent of sensitization by K or Mg deficiency; and 2. whether the morbid changes so induced would be prevented equally with various chlorides.

*Materials and Techniques*

One hundred and seventy rats, with a mean initial body weight of 45 g (range: 40 to 54 g) were subdivided into 17 equal groups and treated as indicated in Table XXVIII. The animals of Groups 2 to 9 were maintained on a K-deficient diet, and those of Groups 10 to 17 on an Mg-deficient diet, respectively, for 5 days prior to as well as during the entire experiment. The composition of these deficient diets is described on pp. 119–120. The control rats, Group 1, were maintained on the normal laboratory food, Purina Fox Chow. All electrolytes were given in 2 ml of water through a stomach tube twice daily. Each individual dose of $NaClO_4$ was 0.5 mM while that of the chlorides or their mixtures consisted of an amount equal to the chloride content of 0.25 mM KCl. The experiment was terminated on the third day (Groups 2 to 9) or on the seventh day (Groups 1, 10 to 17) and the cardiac changes were evaluated on histologic sections stained with hemotoxylin-phloxine.

### *Results and Discussion*

As the data in Table XXVIII show, after sensitization with either a K-deficient or Mg-deficient diet a short period of treatment with $NaClO_4$ sufficed to cause widespread cardiac necroses in the vast majority of the experimental animals. On the other hand, this dietary conditioning to the cardiotoxic effect of $NaClO_4$ was abolished or at least markedly diminished by concurrent administration of various chlorides. Only the prophylactic effect of NaCl was not significant in the K-deficient animals. It is particularly interesting to note that the sensitizing action of K-deficiency was effectively decreased by, among others, $MgCl_2$, and vice versa. Consequently, the anion must play an important role in this preventative reaction, since K and Mg ions are believed to be in many respects even antagonistic (711).

### *Summary*

Experiments in the rat indicated that:

1. K- or Mg-deficiency equally sensitizes the heart to the cardiotoxic effect of $NaClO_4$;

2. The sensitizing effect of both these dietary deficiencies is significantly diminished or abolished by the oral administration of various chlorides; among these, KCl is as active in Mg-deficient animals as is $MgCl_2$ in rats kept on a diet low in K.

*Table XXVIII*

Sensitization with K- or Mg-Deficiency for the Necrotizing Effect of $NaClO_4$: The Role of Chlorides in its Prevention

| Group | Treatment | Cardiac necrosis | |
|---|---|---|---|
| | | (Severity) | (Incidence) |
| 1 | $NaClO_4$ | 0 | 0 |
| 2 | K-Deficient Diet | 0 | 0 |
| 3 | K-Deficient Diet + $NaClO_4$ | 2.8 ± 0.18 | 100 |
| 4 | K-Deficient Diet + $NaClO_4$ + KCl | 0 | 0 |
| 5 | K-Deficient Diet + $NaClO_4$ + $MgCl_2$ | 0.4 ± 0.20 | 30 |
| 6 | K-Deficient Diet + $NaClO_4$ + NaCl | 2.1 ± 0.32 | 80 |
| 7 | K-Deficient Diet + $NaClO_4$ + $CaCl_2$ | 0.6 ± 0.25 | 30 |
| 8 | K-Deficient Diet + $NaClO_4$ + $NH_4Cl$ | 0.1 ± 0.10 | 10 |
| 9 | K-Deficient Diet + $NaClO_4$ + $MgCl_2$ + NaCl + $CaCl_2$ + $NH_4Cl$ | 0.2 ± 0.15 | 10 |
| 10 | Mg-Deficient Diet | 0 | 0 |
| 11 | Mg-Deficient Diet + $NaClO_4$ | 1.5 ± 0.27 | 80 |
| 12 | Mg-Deficient Diet + $NaClO_4$ + KCL | 0.3 ± 0.17 | 20 |
| 13 | Mg-Deficient Diet + $NaClO_4$ + $MgCl_2$ | 0 | 0 |
| 14 | Mg-Deficient Diet + $NaClO_4$ + NaCl | 0.4 ± 0.18 | 40 |
| 15 | Mg-Deficient Diet + $NaClO_4$ + $CaCl_2$ | 0.2 ± 0.15 | 10 |
| 16 | Mg-Deficient Diet + $NaClO_4$ + $NH_4Cl$ | 0 | 0 |
| 17 | Mg-Deficient Diet + $NaClO_4$ + KCl + NaCl + $CaCl_2$ + $NH_4Cl$ | 0 | 0 |

## C. Dietary Deficiencies and Other Desensitizing Factors

### *a) Provocation and Prevention of K-deficiency by Various Ions*

It has long been known that rats kept either on K-deficient (202, 566, 749) or on Mg-deficient (250, 403, 566) diets tend to develop focal myocardial necroses and nephrocalcinosis. In the case of Mg-deficiency, these changes are frequently accompanied by convulsions.

Several observations suggested that an excess of Na can aggravate K-deficiency (213, 411), but in none of these earlier studies were the effects of various Na-salts compared, because at that time there was no reason to suspect a dependence of Na-actions upon anions. The possibility of a replacement of K by Mg was also disregarded. Thus, for example, one group of workers claimed that administration of excess NaCl aggravates the myocardial necroses characteristic of severe K-deficiency (103, 506). They arrived at this conclusion by substituting $MgCl_2$ for NaCl in their control rats. SCHRADER *et al.* (566) postulated that simultaneous Mg-deficiency does not significantly alter the course of K-deficiency in the rat; indeed, some workers believe that there exists an actual antagonism between Mg and K (124, 711, 711a).

In view of our findings concerning participation of electrolytes in production of myocardial necroses by steroids, we wished to dermine: 1. whether the cardiac necroses and other manifestations of dietary K-deficiency would be most markedly aggravated by those Na-salts that sensitize for production of the ESCN and 2. whether the morbid changes usually ascribed to a lack of K are accentuated by a concurrent deficiency in Mg.

## *Materials and Techniques*

In the *first experiment,* sixty rats, with a mean initial body-weight of 49 g (range 43–55 g) were placed on the 'Low Potassium Diet' of the Nutritional Biochemicals Corp. (Cleveland, Ohio) for 7 days. For the composition of the diet see p. 119.

On 7th day, the rats were subdivided into 6 equal groups and treated as indicated in Table XXIX. 0.5 mM of $Na_2HPO_4$, 0.25 mM of KCl and 0.25 mM of $MgCl_2$ were administered in 2 ml of water, twice daily, by stomach tube. The experiment was terminated on the 13th day, that is, after 6 days of electrolyte treatment. In the *second experiment,* fifty rats, with a mean initial body-weight of 51 g (range: 43–55 g), were placed on the same 'Low Potassium Diet' used in the first series. On the 7th day the rats were subdivided into 5 equal groups and treated as indicated in Table XXX. The treatment was the same as in the first experiment except that, here, 0.5 mM of $Na_2HPO_4$ was administered once daily, and 0.5 mM of KCl and of $MgCl_2$ was given twice daily by stomach tube, always in 2 ml of water. Furthermore, a special control group was added which received the same amount of Na, in the form of 1 Mm of NaCl, as was given to the rats treated with $Na_2HPO_4$. This experiment was terminated on the 9th day, that is, after 2 days of electrolyte treatment. In both experimental series the heart and kidneys were fixed in neutral formalin and stained with the acid-fuchsin technic for demonstration of early necrotic changes, and with von Kóssa's silver nitrate technique for histochemical detection of calcium.

*Results*

The most striking change observed in the course of the *first experiment* was the development of intense muscular cramps and convulsions, in the $Na_2HPO_4$-treated rats (Group 2). There was at first a fine fibrillar tremor followed by slow spastic extensions of the hind paws, and, eventually, generalized convulsions with forceful extensor movements in both hind legs. These cramps began 2–3 hours after $Na_2HPO_4$ administration and resulted in 100% mortality within the first 24 hours. Slight transient tremor was also observed in the rats which, in addition to $Na_2HPO_4$, received KCl (Group 4) but in none of the other groups.

*Table XXIX*

Provocation and Prevention of Potassium Deficiency by Various Ions
(First Experiment)

| Group | Treatment | Cardiac necrosis | Nephrocalcinosis | Muscular cramps | Mortality (%) |
|---|---|---|---|---|---|
| 1 | None | 1.1 ± 0.30 | 0 | 0 | 10 |
| 2 | $Na_2HPO_4$ | 2.7 ± 0.10 | 0.3 ± 0.30 | 3.0 ± 0 | 100 |
| 3 | KCl | 0 | 0 | 0 | 10 |
| 4 | KCl + $Na_2HPO_4$ | 0.1 ± 0.10 | 0.1 ± 0.10 | Transient tremor | 30 |
| 5 | $MgCl_2$ | 0.4 ± 0.20 | 0 | 0 | 30 |
| 6 | $MgCl_2$ + $Na_2HPO_4$ | 1.1 ± 0.30 | 0 | 0 | 20 |

Yellowish patches of myocardial necroses were quite evident, even by mere macroscopic inspection, in most of the animals of Group 2. The histologic findings (Table XXIX) indicate that after having been kept on the 'Low Potassium Diet' for 13 days, even the otherwise untreated controls (Group 1) showed moderate cardiac necroses. These lesions were significantly aggravated by $Na_2HPO_4$ (Group 2), but prevented or diminished by KCl (Group 3) or $MgCl_2$ (Group 5). Indeed, even in the event of simultaneous treatment with $Na_2HPO_4$ both KCl (Group 4) and $MgCl_2$ (Group 6) exerted at least a partially protective effect upon the induction of cardiac necroses.

Nephrocalcinosis was negligible in all groups of this series, presumably because the animals most likely to develop it (those of Group 2) died within a few hours after the $Na_2HPO_4$ treatment. The detrimental effect of $Na_2HPO_4$ can definitely be ascribed to conditioning by the 'Low Potassium Diet', because numerous control experiments (613) showed that, under similar circumstances, even fatal doses of $Na_2HPO_4$ produce no cardiac necroses or muscular cramps.

In the *second experiment,* $Na_2HPO_4$ treatment was reduced while the prophylactic administration of KCl and $MgCl_2$ was increased. This was done, in order to prolong survival and, thereby, permit development of morphologic changes in the rats treated with $Na_2HPO_4$ and,

*Table XXX*

Provocation and Prevention of Potassium Deficiency by Various Ions (Second Experiment)

| Group | Treatment | Cardiac necrosis | Nephrocalcinosis | Muscular cramps | Mortality (%) |
|---|---|---|---|---|---|
| 1 | None | 0 | 0 | 0 | 0 |
| 2 | NaCl | 0 | 0 | 0 | 0 |
| 3 | $Na_2HPO_4$ | 2.5 ± 0.20 | 2.8 ± 0.10 | 3.0 ± 0 | 60 |
| 4 | KCl + $Na_2HPO_4$ | 0 | 0 | Transient tremor | 0 |
| 5 | $MgCl_2$ + $Na_2HPO_4$ | 0 | 0 | 0 | 0 |

at the same time, to offer a better chance of protection by KCl and $MgCl_2$. The results summarized in Table XXX indicate, that, under these conditions, marked cardiac necroses and nephrocalcinosis developed after 2 days of $Na_2HPO_4$ treatment following 9 days of the 'Low Potassium Diet'; at this time the controls (Group 1) had not yet developed cardiac necroses. The experiment also shows that $Na_2HPO_4$ was not effective merely by virtue of its Na-content, since equivalent amounts of NaCl (Group 2) were completely ineffective. On the other hand, the somewhat larger doses of KCl and $MgCl_2$ given in this experiment offered virtually complete protection against the mortality as well as the cardiotoxic, nephrotoxic and muscular-cramp-producing effects of combined treatment with the 'Low Potassium Diet' plus $Na_2HPO_4$.

### *Discussion*

The earlier findings reported in our introduction created the impression that Mg-content of the diet is of little if any importance in determining course of K-deficiency (566). This is presumably why the Nutritional Biochemical Co. (Cleveland, Ohio), which prepares the 'Low Potassium Diet'—that we, like so many other laboratories, have used—did not consider it necessary to check the Mg-content of this ration. We found it to contain 52 mg/kg, which is close to the minimal amount necessary for growth according to TUFTS AND GREENBERG (753). On the other hand, the latter investigators claim to have demonstrated, by adding various concentrations of calcium phosphates to Mg-deficient diets, that 'a high content of calcium in the diet increases the severity of magnesium deficiency'. However, they disregarded the fact that when Ca was raised (from 0.39 to 1.66%), phosphorus was also considerably increased (from 0.45 to 1.00%). Although it is quite possible that Ca itself exerts a sensitizing effect, it is also evident from our experiments that $PO_4$ can do so even when not attached to Ca.

### *Summary and Conclusions*

When rats are kept on a 'Low Potassium Diet' that contains only near minimal maintenance levels of Mg, there develop cardiac necroses which can be prevented both by KCl and $MgCl_2$ administration. On the other hand, $Na_2HPO_4$ (unlike equivalent amounts of NaCl) rapidly provokes development of severe cardiac necroses, nephrocalcinosis and muscular cramps before this diet, in itself, produces any obvious morbid changes. The particularly severe K and/or Mg-deficiency syndrome induced by $Na_2HPO_4$-supplements, in animals on this diet, can be prevented by either KCl or $MgCl_2$. These observations highlight the importance of $PO_4$- and Mg-ions in the development of the syndrome usually ascribed to K-deficiency. (We are greatly indebted to Dr. K. Mori for determination of the Mg-content of the diet used in these experiments.)

### *b) Effect of Na-deficiency upon Necrotizing Cardiopathies Produced by Various Agents*

It will be recalled that in one of our earlier experiments (see p. 149) it was observed that certain Na-salts (e.g., $NaHCO_3$, Na-succinate, -pyruvate, -tartrate, -formate, -glutamate) are well tolerated, even by rats simultaneously treated with Me-Cl-COL or neuromuscular stressors. However, these same salts produce massive, and sometimes fatal, cardiac necroses in animals exposed to stress, after conditioning with Me-Cl-COL. It was concluded, therefore, that during stress the metabolism of certain otherwise innocuous Na-salts and/or steroids is so altered that they acquire severe cardiotoxic properties.

These investigations suggested that Na may play a key role in the pathogenesis of certain types of necrotizing cardiopathies that are produced by biochemical means. In the following experiments we wish to report upon the effect of Na-deficiency upon cardiac necroses produced by various agents.

#### *Materials and Techniques*

One hundred and eighty rats, with a mean initial body weight of 50 g (range: 46–58 g), were subdivided into 18 equal groups and treated as indicated in Table XXXI.

The experimental animals in the even-numbered groups were kept on a Na-deficient diet, while the control rats (odd-numbered groups) were maintained on a basic diet, which contained sufficient amounts of Na. In this manner, we hoped to eliminate any possible nonspecific effect that might have been due to the pure synthetic diet. (For the composition of both these diets, see 'General Methodology', pp. 122–123). The rats on the Na-deficient diet received distilled water to drink; those on the basic, tap water.

In a preliminary experiment the rats showed approximatively the same growth rate when they were kept on this diet or on the normal laboratory food, 'Purina Fox Chow'.

The potentially cardiotoxic agents used were the following: *Noradrenaline* was given in doses of 200 µg in 0.2 ml of oil, twice daily, subcutaneously on the 10th and 19th days of the experiment. The rats were then killed on the 21st day. *Vasopressin* was injected on the 18th and following day, in doses of 15 I.U. in 1.5 ml of water, twice daily, subcutaneously. The animals were killed 48 hours after the last injection. *DHT* was always given in the form of a microcrystal suspension, twice daily, through a stomach tube. This treatment was initiated on the 18th day of the experiment (Groups 7–10). The rats in Groups 7 and 8 received 50 µg of DHT daily, in two equal portions (always in 0.5 ml of water) during the first 4 days after initiation of the treatment. This dose was raised on the 22nd day to 100 µg per day and then to 200 µg on the 25th day. This last dose level was given until the 31st day, when the experiment was terminated. In Groups 9 and 10, the DHT was administered in mixture with Ca-acetate, in 2 ml of water, twice daily. The daily amount of DHT was 30 µg from the 18th to the 20th days, inclusive; on the following day the dose was raised to 60 µg. From then on, no further adjustment of the dose was necessary, since the animals died between the 22nd and 25th days of the experiment. *Ca-acetate* was administered (together with DHT) in a concentration of 0.5 mM in 2 ml of water, twice daily, through a stomach tube. Treatment with Ca-acetate was initiated on the 18th day; 4 days later the concentration was raised to 1 mM daily and was not further adjusted. Plasmocid, 6-methoxy-8-(3diethyl-amino-propylamino)-quinoline dihydroiodide was injected on the 18th and 19th days, at the daily dose of 0.30 mg in 0.2 ml of water, intraperitoneally. The three daily injections were so divided that there was a 4-hour interval between each. The rats were killed 48 hours after the last injection. *Papain* (5%, filtered solution) was injected once on the 18th day; 0.15 ml via the jugular vein. The rats were killed 48 hours after the papain injection. *F-COL* was injected subcutaneously, in the form of a microcrystal suspension in 0.2 ml of water, in doses of 500 µg daily, from the 14th to the 19th days of the experiment. *Restraint* was applied on the 18th day, for a period of 17 hours. All animals were killed 48 hours after the initiation of the restraint. *Quadriplegia* was performed on the 18th day; these rats were then killed on the 20th day.

At autopsy, the hearts were fixed in neutral formalin for subsequent embedding in paraffin. The sections were stained with von Kóssa's technique for the histochemical demonstration of calcium (using hematoxylin-phloxine counterstain).

### *Results*

As will be seen from the data in Table XXXI, Na-deficiency markedly inhibited the cardiotoxic effect of some agents and reduced that of others. Only the necrotizing action of a combined DHT + Ca-acetate treatment was not beneficially altered.

Na-deficiency significantly protected the animals against the cardiac lesions normally produced by DHT (Groups 7 and 8), plasmocid (Groups 11 and 12), papain (Groups 13 and 14) and restraint + F-COL (Groups 15 and 16). We note that in the rats kept on a Na-deficient diet, not only was the cardiac muscle protected against the calcifying and necrotizing actions of DHT but, also, the renal tissue of these animals failed to show the exclusively cortical nephrocalcinosis normally induced with overdosage of this vitamin D derivative (Fig. 17). It is especially interesting, furthermore, that the large, patchy myocardial necroses and myocarditic lesions produced with plasmocid in 100% of our control animals were so markedly inhibited in the Na deficient rats (Figs. 18 and 19). It will be recalled that the plasmocid lesions differ from the many other experimental cardiopathies that we studied in that only the former cannot be prevented by KCl or $MgCl_2$ and are not greatly aggravated by pretreatment with corticoids or sensitizing Na-salts (613). The miliary, disseminated cardiac necroses due to the intravenous injection of papain were much milder in the Na-deficient rats; this protective effect is also manifest in the percentage of mortality. In the F-COL conditioned rats, a neuromuscular effort induced by forced restraint constantly elicited small necrotic foci ('micronecroses') within the myocardium. Here again, dietary deficiency in Na was found to protect the heart. However, it is not very remarkable that the occasional mild lesions produced in this experiment with another stressor agent (i.e., quadriplegia) were prevented by Na-deficiency (Groups 17 and 18).

Statistically, it is questionable whether Na-deficiency also offered protection against 'spotty myolysis' induced by noradrenaline (Groups 3 and 4) or by vasopressin (Groups 5 and 6). However, it should be noted that at the time when noradrenaline and vasopressin were injected the Na-deficient rats weighed about 8 to 12 g less than did the controls and, therefore, the former received a somewhat higher dose per gram of body weight.

*Table XXXI*

Effect of Sodium Deficiency upon Necrotizing Cardiopathies Produced by Various Agents

| Group | Treatment* | Cardiac necrosis | | Mortality (%) |
|---|---|---|---|---|
| | | (Severity) | (Incidence) | |
| 1 | None | 0 | 0 | 0 |
| 2 | Na-Deficiency | 0 | 0 | 0 |
| 3 | Noradrenaline | 1.8 ± 0.21 | 90 | 0 |
| 4 | Noradrenaline + Na-Deficiency | 1.1 ± 0.27 | 60 | 0 |
| 5 | Vasopressin | 1.5 ± 0.18 | 80 | 0 |
| 6 | Vasopressin + Na-Deficiency | 1.0 ± 0.20 | 50 | 0 |
| 7 | DHT | 2.8 ± 0.13 | 100 | 30 |
| 8 | DHT + Na-Deficiency | 0.7 ± 0.17 | 40 | 0 |
| 9 | DHT + Ca-acetate | 3.0 ± 0 | 100 | 100 |
| 10 | DHT + Ca-acetate + Na-Deficiency | 3.0 ± 0 | 100 | 100 |
| 11 | Plasmocid | 2.8 ± 0.13 | 100 | 50 |
| 12 | Plasmocid + Na-Deficiency | 0.9 ± 0.25 | 40 | 0 |
| 13 | Papain | 3.0 ± 0 | 100 | 100 |
| 14 | Papain + Na-Deficiency | 1.4 ± 0.23 | 70 | 10 |
| 15 | Restraint + F-COL | 1.6 ± 0.18 | 80 | 0 |
| 16 | Restraint + F-COL + Na-Deficiency | 0.2 ± 0.15 | 20 | 0 |
| 17 | Quadriplegia + F-COL | 0.5 ± 0.10 | 50 | 0 |
| 18 | Quadriplegia + F-COL + Na-Deficiency | 0.1 ± 0.10 | 10 | 0 |

* All the odd-numbered groups were kept on a synthetic (basic) diet, as described in the text.

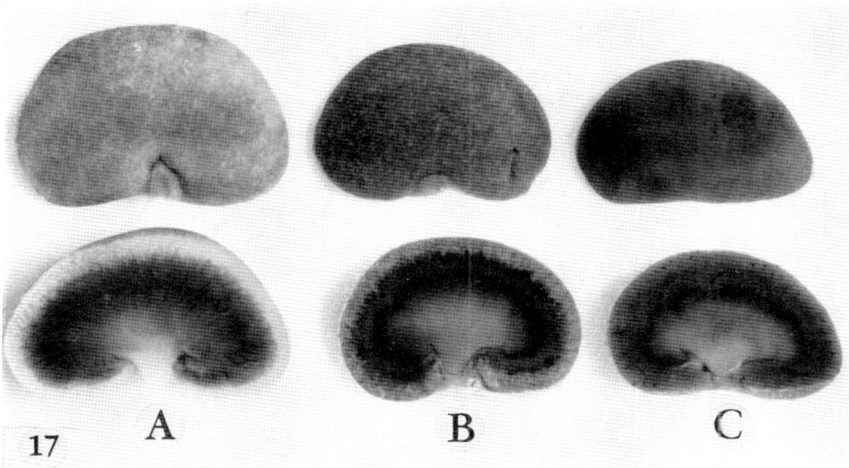


*Fig. 17* (A and B) Macroscopic appearance of cortical nephrocalcinosis produced with DHT and (C) its prevention by Na-deficiency.

On the other hand, it is clear from this experiment that the myocardial and coronary calcification as well as the suppurative myocarditis produced by combined DHT + Ca-acetate treatment were not beneficially influenced by Na-deficiency (Groups 9 and 10) perhaps merely because the damage was too severe to be influenced.

*Discussion*

It is obvious from the results described in the foregoing that dietary deficiency in Na is very effective in desensitizing the heart against various potentially cardiotoxic agents. Nothing is known as yet about the mechanism through which Na-deficiency exerts its protective effect against several types of necrotizing cardiopathies that formed the subject of our investigations. We are equally ignorant concerning the biochemical basis of the protection by Na-deficiency against periarteritis nodosa and hyalinizing myocarditis normally elicited with DOC overdosage in the rat (692).

It is interesting, however, that the cardiotoxic actions of those agents that were significantly synergized in previous experiments by

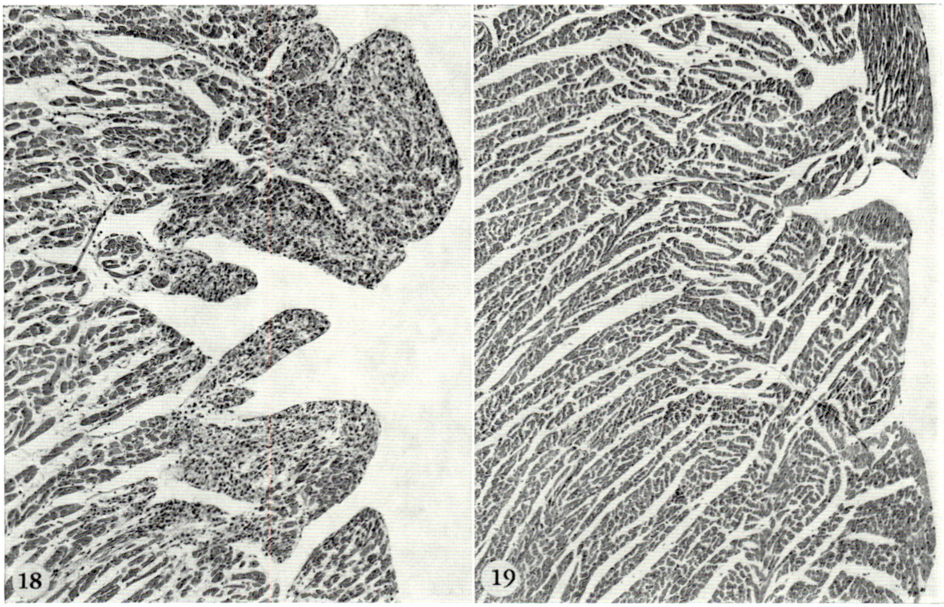

*Figs. 18–19 Prevention by Na-deficiency of the necrotizing cardiopathy normally produced by plasmocid.* Fig. 18: Subendocardial layer of the ventricles of heart of a plasmocid-treated rat, exhibiting diffuse necroses and myocarditic lesions. Fig. 19: Heart of a rat treated with the same dose of plasmocid but maintained on a Na-deficient diet exhibits no structural abnormality (von Kóssa + hematoxylin-phloxine, × 100).

administration of certain Na-salts and/or corticoids were most markedly prevented, here, by the Na-deficient diet. Furthermore, the observation that even the spotty myolytic changes caused by noradrenaline and vasopressin were somewhat reduced and that the plasmocid necroses, which are so resistant to most other agents, were almost completely inhibited in the Na-deficient animals supports the assumption that Na plays an important role in the common biochemical derangement that produces necroses, inflammation and calcification of the heart muscle.

It is especially noteworthy that the Na-deficient animals were entirely protected against the intensive calcinotic effect of DHT. However, when Ca-acetate was administered even with smaller doses of DHT, this protective action of Na-deficiency was not observed. In the latter case the mortality was the same in the control and the deficient animals; all the hearts exhibited an acute, suppurative myocarditis with intensive calcification (Mönckeberg type) of the coronary vessels. However, this resistance to therapy may have been due to the fact that the lesion was too severe to be prevented.

It remains to be established whether similar electrolyte-steroid interactions and, specifically, certain salt constituents of diets also play a role in the spontaneous arteriosclerotic and cardiac diseases of man.

*Summary*

Experiments on rats were performed to examine the effect of Na-deficiency upon various experimental cardiac lesions, which differ widely from each other in both their causative agents and their histologic characteristics.

It was found that sodium deficiency significantly protected the heart against the production of necrosis, inflammation and/or calcification by DHT, plasmocid and papain. In F-COL conditioned, Na-deficient animals the cardiac necrosis eliciting effect of neuromuscular effort was also markedly inhibited. A reduction of the severity and incidence of the 'spotty myolysis' normally due to the administration of noradrenaline and vasopressin was suggestive, but not statistically significant.

On the other hand, combined administration of DHT + Ca-acetate produced fatal, acute suppurative myocarditis of an equal degree in the control and Na-deficient rats. Thus, the protective effect of Na-deficiency against the calcifying and necrotizing actions of DHT was completely abolished by the concurrent administration of calcium acetate.

The importance of Na in the pathogenesis of cardiac necroses and the possible role of electrolyte-steroid interactions in calcifying and necrotizing cardiac diseases are briefly discussed on the basis of these and previous observations.

*c) Effect of Pregnancy Upon Myocardial Lesions Produced by Various Agents*

Several earlier investigators reported that pregnancy appears to protect the experimental animals against some types of morphologic changes that are normally induced by chemical agents. This was illustrated, for example by SELYE (620) concerning the ESCN. In pregnant rats, otherwise effective doses of Me-Cl-COL plus $NaH_2PO_4$ produced little or no myocardial necroses. The development of nephrocalcinosis that normally accompanies such treatment was likewise inhibited by gestation, but not as completely as the ESCN itself. According to HOLMAN AND JONES (305), in dogs, pregnancy can also prevent the induction of the polyarteritis and the myocardial necroses that normally occur following the infliction of renal damage in animals previously maintained on a high-fat diet. Furthermore, during gestation, rats are unusually resistant to the production of cardiovascular calcification by DHT (610).

On the other hand, 'puerperal myocarditis', a disease that appears to be similar to Fiedler's myocarditis, may occur in women during late pregnancy or the early puerperium (92).

In view of these observations, it was interesting to determine the effect of pregnancy upon the development of various experimental cardiopathies that formed the subject of our comparative studies.

### *Materials and Techniques*

Two hundred rats, having a mean initial weight of 270 g (range: 230–300 g), half of them pregnant, were subdivided into 20 equal groups of 10 rats each, and treated as indicated in Table XXXII.

*Noradrenaline* was given twice daily, at the dose of 750 µg in 0.4 ml of oil, subcutaneously, during the first two days. The rats were killed 24 hours after the last injection. *Vasopressin* was injected on the first day, at the dose of 30 I.U. in 3 ml of water, twice daily, subcutaneously. All the surviving rats were killed 48 hours following the last treatment. *Papain* (5%, filtered solution) was injected into the jugular vein, 0.5 ml, once, on the first day. The experiment was terminated 48 hours after the papain injection. *Plasmocid,* 8-(3-diethylaminopropylamino)-6-methoxyquinoline was given at the dose of 1.5 mg in 0.5 ml of water, intraperitoneally, three times on the first day. The animals were killed 48 hours following the last injection. *Me-Cl-COL* was injected subcutaneously, at the daily dose of 500 µg per 100 g body weight, in 0.2 ml of water, during five days. The controls, treated with Me-Cl-COL alone, like the Me-Cl-COL-sensitized and subsequently stressed (quadriplegia, cold baths, restraint) rats, were killed on the 7th day, that is, two days after initiation of exposure to stress. *Quadriplegia* was performed on the 5th day; the rats were then killed on the 7th day. *Cold baths* were applied twice on the 5th day, during 5 minutes in each time. *Restraint*, for a period of 17 hours, was applied on the 5th day; the animals were killed 48 hours after the initiation of the cold baths and restraint. *Nephrectomy:* bilateral total nephrectomy was performed under light ether anesthesia, on the 5th day of the experiment. To prolong the survival time, food and water were then removed. The rats were killed 48 hours following the surgical intervention. We note that bilateral nephrectomy tends to produce foci of necrosis ac-

*Table XXXII*

Effect of Pregnancy upon Myocardial Lesions Produced by Various Agents

| Group | Treatment | Condition | Cardiac necrosis | Mortality (%) |
|---|---|---|---|---|
| 1 | None | Not pregnant | 0 | 0 |
| 2 | None | Pregnant | 0 | 0 |
| 3 | Noradrenaline | Not pregnant | 2.8 ± 0.20 | 20 |
| 4 | Noradrenaline | Pregnant | 1.3 ± 0.27 | 0 |
| 5 | Vasopressin | Not pregnant | 1.4 ± 0.34 | 0 |
| 6 | Vasopressin | Pregnant | 0.2 ± 0.15 | 80 |
| 7 | Papain | Not pregnant | 2.6 ± 0.27 | 60 |
| 8 | Papain | Pregnant | 0.9 ± 0.30 | 40 |
| 9 | Plasmocid | Not pregnant | 2.6 ± 0.17 | 50 |
| 10 | Plasmocid | Pregnant | 2.4 ± 0.23 | 80 |
| 11 | Me-Cl-COL + Quadriplegia | Not pregnant | 0.6 ± 0.30 | 40 |
| 12 | Me-Cl-COL + Quadriplegia | Pregnant | 0.2 ± 0.13 | 40 |
| 13 | Me-Cl-COL + Cold | Not pregnant | 1.4 ± 0.38 | 0 |
| 14 | Me-Cl-COL + Cold | Pregnant | 1.4 ± 0.30 | 0 |
| 15 | Me-Cl-COL + Restraint | Not pregnant | 1.1 ± 0.27 | 30 |
| 16 | Me-Cl-COL + Restraint | Pregnant | 1.1 ± 0.23 | 0 |
| 17 | Me-Cl-COL + Nephrectomy | Not pregnant | 1.0 ± 0.27 | 10 |
| 18 | Me-Cl-COL + Nephrectomy | Pregnant | 0.4 ± 0.30 | 10 |
| 19 | Me-Cl-COL | Not Pregnant | 0 | 0 |
| 20 | Me-Cl-COL | Pregnant | 0.2 ± 0.15 | 0 |

companied by marked inflammatory changes and usually by calcification (628). The object of our investigation was to see whether pregnancy would affect the cardiotoxic actions of some or all of these agents.

The hearts were fixed in neutral formalin and stained with the von Kóssa technique for the histochemical demonstration of calcium (using hematoxylin-eosin counterstain).

### *Results*

As will be seen from the data in Table XXXII, the cardiotoxic effect of some agents was markedly inhibited, while that of others remained uninfluenced by pregnancy.

Pregnancy significantly protected the animals against the cardiac lesions normally produced by noradrenaline (Groups 3,4), vasopressin (Groups 5,6) and papain (Groups 7,8). In view of the comparatively large standard error, it is somewhat dubious, whether pregnancy also offered some protection against the uremic cardiopathy induced by total nephrectomy (Groups 17, 18). It is quite clear, however, that pregnancy offered no protection against the cardiac damage caused by plasmocid (Groups 9, 10), quadriplegia (Groups 11, 12), cold (Groups 13, 14) and restraint (Groups 15, 16). As previously stated, Me-Cl-COL does not produce any cardiac damage in itself, although it is strong conditioner for the potential cardiotoxic action of certain other agents. In the present experiment, the normal controls likewise failed to respond with any detectable cardiac damage to the injection of the comparatively large doses of Me-Cl-COL which were administered here. The very slight damage that was detectable in the hearts of two among the pregnant, Me-Cl-COL-treated rats is of dubious significance.

### *Discussion*

Nothing is known as yet about the mechanism through which pregnancy exerts its protective effect against the various types of cardiopathies that formed the subject of this experimental series. We are equally ignorant of the manner of protection by gestation against the typical ESCN (620), or against the cardiovascular calcification normally elicited by DHT (610). In any event, the increase in body mass—that is due to the development of the embryos and the uterus—cannot satisfactorily explain the protective effective of gestation, because, in the present experimental series, the rats treated with any one agent were of equal mean body weight at the beginning of the experiment, irrespective of whether or not they were pregnant. Such an explanation, based on a pure dilution effect owing to differences in body mass, would also fail to account for the fact that pregnancy offers protection only against some of the cardiotoxic agents that we examined. It is interesting, however, that, in an independent investigation on the influence of age upon the development of various experimental cardiopathies, we found that youth protects the heart essentially against the same cardiotoxic agents against which pregnancy offers protection. Thus young animals proved to be particularly resistant against noradrenaline, vasopressin, papain but not against quadriplegia or restraint (see p. 190).

*Summary*

Experiments on rats indicate that pregnancy offers significant protection against the production of myocardial lesion by noradrenaline, vasopressin and papain. These findings complement earlier observations concerning the prophylactic effect of pregnancy against the induction of cardiovascular calcification by vitamin-D derivatives and against the production of infarct-like myocardial changes by combined treatment with corticoids and certain Na-salts. On the other hand, the present experimental series shows that pregnancy does not protect against the production of cardiac necroses by quadriplegia (induced by motor-nerve transection), cold, or forced restraint, in rats specifically sensitized to the cardiotoxic action of these stressors by Me-Cl-COL.

Pregnancy offers only slight (and perhaps not statistically significant) protection against the uremic type of cardiopathy induced by bilateral nephrectomy in Me-Cl-COL-sensitized animals.

It is known that, although Me-Cl-COL itself produces no significant change in cardiac structure, it 'conditions' the myocardium for the production of infarct-like changes by various stressors. In this connection, it is of interest that pregnancy failed to induce myocardial changes in rats conditioned by Me-Cl-COL for the cardiotoxic effect of stress.

The effects of pregnancy upon the development of structural changes in the myocardium are discussed, on the basis of these observations.

## IV. Development of New Techniques for the Induction of Experimental Cardiovascular Disease

### *a) Simple Techniques for the Surgical Occlusion of Coronary Vessels in the Rat and the ECG Alterations so induced*

Experimental coronary occlusion has been studied extensively in large laboratory animals, but these subjects do not lend themselves well to the large-scale testing of surgical procedures and drugs that may be useful in the prophylaxis or treatment of coronary heart disease. Besides, in the dog—the animal most frequently used for this type of study—the results of coronary ligation are extremely variable as regards both the production of infarcts and mortality, 'Even when the same artery is ligated at the same site in every animal the outcome from one dog to the next is unpredictable' (328) and, according to a recent survey, the mortality statistics reported by different investigators range between 0 and 100% (223). Because of this, studies on the physiology, pathology or pharmacology of the coronary circulation would necessitate using an extraordinarily large number of subjects, to obtain statistically significant results; with large animals, which are costly to maintain and require laborious surgical techniques, this often becomes a virtually insuperable handicap.

In view of these considerations, experimenters interested in cardiovascular pathology have long searched for simple techniques that would permit the production of predictable cardiac lesions by the surgical obstruction of coronary arteries or veins in the most commonly used small experimental animal, the rat. Since 1942, almost all investigations on the biochemical production and prevention of cardiac lesions (by steroids, electrolytes, and exposure to stress) have been performed on the rat (613); we therefore needed techniques that would permit in this same species comparisons between chemically and surgically induced cardiac lesions, particularly as regards their response to treatment.

In the earlier literature, we found only one technique designed for the surgical occlusion of coronary arteries in the rat, namely, that of HEIMBURGER (279), as modified by JOHNS AND OLSON (328). However, this procedure is rather complicated and causes a comparatively high mortality; besides, it was often unsuccessful in producing infarction, even in the hands of its discoverers, so it was never used for solving any physiologic or pharmacologic problem. Indeed—as far as we can establish—since its initial description in 1946 (279) and its modification in 1954 (published as the first of a proposed series [328]), the method was used only for two small experiments limited to the verification of its feasibility and the description of the morphologic changes that occur after infarction in the rat heart (95, 341).

As regards the consequences of isolated coronary vein ligature in the rat, we were able to find only one statement in the literature, namely: 'The left coronary vein was ligated in 5 . . . rats. Examination after 10 days revealed no significant pathologic changes' (279).

In this communication, we wish to describe simple and reliable techniques that permit surgical occlusion at various points of the left or right coronary artery as well as the main coronary veins. In addition, we shall briefly describe some of the consequences and applications of these interventions.

### *Surgical anatomy of the large coronary vessels in the rat*

*The coronary arteries.* Immediately after branching from the aorta, both coronary arteries of the rat enter the myocardial substance and are completely surrounded by cardiac muscle throughout their entire course. In view of this fact, and because of the minute size of these vessels, it is often difficult, if not impossible, to see them, even with the use of a binocular loupe and a strong frontal lamp. Therefore, we first had to familiarize ourselves with the course of these arteries in relation to certain readily visible landmarks. For this purpose, after first washing out the blood with physiologic saline, the coronaries were injected, retrograde from the aorta, with colored materials (e.g., lead oxide suspended in latex to which some kaolin was added to prevent passage of the dye through the capillaries into the veins). The following description and two of our photographs (Fig. 20 and 21) are based upon observations on numerous animals in which the coronary arteries were thus made easily visible.

*The left coronary* artery originates from the aorta, in contact with the left margin of the pulmonary cone, at about 1 mm from the insertion of the left auricular appendage. These adjacent structures are always readily visible by mere inspection and, hence, serve as convenient landmarks. If the left coronary artery is to be ligated near its origin the needle that carries the occluding thread should be introduced into the wall of the pulmonary cone and brought to the surface again at a point somewhere near the middle of the line connecting the pulmonary cone with the insertion of the left auricular appendage (Fig. 20 and 21). The septal artery, the first major branch of the left coronary artery, descends along the right surface of the interventricular septum. The rat has no true equivalent of a circumflex artery. Most of the blood of the left coronary artery is carried by the left descending branch; this courses in an almost straight line from its origin towards the apex of the heart and supplies the left ventricular wall by numerous almost horizontal lateral branches, none of which are particularly prominent. Near the apex the main trunk usually bifurcates, forming two branches of approximately equal size (Fig. 20).

*The right coronary artery originates* from the aorta in close contact with the right margin of the pulmonary cone and at about 2 mm from the insertion of the right auricular appendage. These structures can serve as readily visible surgical landmarks. The right coronary artery supplies the wall of the right ventricle, again through numerous branches that course almost perpendicularly to the main descending trunk. However, this vessel—unlike its counterpart on the left—usually subdivides into two or more, rather irregular principal rami, a few millimeters below its origin.

*The coronary veins.* In the rat, the main coronary sinus enters the right auricle on the posterior aspect of the heart, just above the auriculo-ventricular borderline. It frequently consists of a single vessel arising from the confluence of two large veins that presumably correspond to the posterior vein of the right ventricle and the middle cardiac vein of man. However, these two veins often enter the ventricle separately—occasionally at some distance from each other—so that there is no actual coronary sinus. Additional coronary veins enter the auricle separately at various points of the auriculoventricular borderline, but they are comparatively unimportant and subject to great individual variations, except for one rather constant small coronary vein that runs parallel with the left descending arterial branch near its origin, and may act as an additional landmark for the indentification of the latter vessel. A detailed description of the blood supply to the rat heart was recently presented by HALPERN (264).

*Surgical technique*

*General procedure.* In developing the surgical techniques to be described here we have used a total of 2095 rats, varying in body weight from 25 g (at which time they were still being nursed by their mother) to 350 g. The animals belonged to various breeds, although most of them were descendants of the Sprague-Dawley strain. We found no striking difference in the ability of these rats to withstand coronary ligatures and used essentially the same procedure, irrespective of strain and age; hence, we shall discuss our technique and results mainly on the basis of observations made with females of the Sprague-Dawley, Holtzman, and Quebec Breeding Farm colonies, and weighing 100 to 150 g at the time of operation.

For all types of coronary artery or vein ligatures the rat is prepared by removing the fur from the chest region with electric clippers. Then the animal is placed under a bell jar and lightly anesthetized with ether. After this, it is fastened to an operating board; two strong rubber bands immobilize the legs and pelvis, whereas to hold the head steady, the upper incisors are hooked through a wire loop fastened to the board itself (Fig. 22 and 26). During preparation for thoracotomy, additional anesthesia may be administered if required—by placing an ether-soaked gauze pad over the head (Fig. 22) but no more anesthetic is given once the thorax is open.

It is unnecessary to observe strictly aseptic precautions, but we always cleanse the skin with Metaphen prior to surgery, use sterile instruments and towels, dip the instruments into Metaphen after every two or three operations, and treat the animals with Terramycin during the 5 days following the intervention. As a result of these precautions, infections are quite exceptional.

The small operating board is placed on a table with the rat's tail towards the surgeon who wears a binocular loupe and a strong frontal lamp to improve vision. A craniocaudal incision of about 2 cm is made, parallel with and slightly to the left of the sternum, through the skin and pectoral muscles, to expose the ribs.

Then, a straight needle is inserted near the middle of the lateral margin of the wound and carried through a tunnel of pectoral muscle tissue, around the cranial half of the incision, to emerge again on the

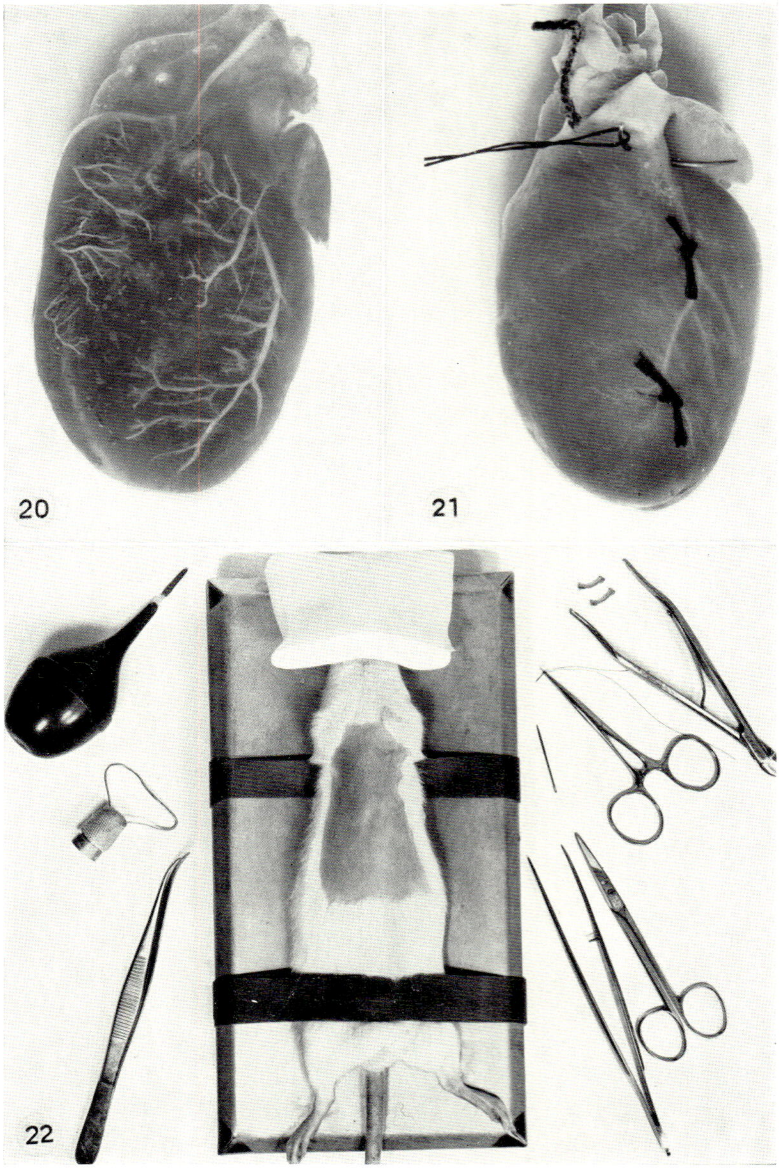

*Figs. 20–26 Illustration of the technique for the surgical occlusion of coronary vessels in the rat.*

wound lip at a point facing that through which the thread was introduced. The ends of this cutaneomuscular ligature are loosely knotted and laid on the neck of the animal, out of the surgeon's way (Fig. 23), so that after the operation, the thoracotomy wound may be closed at once by merely tightening the knot (Fig. 26).

A blunt curved forceps is then plunged between the fifth and sixth ribs, through the intercostal muscle, at a point approximately 2 mm to the left of the sternum. Thereby, bleeding from the internal epigastric artery (which courses just to the left of the sternum) can be avoided. The gap is then widened to about 15 mm by gentle lateral pressure with the perforating forceps, while the sixth rib is held steady with another curved forceps. At this time, the rapidly beating heart becomes visible. Air now enters the chest cavity and respiration becomes impossible, but this does not matter, since the intrathoracic part of the operation takes only 60 to 90 seconds.

The sixth costal cartilage is transected with fine, pointed scissors at about 0.5 cm to the left of the sternum: one forceps holds the sternal end of this cut rib in position, whereas the other enters the thorax to

*Fig. 20* Anterior aspect of the heart in a rat whose coronary arteries have been injected with lead oxide in latex. The superficial myocardial layers have been partially cleared in methyl benzoate to make the intramuscular arteries more readily visible. The left coronary artery originates between the pulmonary cone and the left auricular appendage (right side of picture). After sending a few major branches towards the pulmonary cone, it descends almost directly towards the apex, along the curved surface of the left ventricle. The main trunk of the right coronary artery is not visible, but its perpendicular lateral branches can be seen to advance (from the left side of the picture) towards the anterior part of the heart, within the wall of the right ventricle.

*Fig. 21* Heart of a rat in which the arteries have again been made visible by injection with colored material, but the myocardium has been left opaque to show its surface markings. A curved needle has been introduced between the pulmonary cone and the insertion of the left auricular appendage, to demonstrate the procedure to be followed for the occlusion of the left coronary artery near its origin. Additional ligatures (such as are used for the production of smaller infarcts) have been placed at lower points along the course of this vessel.

*Fig. 22* Operating table, as it appears just prior to skin incisions. The fur is clipped from the chest region and the animal is tied to the operating board by rubber bands. A gauze pad for the application of ether covers the snout and also the metal loop (visible in Figure 26) into which the incisors are hooked to stabilize the head. Note rubber syringe, 'thimble retractor', blunt curved forceps, Michel clips and clip forceps, small hemostat bearing curved needle with black thread (for ligature of cardiac vessels), large straight needle with, here, an almost invisible white thread (for cutaneomuscular stitch), small pointed scissors, and second curved forceps.

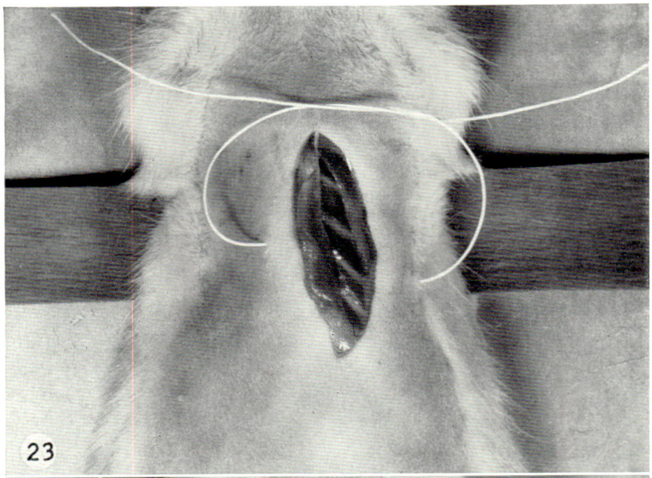

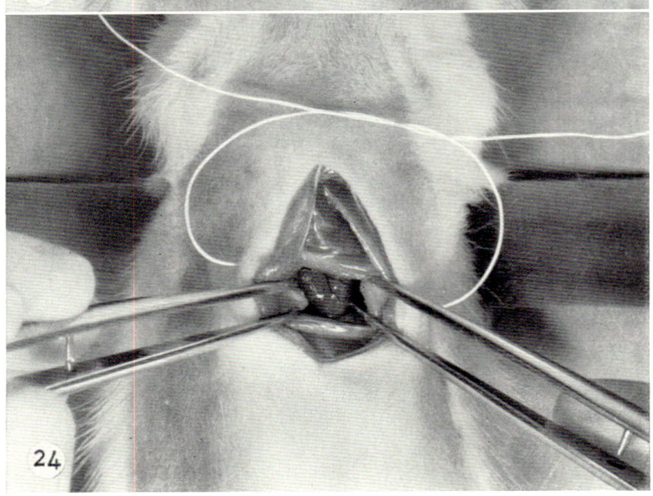

*Fig. 23* Stage 1: The cutaneomuscular stitch is in position and the ribs are exposed.

*Fig. 24* Stage 2: Costotomy has been performed (note sternal stump of cut rib-cartilage between the prongs of the left forceps). The tip of the heart becomes visible between the fourth and sixth ribs; in this position, the heart can be exteriorized by slight pressure with the forceps against the elastic thoracic cage of the rat.

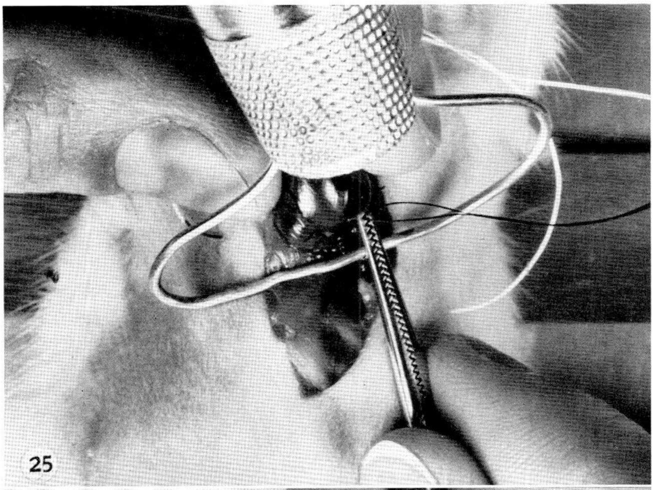

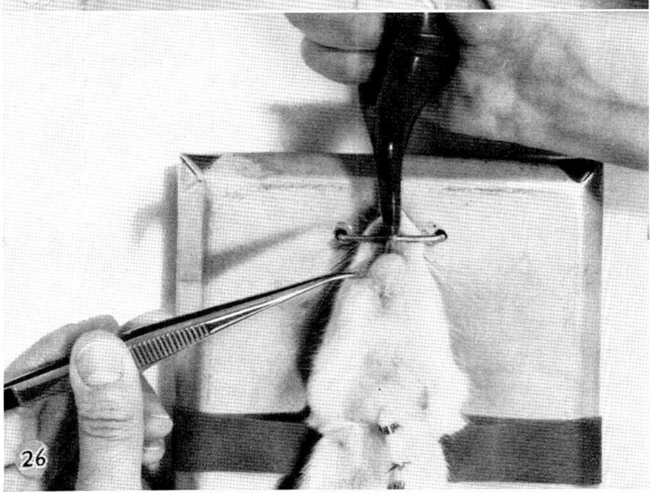

*Fig. 25* Stage 3: The exteriorized heart is held between the surgeon's left thumb and middle finger. The 'thimble retractor' on the index finger of the same hand pushed the left auricular appendage out of the way, while the curved needle (bearing the fine black thread) is pushed through behind the major cardiac veins (arrows) with the hemostat. In this operation, designed to ligate the principal coronary veins, the posterior aspect of the heart is exposed; otherwise, the operation is carried out in the same manner as when the coronary arteries are to be ligated (shown in Figure 21).

*Fig. 26* Stage 4: The operation is completed. The thorax was closed by tying the cutaneomuscular stitch and applying two additional Michel clips (one above and one below the stitch) to ensure perfect wound closure. The tongue is pulled forward with forceps while mucus is being removed from the pharynx with the rubber syringe.

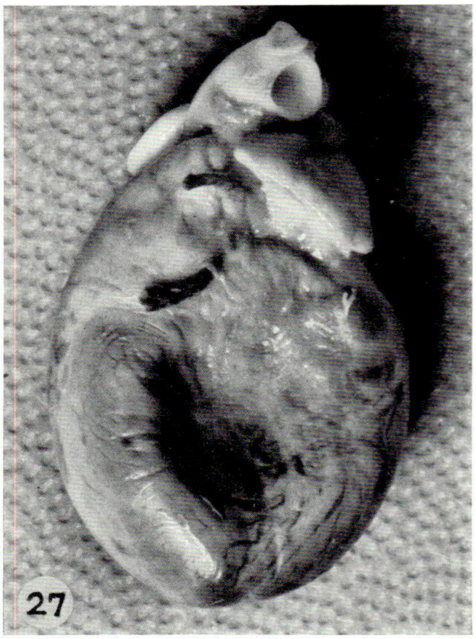

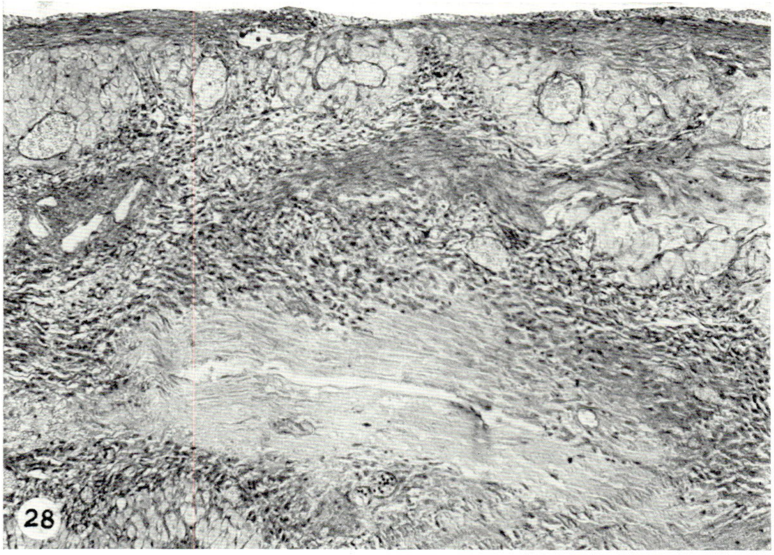

*Figs. 27–28 Morphologic consequences of ligature of the left coronary artery in the rat.*

sever the pericardium and exteriorize the heart (Fig. 24). Light pressure upon the thorax helps bring the heart to the outside without damage. The coronary arteries or veins are then ligated, as described below (Fig. 25), the heart is replaced into the thorax, and the previously placed cutaneomuscular thread is tightened to close the thoracic wall. Slight lateral pressure immediately after tying this ligature squeezes the air out of the thorax and—since the skin, subcutaneous tissue, and muscles act as a valve—breathing immediately becomes possible again. Should respiration be slow to start or impeded by the accumulation of mucus, a rubber syringe is introduced into the throat to remove any blockage (Fig. 26). The operation is then terminated by placing one Michel clip above and one below the cutaneomuscular stitch, to assure perfect closure of the thoracic cavity. After ligature of either coronary artery or of the main coronary veins, the animals usually regain consciousness and walk within a few minutes after closure of the thorax. The Michel clips and the cutaneomuscular stitch are removed on the sixth day after the operation.

The intervention takes approximately 2 to 3 minutes from skin incision to the completion of wound closure. The simplest and most rapid among the operations discussed here are the ligature of the left descending coronary artery near the middle or lower third of the ventricle, and the ligature of the coronary veins (about 2 minutes); the most difficult and time-taking intervention is the ligature of the left coronary artery near its origin (about 3 minutes). Of course, such operations could not be performed if they were more time-taking, since the animal does not breathe during the intervention.

*Ligature of the left coronary artery.* After exteriorization of the heart, the ventricle is held between the thumb and index finger of the left

*Fig. 27* Macroscopic appearance of the heart 14 days after ligature of the left artery near its origin. The knot of the ligature has become surrounded by granuloma tissue, but the two free ends of black thread mark the site of the occlusion between the left margin of the pulmonary cone and the insertion line of the left auricle. Virtually the whole left ventricular wall is transformed into a thin scar tissue which, in this specimen, has caved in into the ventricular lumen.

*Fig. 28* Entire thickness of an infarcted left ventricle on the fifth day after operation. Muscle cells are well preserved near the epicardium (top), especially around the veins. The central, light necrotic area contains virtually no inflammatory cells, but is surrounded by a granuloma. A few residual subendocardial muscle cells are visible near the lower left-hand corner (PAS stain × 120).

hand, with the apex pointing craniad and slightly to the right side of the rat. In this position, a small curved needle (corneal needle $^3/_8$ circle, 9 mm) can readily carry a thread (black braided, nonslipping silk, size oooooo) through, between the point of entry on the left margin of the pulmonary cone and the middle of an imaginary line connecting this point with the closest point on the insertion line of the left auricular appendage (Fig. 20). After this ligature is tied, virtually the whole lateral wall of the left ventricle becomes necrotic.

If small infarcts are to be produced, the ligature may be placed similarly, but lower along the course of the left coronary artery, for example, near the middle or apex of the heart (Fig. 20). Since the artery itself is rarely visible, these ligatures are placed along an imaginary line connecting the point of origin of this vessel (identifiable by the previously described landmarks) with the apex of the heart.

*Ligature of the right coronary artery*. Immediately after exteriorization of the heart, the board to which the animal is fastened should be turned around (the animal's head towards the surgeon). The ventricle is then held between the thumb and middle finger of the left hand, the apex pointing caudad. The right auricular appendage tends to become engorged with blood and to cover the origin of the right coronary artery. To obviate this difficulty we designed a special retractor consisting of a silver thimble to which a silver wire loop has been soldered. When the 'thimble retractor' is placed on the surgeon's index finger, its wire is in just the proper position to keep the auricular appendage out of the way. The small curved needle can now readily carry a thread through underneath the surface of the ventricular wall—just to the right of the right margin of the pulmonary cone, near the aorta—to ligate the right coronary artery close to its origin (Fig. 21). Occlusion of the vessels at this point causes massive infarction of virtually the entire right ventricular wall.

Because of the irregular course of the right descending coronary artery in the rat, it is difficult to identify its course by visible landmarks. Hence, we did not attempt to produce less extensive infarcts by ligatures at lower levels as was done in the case of the left coronary artery.

*Ligature of both main coronary arteries*. Our attempts to ligate both the right and the left coronary arteries near their origin in a single session failed in almost all instances, because the animals died immediately after the operation. Somewhat better results were obtained by ligating the left coronary artery first and the right on the following day. Even so immediate postoperative mortality was close to 80%. However, occasional animals can survive for several weeks; it would appear that as both coronaries are ligated near their origin and both ventricular walls are extensively infarcted, here, most of the ventricular work is performed by the surviving septal and papillary musculature.

*Ligature of the large coronary veins.* This operation is performed with the heart exteriorized and held just as for the ligature of the left coronary artery, except that the ventricle is rotated around its longitudinal axis, so as to expose the posterior aspect where the two main coronary veins enter (separately or after uniting into a single sinus) into the right auricle. These vessels are always readily visible on naked-eye inspection and can easily be ligated by merely passing a curved needle just behind them, without entering deeply into the ventricular musculature. Even when the two veins enter the auricle some distance apart, one length of thread suffices. In this case, it is best to pass the needle first around one vein and then, after drawing it to the outside, around the other; owing to the elasticity of the subendocardial tissue and of the veins themselves, the two loops are easily brought together when the ligature is subsequently tied.

## *Consequences of coronary vessel occlusion in the rat*

*Functional consequences.* It would be difficult to make meaningful statistical studies on the survival rate and the incidence of successful occlusion of the coronary vessels following the interventions just described.

The fate of rats with coronary-vessel ligatures has only been followed up for 1 month; during this period, postoperative mortality was negligible and usually attributable to accidental infections. On the other hand, as we have mentioned already, simultaneous occlusion of both coronary arteries at or near their origin proved to be almost invariably fatal. The same was true of interventions in which the left coronary artery and the large coronary veins were ligated simultaneously near their origin. The ECG alterations caused by ligation of the coronary vessels in the rat will be described later (see p. 253).

*Morphologic consequences.* The pathologic changes induced by the ligature of either of the *main coronary arteries* at any point along its course are essentially the same in quality: in the area deprived of blood supply the entire myocardium becomes necrotic and then gradually disappears (Fig. 27). Curiously, this absorption of dead muscle proceeds with very little inflammatory reaction, except along the line of demarcation between the necrotic and surviving muscle tissue (Fig. 28). In the interior of the infarct the necrotic muscle fibers simply shrink until they disappear. The arteries and veins within the affected area do not become thrombosed, perhaps because some slow circulation continues through collateral channels, although not at a rate sufficient to maintain the integrity of the myocardial tissue.

After the ligature of a main coronary artery, virtually the entire corresponding ventricular wall undergoes massive necrosis, yet a thin layer (about 3 to 5 muscle fibers in width) regularly remains intact underneath the endocardium along the entire inner surface of the infarct. A similar sheet is preserved around the larger veins, but not along the arteries, that traverse the necrotic area. A shell of myocardial tissue also remains preserved beneath the epicardium, but it is usually even thinner and less regular than that bordering the ventricular cavity and the large veins (Fig. 29). Presumably, these surviving muscle fibers are nourished directly from the ventricular blood, the venous blood, and the pericardial vessels, respectively. The veins may receive their blood from more peripheral intact myocardial tissue or retrograde from the cardiac cavities. In the infarcted area, all surviving muscle cells undergo pronounced hypertrophy and presumably contribute towards the maintenance of functional cardiac sufficiency after coronary artery ligature.

The scar that replaces the dead muscle tissue in the infarcted area is extraordinarily rich in elastic fibers; these begin to develop as a reticulum of extremely thin, wavy threads and gradually increase in thickness.

Massive calcium deposition has never been observed in infarcts, following ligature of coronary arteries, but fine granules of calcium salts can occasionally be detected with von Kóssa's stain, especially near the borderline between the living and dead tissue.

The morphologic consequences of *coronary vein* ligature are entirely different. After occlusion of even major peripheral veins, the myocardium remains unaffected. However, following occlusion of both major trunks (or, in the case of confluence between them, of the resulting terminal sinus itself) there immediately develops a pronounced pericarditis over the region drained by the ligated veins. During the next 2 to 4 days massive calcification begins in the affected area. Macroscopically, this manifests itself in the development of white, isolated or confluent subepicardial spots that form a corona at some distance from and surrounding the major occluded venous trunks. Histologically, the affected areas prove to be superficial, quite limited to the subepicardial tissue. The calcium is first deposited within degenerating muscle fibers, but after these disintegrate, it comes to lie within the fibrous and granulomatous stroma. In addition, many muscle fibers (with or without calcified inclusions) are transformed into multinuclear giant cells not unlike those seen in the Aschoff nodules of rheumatic carditis.

In the few instances in which we succeeded in keeping animals alive after concurrent ligature of the left coronary artery and the coronary sinus, the picture was a combination of the usual consequences of arterial and venous ligature: there was massive necrosis of the central portion of the left ventricular wall, with intense calcification of the dead cells. Here again, the subendocardial muscle layers were preserved as they are after ligature of the coronary artery alone, but the subepicardial layers became necrotic and calcified as they are after occlusion of the coronary veins.

### *The ECG alterations in surgically induced cardiopathies in the rat*

As it was pointed out, experimental cardiac infarction resulting from surgical occlusion of coronary vessels has been studied extensively in the rabbit and dog, but in the rat—the animal most suitable for large scale testing of drugs— only a few investigations have been reported. Therefore, we considered it of value to investigate the ECG changes in certain, surgically induced, cardiopathies of the rat. It was interesting to determine whether the ECG alterations registered in rats, following ligature of the main coronary arteries, resemble those of human cardiac infarcts.

*Methods.* Rats with an average initial body weight of 108 g (range: 98–116 g) were used in these investigations. In one group of animals, the right coronary artery (while in another group, the left coronary artery) was ligated at a point 3 mm from its origin. In a subsequent group, the coronary sinus was ligated at its entry into the right auricle. In the last group of animals, the ligature was placed around the ventricles at the level of the lower third of the ventricular muscle. The number of rats examined in each group as well as the specifications of the controls used are given later in the text.

The ECG was registered in unanesthetized animals on a Sanborn Polygraph. (For further details see 'General Methodology', p. 123.) In each case, records were taken before the operation; once, at different intervals, soon after the surgical intervention, and once on the 9th to 11th days following surgery. Immediately after the third ECG record, the animals were killed and the hearts were carefully inspected. Only in some doubtful cases was it necessary to verify the macroscopic findings by histologic examination, using the PAS technique.

*Normal ECG in the rat.* The 'normal' ECG's of unanesthetized rats, that is, records taken before the operations in the std. leads, were the same as those described by ZSOTÉR *et al.* (799) earlier in rats slightly anesthetized with ether. The main differences between these and the human ECG were the rather consistently low, or isoelectric, $P_1$ as well as $T_1$, and an electrical axis deviated to the right, 67° on the average. The precordial records (corresponding to $V_2$, $V_4$ and $V_6$) obtained in various individual animals showed some variations in the height of the T waves.

*Controls.* Two types of controls were used in the present investigation. In 6 rats, the records were repeated 2–5 and 10 days later, without any surgical intervention. These ECG's revealed no significant alterations. In 6 other animals 'sham' operation was performed: the heart was exposed through a thoracic incision and handled gently with two fingers (in a manner similar to that necessary for vessel ligature); the thorax-wound was then closed. Records taken 7 and 11 days after this operation showed slightly decreased heart rate in 5 rats. $T_1$ in two and the precordial T waves in another rat became slightly negative 7 days after the surgical intervention; but on the 11th day they were again isoelectric. No other alterations were seen in the ECG's of the 'sham' operated animals (Fig. 29), and the autopsy findings were negative, except for a few pleuropericardial adhesions.

*Ligature of the right coronary artery.* When the ECG was registered 2–7 and 9–11 days, respectively, after ligation of the right coronary artery, the characteristic picture consisted of a deep QS in the II. and III. std. lead as well as negative $T_3$ (Fig. 29). Posterior necrosis was evident in 7 out of 9 animals, while $T_3$ became markedly negative in 8 rats. $T_2$ and sometimes also the precordial T waves became similarly

*Fig. 29* ECG alterations in surgically induced cardiopathies of the rat.

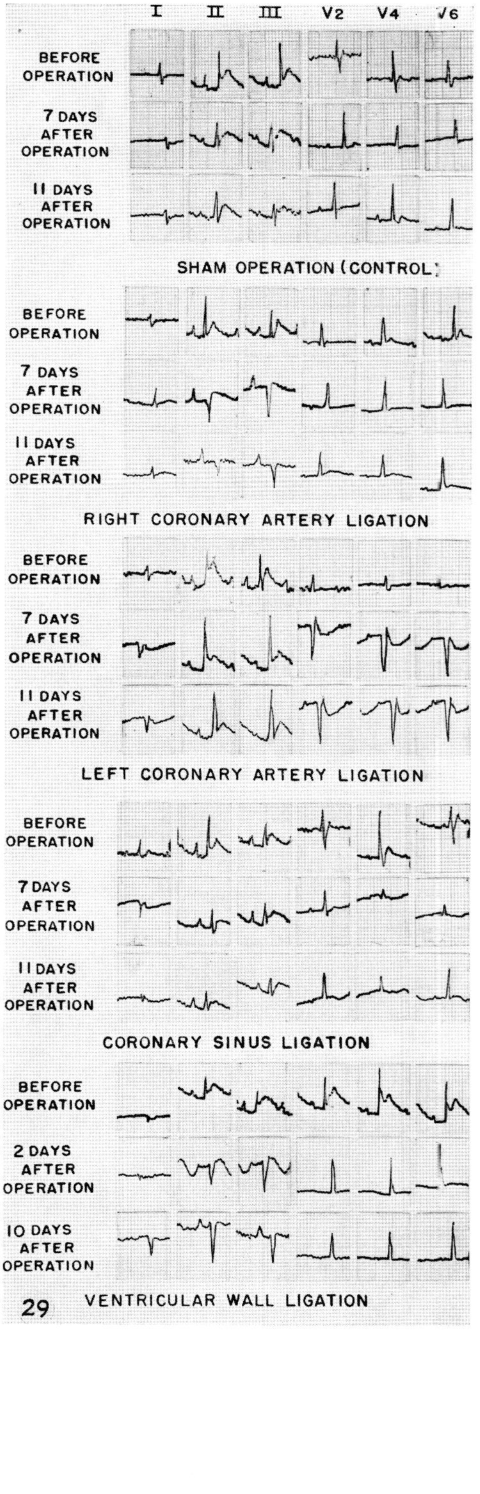
I II III V2 V4 V6
BEFORE OPERATION
7 DAYS AFTER OPERATION
11 DAYS AFTER OPERATION
SHAM OPERATION (CONTROL)
BEFORE OPERATION
7 DAYS AFTER OPERATION
11 DAYS AFTER OPERATION
RIGHT CORONARY ARTERY LIGATION
BEFORE OPERATION
7 DAYS AFTER OPERATION
11 DAYS AFTER OPERATION
LEFT CORONARY ARTERY LIGATION
BEFORE OPERATION
7 DAYS AFTER OPERATION
11 DAYS AFTER OPERATION
CORONARY SINUS LIGATION
BEFORE OPERATION
2 DAYS AFTER OPERATION
10 DAYS AFTER OPERATION
VENTRICULAR WALL LIGATION

29

negative and were proportionally lower than in the control records. Arrhythmia (premature nodal beat) was only registered once, in one rat. The electrical axis, indeterminable when necrosis was present, deviated markedly to the left. It is difficult, if not impossible, to evaluate the ST elevation in the ECG of rats; only in two rats and only 2 days after ligature of the artery was the picture somewhat similar to that characteristic of fresh human coronary occlusions.

Autopsy revealed grade 3 necrosis in 6 rats, in which the entire right ventricular wall became very thin, and in 3 others, small, mostly superficial (grade 1) necrosis was seen. In two of the latter cases, the ECG's did not show necrosis.

*Ligature of the left coronary artery.* ECG's registered on the 3rd–7th and 9th–11th days, respectively, after left coronary artery ligature revealed anterior necrosis in 11 out of 12 animals (Fig. 29). Even a few days after the operation, deep QS was seen in $V_4$ and $V_6$ of 11 rats; in $V_2$ and I. std. leads, 10 animals showed similar alterations. It should be noted that these changes were even more pronounced on ECG's obtained later, i.e., on the 9th–11th days. Markedly low or negative T waves in the I. std. and in the three precordial leads were, however, at least as pronounced 2 days after the operation as 11 days after. ST elevation was 'suspect' 3 days after ligature, but only in three animals. The heart rate became rather consistently lower, on the average from 490.8 to 441.9. Furthermore, in all cases the electrical axis deviated markedly to the right. No arrhythmia or other alterations were observed on the ECG's.

At autopsy, grade 3 necrosis, involving nearly the whole left ventricle, was seen in 10 rats; grade 2 necrosis in 1; and grade 1 necrosis in one other animal In this last rat, the ECG did not show necrosis.

*Ligature of the coronary sinus.* The ECG's failed to demonstrate necrosis in any of the 14 rats in this group, either 3–7 or 9–11 days after the surgical occlusion (Fig. 29). Ischemia was the characteristic finding: T became negative in each animal in the I. std. lead and lower or negative in the other derivations. These alterations were rather less pronounced in the second ECG series (i.e., on the 9th–11th days) than in the first. This was the only group in our studies in which the heart rate did not decrease consistently after surgical intervention. The electrical axis deviated to the right, from 54° to 90°. Wenckebach periodicity appeared in 1 animal three days after the intervention. Negative P in $V_{2\text{-}4}$ was a further finding, but only in 2 animals.

At autopsy, extensive, but only superficial, calcification was observed and was located subpericardially on the dorsal surface of the heart of each animal.

*Ligature of the ventricular wall.* When both ventricles were tied tightly with a firm ligature, deep QS appeared in the II. and III. derivation as soon as in 2 or 3 days after the intervention in each of the 13 rats examined (Fig. 29). QS in lead I. was apparent only in 5 records and in none of the precordial leads. 10–11 days after the intervention QS generally became still deeper. T in the std. leads was negative or markedly lower, in all cases, but in the precordials, however, in 11 animals only. Decrease in heart rate, marked deviation of the electrical axis to the left, and prolongation of the electrical systole were rather consistent findings.

Autopsy revealed intensive necrosis and suppurating abscess formation around the apex, in each animal; thus, the whole ligated one third of the ventricular wall became necrotic.

*Discussion*

*Technical advantages.* We see the principal advantages of our techniques in their reliability, simplicity and speed: they can be easily and rapidly performed with minimal mortality and regularly permit the occlusion of coronary arteries or veins at various points clearly defined by landmarks. Their simplicity and speed make it possible for technicians without previous surgical experience to perform these operations routinely in large numbers of the most common laboratory animal, the rat.

It is difficult to make accurate comparisons between our techniques and those previously used, since none of the few earlier investigators who attempted such operations in rats have published any photographs or drawings to illustrate their procedures. Yet, as far as we can see from the brief earlier descriptions, the advantages of our technique are primarily due to four factors: 1. the establishment (on the basis of vascular injection preparations) of readily visible landmarks, which help in the exact location of vessels that cannot be seen clearly, 2. the use of a binocular loupe and a strong frontal lamp, which greatly increase visibility, 3. the costotomy and the special 'thimble retractor', which assist in exposing the cardiac vessels with a minimum of accidental trauma, 4. elimination of the need for continuous pressure respiration.

*Application to specific research problems.* As previously stated, we became interested in techniques for large-scale experimentation on the coronary vessels of the rat, principally because we wanted to compare chemically and surgically induced cardiac necroses as regards their general characteristics and, particularly, their response to treatment. It is undoubtedly significant that the histologic aspect of the infarcts produced in rats by ligation of the coronary arteries differs in many respects from that of the chemically induced cardiac necroses. Infarcts that follow ligation of even the main coronary arteries always leave the subendocardial and subepicardial muscle layers intact and, usually also, the myocardial fibers that surround the cardiac veins within the necrotic area. Furthermore, these purely occlusive infarcts in the otherwise healthy myocardial tissue of young rats show little tendency to become infiltrated and removed by inflammatory cells. Conversely, the chemically induced cardiac necroses (e.g., those produced by certain electrolytes plus corticoids, stress plus corticoids, vitamin-D derivatives plus phosphates, or intravenous injection of proteolytic enzymes) show no tendency to avoid the superficial and perivenous muscle layers; indeed, they exhibit a definite predisposition for the subendocardial strata and are rapidly infiltrated and removed by inflammatory cells. In all these respects, the chemically induced experimental necroses resemble the usual myocardial infarcts of man more closely than do the infarcts that result from ligature of coronary arteries. Any attempt at a complete interpretation of these differences would be premature, but they suggest that interruption of the arterial blood supply may not be the only factor in the pathogenesis of the typical cardiac infarcts of man. Of course, the latter rarely occur in perfectly healthy young heart muscle and their development may be conditioned by biochemical changes resulting from wear and tear and, particularly, from chronic arteriosclerosis and myocardial fibrosis, which usually precede the development of cardiac infarction in man.

Many of the chemically induced cardiac necroses can be prevented by KCl or $MgCl_2$. Certain preliminary experiments led us to believe that KCl and $MgCl_2$ could also protect the rat against necroses resulting from the surgical obstruction of coronary vessels (47). However, using our new technique we found that the cardiac lesions resulting from complete, sudden occlusion of the major coronary arteries or veins cannot be prevented by these electrolytes. Our preliminary experiments, were based on our interpretation of an earlier report (328), which stated that 'in the rat, the main left coronary artery can be ligated at a point just beneath the left auricular appendage and proximal to any major branch'. The auricular appendage of the rat is a broad, semicircular structure that is about as wide as the auricle itself and constantly changes its size; hence, it is difficult to locate a minute artery by selecting a point 'just beneath' it. In any event, when we tried to follow these directives we obtained superficial calcified necroses such as occur after occlusion of the major cardiac veins. Furthermore, according to the technique of JOHNS AND OLSON (328), the heart must be delivered through the thin slit afforded by an intercostal thoracotomy (without costotomy); this exposes the cardiac muscle to a type of traumatic damage different from that caused by a clean-cut, isolated coronary ligature. Numerous experiments performed in the meantime have convinced us that of all the surgically induced myocardial necroses, only those produced by the technique used for our preliminary experiments can be consistently inhibited by KCl and $MgCl_2$. It is hoped that, with the improved techniques, it will be possible to identify the components of such traumatic interventions (mechanical injury to the heart, inflammation, incidental ligature of adjacent minor coronary arteries and veins) that are particularly sensitive to electrolyte treatment.

Finally, we hope that our techniques will help in the large scale testing of various factors that may affect the changes normally caused by the selective occlusion of certain coronary vessels, such as: the absorption of necrotic muscle, the proliferation of collagenous and elastic tissue, calcium deposition, ECG-changes, and the functional sufficiency of the myocardium.

*Conclusions drawn from the ECG studies.* The first conclusion that can be drawn from our studies is that it is not necessary to anesthetize a rat in order to register the precordial ECG. The precordial leads were particularly useful for demonstrating the extensive anterior necroses produced by ligature of the left coronary artery. It is important to note, however, that it is difficult to place the electrodes consistently in the same intercostal space, and so some variations may occur in the records. Comparing the localization of necroses in rats with that in humans the former would correspond to the localization in a heart rotated to right; while deep QS was present in $V_2$, we always found an intact ventricular septum at autopsy. We agree with SAMBHI AND WHITE (547) in that the ST segment in the rats' ECG is absent, but not that it must always be so. Using a higher paper speed, in occasional cases a more or less pronounced ST 'segment' could be detected.

In each group of animals, the ECG alterations were remarkably uniform. We feel that cardiac necrosis produced by ligature of coronary arteries according to the methods described on the preceding pages did result in ECG records corresponding to those characteristic of human cardiac infarcts. On the other hand, the differences between the ECG's of surgically induced experimental cardiopathies and those of the so-called electrolyte-steroid-cardiopathy (which can be produced by the combined administration of certain corticoids plus Na-salts) are quite marked. In the latter case no necrosis but arrhythmia as well as consistent prolongation of the QT were the characteristic findings (799).

As regards functional consequences of the surgically induced cardiopathies, it is important to point out again the absence of arrhythmia or of any disturbance of conduction, and the presence of a rather consistent decrease in the heart rate. It is probable that the first, i.e., control, recordings caused a certain tachycardia. Finally, with regard to 'time factors' we may say that the development of necrosis was already clearly demonstrable on ECG's 2 days after ligature of either coronary artery or of the ventricular wall. Later on, the alterations were, however, more pronounced. On the other hand, 'sham' operation and ligature of the coronary sinus produced only rather temporary changes.

*Summary*

Surgical techniques are described that regularly permit the occlusion of coronary arteries or veins at precisely defined points in the rat. The simplicity and speed of these procedures make it possible for technicians, even without previous surgical experience, to perform such operations routinely in large series, for the screening of factors that might influence the course of coronary infarction.

The advantages of these methods are ascribed principally to four factors: 1. establishment (on the basis of vascular injection preparations) of readily visible landmarks that help to locate vessels that cannot be seen clearly; 2. use of binocular loupe and a strong frontal lamp; 3. exposure of the cardiac vessels with a minimum of accidental trauma, owing to the use of costotomy and a special 'thimble retractor'; 4. elimination of the need for pressure respiration.

The infarcts thus produced in healthy, young cardiac muscle by the selective, sudden occlusion of certain coronary vessels differ in many respects from those elicited in experimental animals by chemical means; these differences, as well as the application of the new techniques to further research, are briefly discussed.

Finally, the ECG, in standard and precordial leads, was registered on unanesthetized rats before and after the surgical induction of different experimental cardiopathies. While 'sham' operation produced little alteration, ligature of the right or left coronary artery resulted in extensive posterior or anterior necrosis, respectively. The ECG's so obtained are quite comparable to the human patterns in coronary occlusion. ECG records showed only ischemia, following the ligature of the coronary sinus; at autopsy, superficial calcification was seen around the occluded vessels. When the ventricular wall is tightly ligated, the ECG picture shows the presence of posterior necrosis.

### *b) Production of Dissecting Aneurysms by Chronic Isoproterenol Treatment*

Repeated intravenous injection of adrenaline is a standard procedure for the production of arterial calcification in the rabbit. In addition, this treatment often produces disseminated myocardial necroses (182, 194, 489, 798). Essentially similar cardiac lesions have also been produced by the catecholamines, particularly ephedrine and noradrenaline, in the rabbit, adrenaline and noradrenaline in the rat (Lit.: 613, 802, 803). Of all the adrenergic catecholamines so far tested, isoproterenol appears to produce the most severe and constant focal cardiac necroses in the rat (534). However, at the dose levels suitable for this type of experimentation isoproterenol causes very pronounced necroses at the site of injection; hence, it has not been possible to explore the results of chronic isoproterenol treatment by administering this substance subcutaneously as is customary. Recently, we succeeded in overcoming this technical difficulty: it was found that, in the peritoneum, isoproterenol produces no obvious topical damage and is tolerated even when given twice daily in large amounts for several weeks. It is the purpose of this experiment to show that, under these circumstances, isoproterenol quite regularly produces dissecting, fatal aneurysms of the aorta and, sometimes, nephrocalcinosis.

### *Materials and Techniques*

Forty rats, with a mean initial body weight of 100 g (range: 90 to 110 g), were subdivided into 4 equal groups and treated as indicated in Table XXXIII. The individual dose of isoproterenol was invariably injected in 0.5 ml of water, intraperitoneally, twice daily. During the course of the experiment, the majority of the animals died as a result of hemothorax formation due to ruptured aneurysms of the thoracic aorta. The experiment was terminated after 27 days. The hearts and aortas of all animals were fixed in Susa solution saturated with picric acid, for subsequent staining with the PAS procedure, while the kidneys, which exhibited macroscopic evidence of nephrocalcinosis, were fixed in neutral alcohol formol as recommended by RENAUD (517) for the histochemical demonstration of calcium with the von Kóssa procedure.

### *Results and Discussion*

It will be noted from Table XXXIII that the great majority of the animals that succumbed during treatment died as a result of rupture of aortic aneurysms, with consequent homothorax formation. All aneurysms were situated in the thorax—usually at the aortic arch at the very beginning of the descending aorta—while the abdominal aorta remained essentially normal.

*Table XXXIII*

Production of Dissecting Aneurysms by Chronic Isoproterenol Treatment

| Group | Isoproterenol (mg/day) | Aortal aneurysms (%) | Mortality (%) |
|---|---|---|---|
| 1 | 25 | 0 | 10 |
| 2 | 50 | 90 | 90 |
| 3 | 2 × 25 | 70 | 70 |
| 4 | 2 × 50 | 100 | 100 |

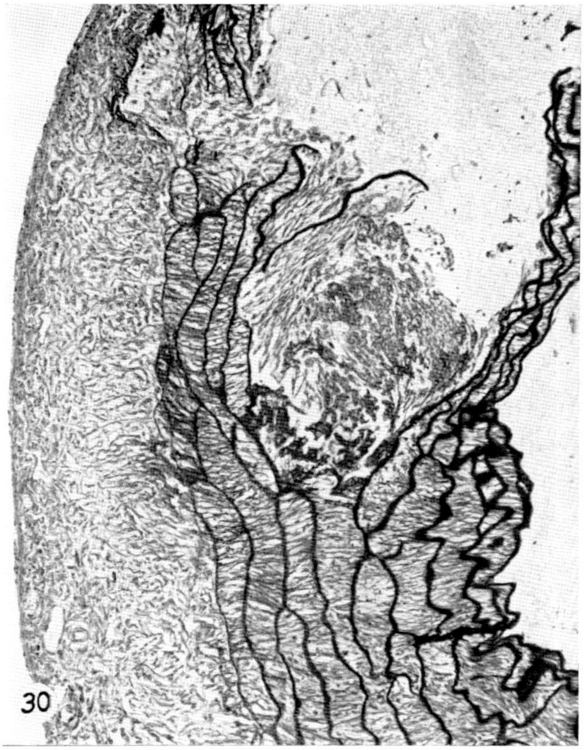

*Fig. 30* Dissecting aneurysms of the aorta in a rat treated with isoproterenol. Necrosis and hemorrhagic infiltration of the wall with disintegration of the elastic membranes and inflammatory infiltration of the adventitia (Aldehyde fuchsin—PAS, × 120).

Histologic examination confirmed that the thoracic hemorrhages were, in fact, due to dissecting aneurysms. These began with partial hyaline necrosis of the wall, then the circulating blood began to infiltrate and to dissect the elastic laminae until even the adventitia yielded to pressure (Fig. 30). Except in a few animals which died during the first week, the cardiac muscle remained essentially free of focal necrosis in these chronically treated rats, perhaps owing to the phenomenon of protection by earlier necroses (694). We know from previous experiments that the daily doses of isoproterenol administered in this series suffice to produce disseminated myocardial necroses constantly in short-term experiment; hence, it is to be assumed that during the first few days such lesions were also present in the surviving rats of this series. However, apparently these healed, while at the same time, the myocardium became resistant to the subsequent induction of new necrotic foci.

In many animals, the kidneys, as stained with the von Kóssa technique, revealed extensive nephrocalcinosis largely limited to the cortical region.

The experimental model-disease just described may be helpful in studying the pathogenesis of dissecting aneurysm of the aorta. As known, the highest incidence of dissecting aneurysm of the aorta occurs in patients beyond the fifth decade of life. Weakening of the media is the predisposing factor in this regard. The defect may be congenital (as in Marfan's disease and congenital narrowing of the aorta), but in most cases the etiology is not known. Recently, HOLESH (304a) pointed out that arteriosclerosis, hormonal abnormalities, collagen disease, and lipoid dystrophies may play a conditioning role in the development of dissecting aneurysms of the aorta.

*Summary*

When administered intraperitoneally, large doses of isoproterenol can be given to rats bidaily over long periods. The most striking change induced by such chronic overdosage is the virtually constant appearance of dissecting aneurysms of the aortic arch. In addition, nephrocalcinosis frequently occurs.

## V. General Summary and Conclusions

Experimental cardiopathies that are widely different in their histologic characteristics were studied in the albino rat. The main purpose of these comparative investigations was to determine whether there are conditioning factors capable of uniformly influencing (aggravating or preventing) the potentially cardiotoxic action of various agents.

It was observed that the development of necrotizing cardiopathies induced by biochemical means depends more or less largely upon conditioning factors some of which (corticoids, Na-salts, dietary deficiency in K, Mg and Cl, acute stress, coronary sclerosis, age) sensitize, while others (Na-deficiency, chlorides, pretreatment with stressors, hemodynamic changes, pregnancy) desensitize the heart to the production of cardiac lesions by most diverse agents.

*Positive conditioning factors* (Table XXXIV). Among the sensitizing agents, *corticoids* appeared to be particularly active conditioning factors in the production of cardiac necroses with different agents. The administration of a combination of both mineralo- and glucocorticoids, or of a single compound possessing both these activities (e.g., Me-Cl-COL, F-COL) is most effective in this respect. For instance, in the conditioning to the cardiotoxic effect of $Na_2HPO_4$-overdosage, a principally mineralocorticoid-acting halogenated corticoid (6α-methyl-9α-21-desoxycortisol) combined with another active mineralocorticoid (DOC) is far less active in its sensitizing ability than a gluco- plus mineralocorticoid mixture (cortisol plus DOC) or Me-Cl-COL. However, even a pure glucocorticoid (e.g., triamcinolone) was found to be active in the production of 'spotty myolysis', when given simultaneously with noradrenaline to intact or adrenalectomized animals.

It was also observed that following suitable conditioning with corticoids otherwise innocuous agents may become cardiotoxic. For example, after pretreatment with Me-Cl-COL, pentamethylentetrazol, Na-arsenate, or diisopropylfluorophosphate all consistently elicited cardiac necroses in the rat, although none of these compounds nor the steroid hormone showed any cardiotoxic properties when given alone. As regards their sensitizing ability, a synergism exists between corticoids and steroids of the vitamin-D group (e.g., DHT). On the other hand, studies on the interactions between steroid hormones did not provide any evidence to show that the conditioning action of one steroid could be prevented by another. Yet, the many antagonisms between steroids in other respects and the fact that pretreatment with stressor agents as well as pregnancy offers considerable protection against most of the cardiopathies studied suggest that research along these lines may be profitable.

Experiments dealing with the participation of *electrolytes* in the production of cardiopathies have given a number of interesting results. Like Me-Cl-COL, $Na_2HPO_4$ greatly predisposes the cardiac muscle to the necrotizing effect of proteolytic enzymes (papain, ficin), as well as to that of stressor agents following conditioning with corticoids, while the cardiotoxic actions of other agents (noradrenaline, vasopressin) were not significantly influenced by this electrolyte. It was also noted that Ca-acetate can alter the calcifying and slight necrotizing actions of DHT, so that a suppurative acute myocarditis results.

Since only Na-salts (phosphates, sulfates and perchlorate) were effective in inducing cardiac necroses (ESCN) with corticoids, it was previously concluded that both the anion and the cation are important factors in the pathogenesis of this type of experimental cardiac disease (613). It was then observed that the same Na-salts ($Na_2HPO_4$, $Na_2SO_4$, $NaClO_4$), previously shown to produce an ESCN, have the same effect in animals briefly sensitized by a K-deficient diet. This similarity in the conditioning influence of K-deficiency and of corticoid overdosage is further emphasized by the fact that equivalent amounts of NaCl were ineffective in both these experimental conditions. However, following conditioning with Me-Cl-COL plus DHT, severe cardiac lesions can be induced by many electrolytes, not only by the classical 'sensitizing Na-salts'. Under these conditions, the cardiotoxic effect cannot be ascribed to Na as such, since several Na-salts are inert in this respect, while others in which the cation is not Na (e.g., $K_2HPO_4$, Ca-acetate) exhibit severe necrotizing properties. Conversely, NaCl, which does not enhance the cardiotoxicity of either DHT or Me-Cl-COL, remains ineffective even when both these sterols are administered. Apparently, electrolytes sensitize the heart to the toxic effects of corticoids and of sterols of the vitamin-D group through some closely related mechanisms; consequently, these two types of steroids can potentiate each other's electrolyte-dependent actions.

Experiments performed on rats kept on *diets* deficient in certain electrolytes give the most uniform results. A brief sensitization with a K-deficient diet enhanced the potentially cardiotoxic actions of all of the agents tried. Mg-deficiency acts similarly in this respect (see also Ref. 448). Interestingly, our experiments suggested that not only the variations in dietary intake of certain cations (such as K and Mg) but also of the anions (i.e., Cl) play an important conditioning role in the pathogenesis of various necrotizing cardiopathies. Cl-deficiency significantly enhances the susceptibility of the heart to the production of cardiac lesions (necroses, inflammation and/or calcification) by plasmocid, papain, DHT, Ca-acetate + DHT, Na-acetate + F-COL, as well as by the stressor effect of forced restraint or quadriplegia after conditioning with F-COL. Only the cardiotoxic action of noradrenaline and vasopressin was not influenced by lowering the Cl-intake.

*Table XXXIV*

Positive Conditioning Actions (Sensitization)

| Cardiotoxic agents | Types of cardiac lesions | Positive conditioning factors* | | | | | | | |
|---|---|---|---|---|---|---|---|---|---|
| | | Corticoids | Cl-deficiency | K-deficiency | Mg-deficiency | Stressor agents | Aging | DHT-arteriosclerosis | Other agents |
| DHT | Small necrotic foci with intensive calcification; arteries also calcified | + Me-Cl-COL | + | + | (+) 448 | + | + | × | (+) Na-salts 664 |
| DHT + $NaH_2PO_4$ (or Ca-acetate) | Suppurating myocarditis | + Me-Cl-COL | + | × | × | + | (+) 613 | × | (+) Corn oil, Glucose |
| Me-Cl-COL (or F-COL) + $NaH_2PO_4$ | Large, infarct-like foci of cardiac necroses with inflammation (ESCN-type) | × | + | × | (+) 448 | (+) 689 | + | + | (+) Corn oil, Glucose 613 |
| Me-Cl-COL (or F-COL) + Stress | Usually small necrotic foci, but sometimes ESCN-type | × | + | × | × | × | ○ | + | + Na-salts |
| F-COL + Na-acetate + Stress | ESCN-type | × | + | × | × | × | × | × | |
| Noradrenaline | Spotty myolysis without extensive necrosis or inflammation | + DOC, Triamcinolone | ○ | + | × | + | + | + | ○ $Na_2HPO_4$ |
| Papain | Miliary, disseminated cardiac necroses | + Me-Cl-COL | + | + | + | (+) 613 | + | + | + $Na_2HPO_4$ |
| Plasmocid | Large, patchy myocardial necrosis and myocarditis | × | + | + | × | (+) 628 | ○ | + | (○) $Na_2HPO_4$ 613 |
| Stress (sudden) | Minute disseminated foci of myocardial necrosis and myolysis | + Me-Cl-COL | × | + | (+) 448 | × | × | + | (+) Antibiotics 517 |
| Vasopressin | Spotty myolysis | + Me-Cl-COL | ○ | + | × | × | + | + | |

* Explanation of symbols used: + aggravated; (+) with number refers to literature data; ○ not influenced; × not investigated, or no published data available.

The importance of anion-cation interactions is further supported by the observations that, when rats are kept on a K-deficient diet, $Na_2$-$HPO_4$ (unlike equivalent amounts of NaCl) rapidly provokes development of severe cardiac necroses before this diet, in itself, produces any obvious morbid changes. This particularly severe syndrome induced by $Na_2HPO_4$ can be prevented by either KCl or $MgCl_2$. These observations highlight the importance of $PO_4$- and Mg-ions in the development of the syndrome usually ascribed to K-deficiency.

We were especially impressed by the observation that sensitization by K- or Cl-deficient diets greatly increases the susceptibility of the heart muscle to the potentially cardiotoxic actions of *stressors*. Administration of Me-Cl-COL, DHT, or DHT + Ca-acetate exerts a similar positive conditioning effect to the cardiac necrosis-eliciting effect of restraint, quadriplegia, hot and cold baths, noradrenaline overdosage, etc. Thus, the precipitating effect of neither of these agents is specific, since all invariably produce cardiac necroses in the suitably conditioned rats. Other experiments then showed that various Na-salts (NaCl, $NaHCO_3$ and many inorganic Na-salts tried) are well tolerated even by rats simultaneously treated with Me-Cl-COL or a neuromuscular stressor (i.e., restraint). However, these same salts produce massive, and sometimes fatal myocardial necroses in rats exposed to stress after conditioning with Me-Cl-COL. It appears that during stress the metabolism of certain otherwise innocuous Na-salts and/or steroids is so altered that these substances acquire severe cardiotoxic properties. Studies have not yet been performed on the biochemical mechanism through which stress predisposes the cardiac muscle to the necrotizing effect of Na-salts and/or steroid hormones. It is of considerable interest, however, that by lowering the Cl-content of the diet from a basic 0.935% to 0.035% all otherwise ineffective Na-salts produce extensive necroses in the F-COL conditioned rats, even without exposure to stressful stimuli. Thus, Cl-deficiency replaces the cardiac necrosis-eliciting effect of stress in the electrolyte-steroid conditioned animals.

Subsequent studies were performed to examine the role of the *age factor* in the production of various experimental cardiac lesions. It was shown that papain, noradrenaline, vasopressin, DHT, and combined treatment with Me-Cl-COL + $Na_2HPO_4$ induce much more pronounced cardiac lesions in old than in young rats when the dose of these substances is adjusted to body weight. On the other hand, stressors, such as restraint and quadriplegia, as well as plasmocid were

*Table XXXV*

Negative Conditioning Actions (Desensitization)

| Cardiotoxic agents | Types of cardiac lesions | Negative conditioning factors* | | | | | | |
|---|---|---|---|---|---|---|---|---|
| | | Na-deficiency | High Cl-intake | KCl | $MgCl_2$ | Stress (pretreatment) | Hemorrhage | Pregnancy |
| DHT | Small necrotic foci with intensive calcification; arteries also calcified | + | + | (○) 613 | (○) 613 | (+) 680 | × | (+) 610 |
| DHT + $NaH_2PO_4$ (or Ca-acetate) | Suppurating myocarditis | ○ | + | (+) 614 | (+) 614 | + | + | + |
| Me-Cl-COL (or F-COL) + Na $H_2PO_4$ | Large, infarct-like foci of cardiac necroses (ESCN-type) | + | + | (+) 648 | (+) 648 | × | + | (+) 620 |
| Me-Cl-COL (or F-COL) + Stress | Usually small necrotic foci but sometimes ESCN-type | + | + | + | + | + | + | ○ |
| F-COL + Na-acetate + Stress | ESCN-type | × | + | × | × | + | × | × |
| K-deficiency + Na-salts | ESCN-type | × | × | + | + | × | × | × |
| Mg-deficiency + Na-salts | ESCN-type | × | × | + | + | × | × | × |
| Noradrenaline | Spotty myolysis | ○ | ○ | (○) 628 | (○) 628 | ○ | + | + |
| Papain | Miliary, disseminated cardiac necroses | + | + | + | + | (+) 48 | + | + |
| Plasmocid | Large, patchy myocardial necrosis and myocarditis | + | + | (○) 660 | (○) 660 | (+) 659 | ○ | ○ |
| Stress (sudden) | Minute disseminated foci of myocardial necrosis and myolysis | × | × | + | + | × | × | × |
| Vasopressin | Spotty myolysis | ○ | ○ | × | × | × | × | + |

* Explanation of symbold used: + prevented; (+) with number refers to literature data; ○ not influenced; × not investigated, or no published data available.

about equally effective in young and old animals. Still, in view of the enormous importance of cardiovascular disease in gerontology, it is of interest that a variety of experimental cardiac lesions depend to such a large extent upon the age factor.

In order to observe the conditioning role of *coronary medial sclerosis,* rats were pretreated with DHT, thus sclerosis and hardening of the coronary system (Mönckeberg-type) was induced. It was found that in these artificially 'aged' animals, otherwise ineffective doses of noradrenaline, vasopressin, papain, or cold baths all produce particularly extensive, macroscopically visible patches of cardiac necrosis throughout the heart. Quite unexpectedly, it was also noted that after sensitization with DHT intense proliferative and eventually obstructive changes developed in all parts of the coronary tree during the action of the cardiotoxic agents enumerated above.

*Negative conditioning factors* (Table XXXV). One of the most interesting results of our experiments was the demonstration that exposure to *stressors* can both elicit and prevent various types of cardiopathies in suitably conditioned animals, depending primarily upon the time, intensity and duration of stress. It was demonstrated that forced muscular exercise, restraint, and bone fractures, if applied before the animal is humorally conditioned for the development of the cardiac necrosis, can all prevent the necrotizing lesions normally elicited when the above stressors are applied after suitable conditioning (e.g., by F-COL + Na-acetate or DHT + $NaH_2PO_4$). Furthermore, the development of true cross-resistance to the cardiotoxic action of various stressors was demonstrated under these experimental conditions; the cardiac necrosis-producing effect of muscular exercise could be prevented by pretreatment with cold, that of cold by muscular exercise, that of noradrenaline by restraint, that of bone fracture by muscular exercise. Even the cardiotoxic actions of other agents (e.g., DHT, papain, plasmocid, oil-feeding) that presumably act through specific mechanism could be abolished by pretreatment with stressor agents (see also Refs. 48, 659, 680). The pathways through which adaptation to stressors protect against otherwise pathogenic actions of various cardiotoxic agents are not yet elucidated. It is, however, remarkable that stress fails to exert this protective effect upon the myocardium if the dietary Cl-intake is markedly lowered. On the other hand, sensitization with a Mg-deficient ration—also known to enhance the disease-susceptibility of the heart muscle—does not influence the normal development of cross-resistance.

Like many other stressor agents, *hemorrhage* also protects against the induction of cardiopathies by various agents. Some of our observations, however, suggest that in this respect hemorrhage does not act merely through its nonspecific stressor effect. For example, the cardiac necrosis normally produced by plasmocid is prevented by pretreatment with restraint, muscular exercise, cold baths, reserpine (659), but not by hemorrhage. Furthermore, the 'spotty myolysis' resulting from noradrenaline-overdosage cannot be prevented with previous exposure to restraint or to other stressors, but it is easily prevented by hemorrhage. It is not completely proven—but we believe it highly probable—that the effect of hemorrhage is due mainly to a decrease in cardiac work.

Synthetic *diets* low in Na- or high in Cl-content proved to be very effective in protecting the rats against diverse cardiotoxic agents. Na-deficiency abolished or at least markedly diminished the pathogenic actions not only of those agents (i.e., papain, DHT, F-COL + stressors) that are otherwise aggravated by the administration of Na-salts, but even that of plasmocid which is singularly resistant to electrolytes. However, the potential cardiotoxic effect of noradrenaline, vasopressin, and DHT + Ca-acetate could not be influenced by this Na-deficient diet. An increase in the Cl-content of the diet (from a basic 0.935% to 1.62%) with no change in the ratio of cations resulted in marked inhibition of various cardiotoxic actions; but here again the development of 'spotty myolysis' normally due to the administration of noradrenaline and vasopressin remained uninfluenced. Yet, the observation that an excess of dietary Cl-intake effectively desensitizes the heart against the most diverse potentially cardiotoxic agents (like papain, plasmocid, DHT, F-COL + $Na_2HPO_4$, F-COL + stress) is in keeping with earlier findings in which, among the various electrolytes tried, no salts of anions other than chlorides offered significant protective action against the ESCN (613).

Experiments studying desensitization by various *chlorides* showed that KCl and $MgCl_2$ prevent the occurrence of not only the necrotizing cardiopathies normally elicited by exposure to stressors with or without corticoid conditioning, but also the cardiac necroses that follow, presumably as a direct result of intravenous treatment with a protease (i.e., papain). The fact that various other types of necrotizing cardiopathies could be prevented by these electrolytes was previously established (613, 628). Our additional experiments then indicated that chlorides of other cations (e.g., NaCl, $NH_4Cl$, $CaCl_2$), as well as a mixture of these electrolytes containing equivalent amounts of the anion, are to a certain extent all effective inhibitors of the ESCN-type, infarctoid cardiac changes normally elicited with $NaClO_4$ after sensitization by diets deficient in K or Mg. From these findings we concluded that both the cations ($K^+$ and $M^{++}$) and the anion ($Cl^-$) play an important role in the yet unclarified biochemical processes that desensitize the myocardium against diverse, potentially cardiotoxic agents.

It is particularly interesting to note that in rats conditioned by a K- or Mg-deficient diet to the cardiotoxic actions of papain, $Na_2HPO_4$, or $NaClO_4$, the sensitizing effect of both these dietary deficiencies was significantly diminished by oral administration of KCl or $MgCl_2$; KCl was as active in Mg-deficient animals as was $MgCl_2$ in rats kept on the diet low in K. Consequently, the anion must play an important role in this preventative reaction, since K- or Mg-ions are believed to be in many respects even antagonistic (711). The importance of chlorides for the maintenance of normal cardiac function and structure was further supported by studies on ESCN-type cardiac lesions, using various ion exchange resins (especially K-, Mg-, and Cl-releasing polystyrene compounds) for prevention (51).

Independent investigations on the influence of age as well as that of *pregnancy* upon the development of various necrotizing cardiopathies revealed that youth protects the heart against essentially the same cardiotoxic agents as does pregnancy. Thus, pregnant animals proved to be particularly resistant to noradrenaline, vasopressin and papain, but not to plasmocid or to the cardiac necrosis-eliciting effect of stressors (i.e., restraint, cold baths and quadriplegia) following Me-Cl-COL conditioning.

*Are all cardiotoxic agents potential pathogens?* The observations just summarized above clearly reveal that most of the agents that are capable of inducing cardiac lesions through some biochemical mechanism are potentially (or conditionally) acting pathogens, whose cardiotoxic action largely depends upon conditioning influences. On the other hand, the cardiac infarct that can be produced by surgical occlusion of coronary arteries in the rat differs basically from all metabolic cardiopathies studied. Ligature of a coronary artery at a given level always produces an infarct of the same extent, irrespective of concurrent treatment or pretreatment with any agents so far examined (see also Ref.: 628). Even the differences between the ECG-alterations of surgically induced cardiopathies and those produced by biochemical means (e.g., by combined administration of corticoids and Na-salts) are quite marked. Apparently, the occlusion of a coronary vessel is a prototype of primary (or unconditionally) acting pathogens that induce cardiac necroses under any circumstances.

As regards their cardiotoxic actions, noradrenaline and vasopressin occupy a mid-position between the two extremes: of potential pathogens and absolutely unconditional pathogens. The development of the spotty myolytic changes normally produced by noradrenaline or vasopressin is singularly resistant to chlorides, Na-deficiency as well as to pretreatment with stressor-agents. Consequently, it would be tempting to assume that noradrenaline and vasopressin act at the final stage of the biochemical chain-reaction that results in necroses, whereas all other agents (electrolytes, steroids, stress) exert their influence at intermediate points. However, it will be recalled that pregnancy offered significant protection against both noradrenaline and vasopressin overdosage and that the cardiotoxic action of noradrenaline was inhibited by hemorrhage. Furthermore, as with the many other cardiopathies studied, the induction of 'spotty myolysis' was greatly enhanced by corticoids, DHT, and by sensitization with a K-deficient diet. These observations suggest that there may be some-common factor in the mechanism through which various humoral agents produce cardiac necroses.

*Theoretical implications.* Our studies, at present, do not permit elaboration of a detailed biochemical theory of necrotizing cardiopathies. It is obvious from the experiments described in this monograph that electrolyte shifts are important, and it may be that corticoids condition the cardiac cell by altering its affinity for certain ions—perhaps through changes in cell permeability.

An overdosage with Na-salts, administration of corticoids, exposure to stressors, and feeding with a low-K diet are all known to result in a positive Na- and negative K-balance. Consequently, it would be tempting to assume that the metabolic cardiopathies are, in all instances, hypokalemic. In this event, the Na-salts could act simply because of the well-known antagonism between Na and K, and exposure to stressors merely by increasing mineralocorticoid activity. In fact, this reasoning is in keeping with the general hypothesis in which, in the final analysis, the disturbance of intra- and extracellular equilibrium of Na- and K-ions (more precisely, a continuous inflow of Na into cell and the concomitant loss of K) would explain the pathogenic actions of stress and/or corticoids at the cellular level (see pp. 90–91).

Although, it seems to be well established that hypokalemia is an important factor that sensitizes the heart to the potentially cardiotoxic actions of various agents, it is not possible to explain all our observations by the over-simplified theory that the conditioning agents examined predispose to the hypokalemia, and that the cardiac lesions precipitated by different means are merely the consequences of an aggravation of K-deficiency.

For example, our experiments revealed that a diet low in Cl-content is just as active in sensitizing the myocardium as is dietary K-deficiency, although lowering the dietary Cl intake does not alter the Na/K ratio in rats tissues (745). It was observed, furthermore, that when rats are kept on K- or Mg-deficient diet for a brief period, the sensitizing effect of both these diets can be abolished by the administration of KCl or $MgCl_2$ as well as even by a mixture of chlorides of other cations. Notably, in this respect $MgCl_2$ was just as active in rats maintained on a K-deficient diet, as KCl in animals kept on a Mg-deficient ration. Although it is known that Mg-deficiency can result in secondary K-depletion, this is only true if rats are fed a deficient diet for one month or more and not for seven days only as in our experiments (405). Further investigations will be necessary to elucidate the mechanism of these complex ionic interactions.

The observation that exposure to stressor agents can either elicit or prevent cardiac necroses in suitably conditioned rats clearly shows the existence of adaptation mechanisms that basically alter the disease-susceptibility of the heart muscle. Thus, adaptive reactions occupy a key position in the pathogenesis of certain necrotizing cardiopathies, but we are ignorant at present of the precise mechanisms involved. Progress along these lines is handicapped by the fact that the neuroendocrine relationships and interactions in adaptive reactions are not only extremely complex, but as yet poorly understood. Furthermore, our knowledge of the metabolic actions of stress and corticoids is not extensive enough to allow for any definite conclusion.

It will be recalled that in reviewing the literature we pointed out (see pp. 97–104) that stress can affect both the function and metabolism of the heart through trans- and extra-adrenal humoral and neural pathways. An increased secretion of corticoids may influence cardiac metabolism directly, or indirectly by altering the ionic equilibrium via the kidneys.

It was shown that an antimineralocorticoid steroid-spirolactone ('Aldactone') offers considerable protection against the induction of cardiac necroses normally produced by stress in rats conditioned by F-COL plus Na-salts (627). This finding may suggest that an increased mineralocorticoid activity upon the kidney is involved. It should be considered, furthermore, that stress, through increasing vasopressin secretion, is a proper antidiuretic agent and, thus, may also contribute in this way to the misregulation of water and electrolyte balance. At any rate, whenever the mineralocorticoid activity increases—which in turn enhances the excretion of K and the retention of Na and Cl—we would expect that the kidney would immediately balance the changes induced in order to keep the body composition normal. Our observations suggest, however, that in certain conditions (e.g., during or consequent to severe stresses) the kidney may not do this, indicating that it has lost its adaptive ability to maintain or restore selective function and that the physiological stimuli to the kidneys are not operating in a proper manner. Interestingly, exposure to stressors does not elicit the typical necrotizing cardiac lesions in the electrolyte-steroid conditioned rat following nephrectomy. Moreover, pretreatment with restraint markedly inhibits the development of the uremic cardiopathy normally produced by bilateral nephrectomy, even if sensitizing amounts of $Na_2HPO_4$ are administered (528). It may be concluded, therefore, that the presence of the kidneys is necessary for the cardiac necrosis-eliciting actions of stress. However, it is equally possible that the phenomenon of cross-resistance does not depend upon the presence of renal tissue.

It was also observed that exposure to stressors elicits cardiac necroses even in adrenalectomized animals sensitzed by Na-salts while maintained on small amounts of corticoids (686). This finding suggests the participation of some extra-adrenal mechanisms. In fact, neuroleptic phenothiazine derivatives (e.g., chlorpromazine, cyamepromazine) were found to block certain, presumably neural, pathways through which various stressors either elicit cardiac lesions or induce cross-resistance of the heart muscle (52).

As a final conclusion, we may say that our investigations suggest that there may be some common mechanism through which various agents influence the heart muscle, thereby producing necroses and/or inflammation. The observation that certain factors uniformly sensitize, while others desensitize the myocardium for the production of structural lesions by a great variety of agents could be interpreted in this manner. The experiments described not only reveal the existence of principal interactions between conditioning factors that basically alter the disease-susceptibility of the heart muscle, but also suggest the directions in which future research could be extended.

*Addendum*

Since this book was completed, a great number of related studies have been carried out and some additional salient points have come to light. Let me briefly review, therefore, our most recent observations in this last section, to make the present volume a truly up-to-date guide.

Several findings described on the previous pages drew our attention to the great *differences in the extent* to which the cardiac and skeletal muscles participate in various disease processes. Interestingly, in many instances toxic actions of compounds (e.g., plasmocid, isoproterenol) or of dietary deficiencies (e.g., K-deficiency) attack the cardiac much more severely than the skeletal muscle, but in other cases (e.g., paraphenylenediamine overdosage in animals, or infectious diseases, such as diphtheria, typhus, in man) inflammatory and necrotic lesions may develop with equal intensity in both structures. As another example it may be recalled that the degenerative changes in hereditary muscular dystrophies of man are most pronounced in the skeletal muscle, and are only occasionally seen in the cardiac muscle. Consequently, it was interesting to observe that in inbred strain 129 mice (which are afflicted with a hereditary myopathy resembling in many respects human muscular dystrophy), structural changes in the myocardium, having some morphologic resemblance to those seen in the skeletal muscle, do occur, although infrequently (820). Further studies then showed that certain dietary factors greatly alter the disease susceptibility of the myocardium and, in fact, determine whether only the skeletal muscle or also the cardiac muscle will be involved in the dystrophic processes (815). For example, a high protein (casein) intake and the feeding of a synthetic high-fat diet both significantly increase the intensity of myocardial involvement in the dystrophic mice. Nevertheless, it is still uncertain whether the biochemical differences demonstrated between the cardiac and skeletal muscle structures (e.g., in the content of electrolytes or amino acids, in substrate utilization and metabolic rate) play the decisive role in this regard and the dietary factors only condition for the site of the degenerative involvement.

The important role of *nutritional factors* (especially of dietary electrolytes) in the pathogenesis and prevention of necrotizing cardiopathies has been the subject of several recent publications (802, 803,

807), in which the related world-literature was discussed at length and correlated with our experimental findings. It may be recalled, here, that the induction of *cross-resistance* by adaptation to stressors continues to be one of the most effective protectors against the development of cardiac necroses (824, 826). Despite extensive studies, the mechanisms involved in this adaptive phenomenon are not yet clearly established. Nevertheless, it is remarkable that the reactivity of the myocardium, as regards defensive reactions, largely depends upon the adequate intake of certain anions (823). The relationship of the general adaptive reactions to cardiovascular pathology has also been extensively analyzed (804) and the governing role of *neuroendocrine systems* in this regard has been discussed (805, 806, 808).

Among the chemicals that were shown to be more or less effective against the induction of experimental cardiac necroses, *serotonin* may be especially important. Our findings on the pathogenesis and prevention of necrotizing cardiopathies are not incompatible with the hypothesis that, in the final analysis, some neurohumoral or other tissue substance is liberated and acts within the myocardium, resulting in metabolic damage and, consequently, degeneration. This hypothesis may be supported by findings repeatedly showing, on the one hand, that an overdosage of catecholamines actually results in cardiac necroses (646), and on the other hand, that a number of antiadrenergic compounds offer protection against the induction of myocardial damage by the most diverse agents (52, 504, 819). Notably, reserpine, which is known to liberate both noradrenaline and serotonin, was found to be one of the most active protective agents. The possibility thus arose that, among the sympathomimetic amines, serotinin may also play a role in the genesis of certain cardiac necroses as well as in the physiological mechanisms that are involved in the prevention of such myocardial damage. In view of the considerations just mentioned, it was interesting to observe that by influencing the metabolism of the highly vasoactive serotonin in different ways, i.e., by administering its precursor 5-hydroxytryptophane, which is readily converted into serotonin in the organism; by injecting a monoamine oxidase inhibitor hydrazine derivative, nialamide, which is known to increase serotonin levels by inhibiting its degradation; or by giving serotonin itself, protection can be obtained against the induction of diverse necrotizing cardiopathies (809, 813, 814). It is reasonable to believe that all these substances act, in the final analysis, through increased serotonin activities, an assumption that is further supported by the observation that the most active prevention can be obtained by combined administration of serotonin plus nialamide. But even if this assumption is correct, it is still difficult to draw definite conclusions regarding the mechanism involved. It was, nevertheless, shown that under certain experimental conditions serotonin is a potent vasodilator; yet it is questionable that our results can be explained simply on this basis. It may be that serotonin actively constricts large vessels and at the same time dilates small vessels, that some interaction takes place between serotonin and other neurohormones (e.g., catecholamines, acetylcholine), or that serotonin decreases the oxygen requirements of the myocardium, etc. It is, thus, a simple matter to suggest diverse pathways that may all be involved, but the design of experiments to test these various theories remains a continuing challenge.

Calcifying cardiopathies react somewhat differently to serotonin administration. This amine prevents the cardiac calcification normally produced by DHT-overdosage and by ligature of the coronary veins; however, the degenerative and necrotic lesions associated with these calcifications are by no means prevented but merely diminished. In this respect, serotonin seems to act directly on the cells and independently of the blood calcium level (821). Thus, a dissociation between necrosis and calcification occurs following serotonin administration, a finding that may open new avenues for research, since actually nothing is known about factors that determine whether the structural alterations of the cardiac muscle (and of other tissues) will or will not be accompanied by calcium deposits. Studies performed along these lines now indicate hypophysectomy as well as the administration of triamcinolone (or other antiphlogistic corticoids) prevents calcification mainly, not the accompanying cardiac lesion itself (816).

As was emphasized on the preceding pages, some of the experimentally induced necrotizing cardiopathies (e.g., those produced by proteolytic enzymes, bilateral nephrectomy, sulfa drugs, polymyxin) steadily calcify, while in others (e.g., those elicited by noradrenaline, isoproterenol, vasopressin, cardiac glycosides), calcification rarely occurs. Nevertheless, a classification based on calcifying and non-calcifying cardiopathies cannot easily be made, since the cardiac lesion that does not calcify under certain experimental conditions may do so under other, apparently similar, circumstances (809, 822), and this variable result depends on some, as yet undetermined, factors. A new approach to the problem was provided by the observation that while the massive cardiac infarcts that follow coronary artery ligature never calcify, the less extensive but still marked necrosis resulting from coronary vein obstruction is always heavily filled with calcium granules (662). Since in the cases of sulfonamide-induced and renoprival cardiopathies a positive correlation was established between parathyroid stimulation and myocardial calcification (391), it was interesting to determine the role of the *thyro-parathyroid system* in the development of myocardial calcification normally due to coronary vein obstruction.

Experiments in the rat indicate that following ligature of the two main coronary veins at the point where they enter (separately or after uniting into a single sinus) the right auricle, necrotic foci occur in the subepicardial muscle layers and massive calcification begins in the affected areas. This type of myocardial calcification—unlike the onset of necrosis—was greatly enhanced by parathyroidectomy performed three days before ligature of the coronary veins. On the other hand, the aggravating action of parathyroid deficiency was counteracted by simultaneous thyroidectomy and could not be restored by replacement therapy with thyroxine (5, 50, 100 or 500 µg/100 gm body weight/day). In fact, following coronary vein ligature, there was less myocardial calcification in the thyro-parathyroidectomized than in the intact animals. However, the steadiest and most marked calcification was observed in those parathyroidectomized rats that were injected with thyroxine, although the administration of the thyroid hormone alone to intact animals did not significantly influence the occurrence and intensity of calcification (817). From all these observations, it is postulated that parathyroid deficiency enhances myocardial calcification, only in the presence of both thyroxine and another, as yet unidentified, thyroid factor. It is likely that these thyroid principles are responsible for promoting the entry of various ions (calcium, phosphorus, carbonate) in excess into the damaged tissue areas and that they are more important detrimental factors in this regard than is the serum level of calcium and/or inorganic phosphorus. This conclusion is further supported by the observation that alterations in serum calcium and inorganic phosphorus levels normally due to parathyroidectomy were not further changed by removal of the thyroids and/or administration of thyroxine. In other words, the great difference in myocardial calcification seen between the parathyroidectomized and thyroparathyroidectomized animals could not be explained simply through an alteration of the electrolyte balance of the organism. Further studies then showed that the administration of DHT—a sterol of the vitamin D group that is a well-known calcifying agent and acts in many respects similarly to parathyroid hormone—can actually prevent the occurrence of myocardial calcification normally due to coronary vein obstruction in intact, parathyroidectomized, and thyroparathyroidectomized rats (818). It is perhaps not surprising that DHT prevents myocardial calcification in parathyroidectomized and thyroparathyroidectomized animals, if we assume that the high serum inorganic phosphorus level that follows removal of the parathyroids plays some role in this regard. We found that in such rats the lowered serum calcium and elevated phosphorus levels were normalized by the administration of DHT. However, in the intact rats daily administration of 50 μg of DHT did not result in any significant alteration in the electrolyte values, yet the calcification of the myocardium was completely prevented. This interesting observation awaits further clarification and only serves to show the complexity of factors that are involved in the processes of tissue calcification.

Finally, I would like to mention some of our *histochemical observations,* as they may be helpful at the formulation of future studies. A great many experiments discussed in this book showed that apart from by direct interference with coronary circulation cardiac necroses can also be regularly induced in laboratory animals by injection of certain chemicals (e.g., plasmocid, isoproterenol, paraphenylenediamine, proteolytic enzymes, cardiac glycosides, vasopressin) as well as by exposure to noxious stimuli (e.g., cold, surgical trauma, forced muscular exercise), especially following suitable pretreatment with corticoids and/or Na-salts. Since these two last-mentioned groups of potentially cardiotoxic agents do not produce any histologically detectable changes in the normal structure of coronary vessels, it may be assumed that the necrosis so induced is the consequence of some biochemical alteration that affects the normal metabolism of myocardial cells. On this basis, a distinction is possible between occlusive and metabolic cardiac necroses that can be produced experimentally in animals; and, indeed, it is likely that some forms of human interstitial myocarditis and cardiac necroses represent reactions to direct metabolic injury in hearts with normal blood supply. Nevertheless, the possibility still exists that even such non-occlusive or metabolic type cardiac lesions are produced through some, as yet unrecognized, vascular mechanism (by resulting in spasm of the small coronary vessels or altering capillary permeability) that cannot be recognized by the usual histologic techniques. It is also true that in many cases, at autopsy, no clear pathologic distinction can be made between the presumably metabolic type of myocardial necroses and those resulting from coronary thrombosis.

Our recent studies indicated that, even in an early stage of development, the occlusive type of necroses (induced by surgical occlusion of a coronary artery) can easily be distinguished from the metabolic necroses (induced by plasmocid administration) by enzyme histochemistry. In the first case, there is a rapid and marked decline in certain oxidative enzyme activities (i.e., cytochrome oxidase, succinic dehydrogenase), normally retained 5-nucleotidase activity, and absence of proteolytic activity (as evidenced by leucine aminopeptidase). In the second case, the oxidative enzymes show no significant change (except in the already necrotic areas), but there is a reduced 5-nucleotidase activity, and an intense reaction for leucine aminopeptidase (811, 822). In addition, in hearts with metabolic cardiac lesions a significant increase in lactic dehydrogenase activity is usually seen, especially in places where the reaction for cytochrome oxidase and succinic dehydrogenase has declined. This phenomenon most probably reflects an adaptive alteration in enzymatic pathways. Since similar enzymatic aberration does not occur in the affected areas following artery ligature, the activation of lactic dehydrogenase is most probably not related to anoxic changes. Among the other histochemically demonstrable changes, the loss of the stainable, labile fraction of glycogen is the most remarkable. It occurs independently of whether the myocardial lesion is induced by chemical or surgical means. But while in the case of occlusive infarct the glycogen content of the fibers begins to decrease already after 1 to 3 minutes following interruption of the blood-supply and then rapidly disappears, after plasmocid administration there is usually a transitory increase in the myocardial glycogen accumulation; this is followed by a decrease, only after 2–3 hours and only in places where necrotic foci actually develop. It should be noted, here, that certain differences between the metabolic and occlusive type of experimental necroses could also be shown with ECG studies (827).

Any attempt at a complete interpretation of the findings just outlined would be premature at present; but is appears that some vascular factors may be involved in the genesis of metabolic lesions and it is likely that the interruption of the arterial blood supply is not the only factor in the pathogenesis of ischemic infarcts. It is in this connection that further comparative histochemical studies on the relation between purely occlusive and metabolic myocardial necroses hold great promise for both pathology and clinical cardiology.

## VI. References

1. Abbou, R. et Vallière, M.: Etude de l'action hypoglycémiante de l'insuline au cours de l'hypothermie provoquée par réfrigération externe. C. R. Soc. Biol. *150:* 1697 (1956).
2. Abrams, W. B. and Harris, T. N.: The effect of cortisone on the electrocardiograms of normal rabbits. Amer. Heart J. *42:* 876 (1951).
3. Ahn, B. von: The acute effect of tobacco smoking and nicotine on the electrocardiogram especially during induced hypoxia. Acta med. scand. (Suppl.) *292:* 1 (1954).
4. Akada, J.: Effect of the administration of thyroid stimulating hormone on the hypothalamo-hypophyseal thyroidal system. Endocrin jap. *6:* 233 (1959).
5. Albeaux-Fernet, M.; Chabot, J. et Gelinet, M.: Etude des fonctions hormonales dans 29 cas d'anorexie mentale et de maigreur fonctionnelle des jeunes filles. Sem. Hôp. Paris *35:* 1000 (1959).
6. Albright, E. C.: Thyroid: fundamental considerations. Amer. J. clin. Nutrit. *8:* 77 (1960).
7. Allen, F. M. and Lisa, J. R.: 'Scottie'—twelve years diabetic. Endocrinology *46:* 282 (1950).
8. Amand, A. E.: The hypothalamus and diabetes mellitus. Marquette M. Rev. *25:* 227 (1960).
9. Anderson, J. M. and Brunson, J. G.: The influence of acute stress on the response of rabbits to intravenous endotoxin. Circulation *7:* 34 (1959).
10. Anderson, B. and Jewell, P. A.: Observations on the hypothalamo-hypophysial neurosecretory system and on variations in the structure of the pituitary of the goat. Acta anat. *35:* 1 (1958)
11. Applezweig, M. H. and Moeller, G.: The pituitary-adrenocortical system and anxiety in avoidance learning. Proc. 15th int. Congr. Physiol., Brussels 1957, p. 602 (North Holland, Amsterdam 1959).
12. Arizono, H.; Iwasaki, M.; Ihara, Y. and Okamoto, S.: Hypothalamohypophyseal neurosecretory responses to pain. J. Osaka Univ. *9:* 339 (1958).
13. Armstrong, D. T.; Schmidt, G. H. and Hansel, W.: Neurohypophyseal regulation of bovine ovarian function. Proc. canad. Fed. Biol. Soc. *2:* 4 (1959).
14. Asburn, L. L.; Daft, F. S.; Endicott, K. M. and Sebrell, W. H.: Lesions in rats given sulfaguanidine in purified diets. Publ. Hlth Rep., Wash. *57:* 1883 (1942).
15. Ashwin, J. G.: Effect of reserpine on adrenalectomized rats. Proc. Soc. exp. Biol. N. Y. *104:* 188 (1960).
16. Assenmacher, I.: Recherches sur le contrôle hypothalamique de la fonction gonadotrope préhypophysaire chez le canard. Arch. Anat. micr. *47:* 447 (1958).
17. Arvay, A.; Balázsy, L.; Jakubecz, S. und Takács, I.: Die Wirkung belastender Nervenreize auf die Struktur und Funktion der Nebennierenrinde. Endokrinologie *39:* 15 (1960).
18. Arvay, A.; Kertész, L. and Lampe, L.: The effect of severe nervous stimulation on pituitary, adrenal and ovarian function. Studies with $P^{32}$. Acta endocrin., Kbh. *30:* 585 (1959).
19. Bachrach, D.: A hypothalamus neurosecretiós müködése néhány föbb kérdéséröl (patkánykisérletek alapján). Kisérl. Orvostud. *10:* 256 (1958).
20. Bahn, R. C.; Storino, H. E. and Schmit, R. W.: The mass of the zona glomerulosa following complete anterior and posterior hypophysectomy and subtotal removal of the pars tuberalis in the dog. Endocrinology *66:* 403 (1960).
21. Bajusz, E.: Über Balneo- und Klimatoreaktionen der Muskeln: Angaben zum Problem der organismischen Verteidigungsregulation. Arch. phys. Ther. *7:* 333 (1955).

22. Bajusz, E.: Blutdruck bei Phosphat-Steroid-Kardiopathie. Z. ges. exp. Med. *130:* 13 (1958).
23. Bajusz, E.: Hormonal production of muscular atrophy in limited vascular territories. Rev. cand. Biol. *17:* 483 (1958).
24. Bajusz, E.: Hormonal bedingte lokale Muskelatrophie. Naturwissenschaften *45:* 271 (1958).
25. Bajusz, E.: Disuse atrophy of skeletal muscle in the rat, aggravated by cortisol and various stress conditions. Canad. J. Biochem. *36:* 825 (1958).
26. Bajusz, E.: Prevention and aggravation of a proteolytic enzyme produced myocardial necroses. Symp. Infarctoid Cardiopathy, ann. Meet. Montreal Phys. Soc., Montreal 1959.
27. Bajusz, E.: Stress und Stress-Therapie. Übersicht mit besonderer Berücksichtigung der Herzschädigung im Sinne von Nekrose oder Entzündung. Z. angew. Bäder-Klimaheilk. *5:* 446 (1958).
28. Bajusz, E.: Neuromuscular atrophy and regeneration, as influenced by hormones. Proc. canad. Fed. Biol. Soc. *1:* 4 (1958).
29. Bajusz, E.: Effect of hormones upon regression of muscle atrophy of nervous origin. Endocrinology *64:* 262 (1959).
30. Bajusz, E.: A study concerning the actions of hydrocortisone acetate on the complex neuromuscular recovery. Acta neuroveg. *20:* 219 (1959).
31. Bajusz, E.: Influence of humoral agents upon recovery of sensory and motor function after nerve lesion. I. Effect of cortisol, desoxycorticosterone, somatotrophic hormone and methyltestosterone. Z. Vitamin-, Hormon-, Fermentforsch. *10:* 81 (1959).
32. Bajusz, E : Influence of humoral agents upon recovery of sensory and motor function after nerve lesion. II. Effect of estradiol, thyroxin, dihydrotachysterol, aminoacetonitrile, vitamin-A and $NaH_2PO_4$. Z. Vitamin-, Hormon, Fermentforsch. *10:* 212 (1959).
33. Bajusz, E.: Unspecific systemic stress reactions and necrotizing cardiopathies. Amer. J. phys. Med. *39:* 153 (1960).
34. Bajusz, E.: Neuroendocrine relationships; in: Progr. Neurol. Psychiat., vol. XV, p. 233, ed. E. A. Spiegel (Grune & Stratton, New York 1960).
35. Bajusz, E.: Neuroendocrine relationships; in: Progr. Neurol. Psychiat., vol. XVI (p. 233), ed. E. A. Spiegel (Grune & Stratton, New York 1961).
36. Bajusz, E. and Fitko, R.: Rola stressu i hormonov kory cadnerezy w powstawaniu doswiadezalnej martwicy micania serca. Fol. Tyg. Lekarski *15:* 6 (1960).
37. Bajusz, E. and Fitko, R.: Udzial hormenow w scherzoniach aiezaleznych od zaburzen w nkladzie dokrewnym. Pol. Tyg. Lekarski *15:* 201 (1960).
38. Bajusz, E. und Kövary, L.: Korrelation zwischen Umgebungstemperatur und Toxizität des Reduktionsindikators Triphenyltetrazoliumchlorid (TTC). Naturwissenschaften *42:* 561 (1955).
39. Bajusz, E. and Nádasdi, M.: Interactions between steroid hormones in the production of experimental myocardial necroses. Folia Endocrin. *11:* 446 (1958).
40. Bajusz, E. and Selye, H.: An experimental type of muscular dystrophy and role of chloride in its prevention. Proc canad. Fed. Biol. Soc. *2:* 5 (1959).
41. Bajusz, E. and Selye, H.: Convulsive neuromuscular disorders as influenced by hormones and stress conditions. IX. int. Congr. Paediatr., Montreal 1959.
42. Bajusz, E. and Selye, H.: Conditioning factors for cardiac necroses. Trans. N. Y. Acad. Sci. *21:* 659 (1959).
43. Bajusz, E. and Selye, H.: Effect of various hormones upon the muscular contractions induced by sodium perchlorate. Acta pharmacol. *15:* 235 (1959).
44. Bajusz, E. and Selye, H.: Influence of variations in dietary intake of chlorides upon diverse necrotizing cardiopathies. Amer. Heart J. *60:* 268 (1960).

45. Bajusz, E. and Selye, H.: Adaptation to the cardiac necrosis-eliciting effect of stress. Amer. J. Physiol. *199:* 453 (1960).
46. Bajusz, E. and Selye, H.: Como alteran las reacciones inespecificas de adaptacion, la susceptibilidad para enfermedades renales y cardiovasculares? Un estudio experimental de la resistencia cruzada. Folia clin. int. *10:* 260 (1960).
47. Bajusz, E. and Selye, H.: The chemical prevention of cardiac necroses following occlusion of coronary vessels. Canad. med. Ass. J. *82:* 212 (1960).
48. Bajusz, E. und Selye, H.: Über die durch Stress bedingte Nekroseresistenz des Herzens. Ein Beitrag zum Phänomen der gekreuzten Resistenz. Naturwissenschaften *47:* 520 (1960).
49. Bajusz, E. and Selye, H.: The role of dietary chloride in the pathogenesis of cardiac necroses. 5th int. Congr. Nutrit., Washington, D. C. 1960.
50. Bajusz, E. and Selye, H.: Neuromuscular disorders as elicited by dietary chloride excess or deficiency. Fed. Proc. *19:* 295 (1960).
51. Bajusz, E. and Selye, H.: Anion-kation kölcsönhatások a szivizominfarctus kémiai megelözésénél. Kisérletes vizsgálatok ioncserélö polisztirol-gyantákkal. Kisérl. Orvostud. *12:* 283 (1960).
52. Bajusz, E.; Selye, H. and Strebel, R.: Neuroleptic phenothiazine derivatives and stress-induced cardiac necroses. 3rd World Congr. Psychiatr., Montreal 1961.
53. Bajusz, E. and Selye, H.: Sensitization by chloride deficiency to corticoid-induced cardiac necroses. Acta endocrin., Kbh. *36:* 295 (1961).
54. Baker, B. L. and Whitaker, L. W.: Interference with local wound healing by the local action of adrenocortical steroids. Endocrinology *46:* 544 (1950).
55. Baker, G. D.: Electrolyte metabolism in the rat exposed to a low environmental temperature. Canad. J. Biochem. *38:* 205 (1960).
56. Baker, W. J.: Intradermal salt solution test in scarlet fever and diphtheria patients. J. amer. med. Ass. *83:* 1566 (1924).
57. Baló, J. and Banga, I.: Elastolytic activity of pancreatic extracts. Biochem J. *46:* 384 (1950).
58. Bansi, H. W. und Olsen, J. M.: Das antidiuretische Prinzip (ADH) und die Osmolarität im Serum bei der Adipositas. Acta endocrin., Kbh. *31:* 426 (1959).
59. Bard, P. A.: A diencephalic mechanism for the expression of rage with special reference to the sympathetic nervous system. Amer. J. Physiol. *84:* 490 (1928).
60. Bard, P.: Anatomical organization of the central nervous system in relation to control of the heart and blood vessels. Physiol. Rev. (Suppl. 4) *40:* 3 (1960).
61. Bargerson, L. M.: Ehmke, D.; Gonlubol, F.; Castellanos, A.; Siegel, A. and Bing, R. J.: Effect of cigarette smoking on coronary blood flow and myocardial metabolism. Circulation *15:* 251 (1957).
62. Barlow, J. C. and Sellers, E. A.: Effect of exposure to cold on response of the rat to whole body radiation. Amer. J. Physiol. *172:* 147 (1953).
63. Bartter, F. C.; Mills, I. H.; Biglieri, E. G. and Delea, C.: Studies on the control and physiologic action of aldosterone. Proc. Laurentian Hormone Conf., 1958; Recent Progr. Hormone Res. *15:* 311 (1959).
64. Basowitz, H.; Persky, H.; Korchin, S. J. and Grinker, R. R.: Anxiety and stress (McGraw-Hill, New York 1955).
65. Bauer, H. G.: Endocrine and metabolic conditions related to pathology in the hypothalamus: a review. J. nerv. ment. Dis. *128:* 323 (1959).
66. Bauer, K. F.: Die Neurohypophyse als Resorptionsorgan. Fortschr. Med. *76:* 621 (1958).
67. Beals, R. and Heijer, H.: An introduction to anthropology, p. 249 (Macmillan, New York 1959).
68. Beau, J. le et Foncin, J. F.: Régénération des vaisseaux du système porte hypo-

thalmo-hypophysaire chez l'homme après hypophysectomie et section de la tige pituitaire. Rev. neurol. *100:* 58 (1959).

69. Beau, J. le and Foncin, J. F.: Anatomical study of anterior pituitary remnants after (1)—stalk section, (2)—hypophysectomy. Acta psychiat. scand. *35:* 13 (1960).

70. Beaulnes, A. and Poirier, L. J.: Effect of tranquilizers on the glycemic and leucocytic response to immobilization in the monkey. Proc. canad. Fed. Biol. Soc. *2:* 8 (1959).

71. Beck, E. and Daniel, P. M.: Some changes in the hypothalamus and proximal pituitary stalk after stalk section. Proc. Soc. physiol., 1959. – J. Physiol., Lond. *146:* 22 (1959).

72. Becker, R. M.: Suppression of local tissue reactivity (Shwartzman phenomenon) by nitrogen mustard, benzol and X-ray irradiation. Proc. Soc. exp. Biol., N. Y. *69:* 247 (1948).

73. Beecher, H. K.: The use of morphine as a therapeutic agent Surg. Gynec. Obstet. *81:* 461 (1945).

74. Beecher, H. K.: Treatment of the state of shock XVI. Problems of sedation and anesthesia in the shock patient. Symp. on Shock, Washington 1951.

75. Bell, E. T.: A post mortem study of vascular disease in diabetics. Arch. Pathol. *53:* 444 (1952).

76. Bellet, S.; West, J. W.; Manzoli, U. C.; Muller, O. F. and Rossi P.: Effect of nicotine on the coronary blood flow in the presence of coronary insufficiency: an experimental study in dogs Ann. N. Y. Acad. Sci. *90:* 317 (1960).

77. Bennett, H. S.; Bassett, D. L. and Beecher, H. K.: Influence of anesthesia (ether, cyclopropane, sodium evipal) on circulation under normal and shock conditions. J. clin. Invest. *23:* 181 (1944).

78. Benoit, J. and Assenmacher, I.: The control by visible radiations of the gonadotropic activity of the duck hypophysis. Proc. Laurentian Hormone Conf., 1958; Recent Progr. Hormone Res. *15:* 143 (1959).

79. Benoit, J. et Assenmacher, I.: Système nerveux central et contrôle de la fonction gonadotrope préhypophysaire. Acta endocrin., Kbh. (Suppl. 50) *34:* 9 (1960).

80. Berger, E. Y.; Quinn, G. P. and Homer, M. A.: Effect of desoxycorticosterone on the colon: its relation to the action of cation exchange resins in man. Proc. Soc. exp. Biol., N. Y. *76:* 601 (1951).

81. Bernard, C.: Introduction à l'étude de la médecine expérimentale (Flammarion, Paris 1876).

82. Berthrong, M.; Rich, A. R. and Griffith, P. C.: Study on the effect of adrenocorticotropic hormone upon the experimental cardiovascular lesions produced by anaphylactic hypersensitivity. Bull. Johns Hopk. Hosp. *86:* 131 (1950).

83. Bierwagen, M. E. and Smith, D. L.: A mechanism of action for antithyroid activity of reserpine. Proc. Soc. exp. Biol., N.Y. *100:* 108 (1959).

84. Bishop, J. S. and Marks, P. A.: Studies on carbohydrate metabolism in patients with neoplastic disease. II. Response to insulin administration. J. clin. Invest. *38:* 668 (1959).

85. Blanquet, P. and Tobias, C. A.: Hypothalamic irradiation in the rat. J. clin. Invest. *37:* 878 (1958).

86. Bogdanove, E. M. and D'Angelo, S. A.: The effects of hypothalamic lesions on goitrogenesis and pituitary TSH secretion in the propyl thiouracil-treated guinea pig. Endocrinology *64:* 53 (1959).

87. Bogdanove, E. M. and Schoen, H. C.: Precocious sexual development in female rats with hypothalamic lesions. Proc. Soc. exp. Biol., N. Y. *100:* 664 (1959).

88. Bonnycastle, D. D. and Bradley, A. J.: Diphenylhydantoin and the release of adrenocorticotropic hormone in the albino rat. Endocrinology *66:* 355 (1960).

89. Booker, W. M.; DaCosta, F.; Mitchell, S. C. and Robinson, E. J.: The effects of cortisone on the perfused rabbit heart. J. Pharmacol., Baltimore *116:* 8 (1956).

90. Boulanger, J. B.: Neurobiologie et psychopathologie. Un. méd. Canada *89:* 590 (1960).
91. Brettschneider, H.: Die Feinstruktur des nervösen Parenchyms von Infundibulum und Neurohypophyse. II. Die Neurosekretion. Z. mikr.-anat. Forsch. *64:* 575 (1958).
92. Brigden, W.: Uncommon myocardial diseases. The non-coronary cardiomyopathies. Lancet, p. 1179 (1957).
93. Brown, H.; Willardson, D. G.; Samuels, L. T. and Tyler, F. H.: 17-hydroxy-corticosteroid metabolism in liver disease. J. clin. Invest. *33:* 1524 (1954).
94. Brown-Grant, K.: The hypothalamus and the thyroid gland. Brit. med. Bull. *18:* 165 (1960).
95. Bryant, R. E.; Thomas, W. A. and O'Neal, R. M.: An electron microscopic study of myocardial ischemia in the rat. Circulation *6:* 699 (1958).
96. Bunim, J. J.: Corticotropin and corticosteroids: chemistry, physiology and metabolic effects; in: Arthritis and allied conditions, 6th edition, p. 342, ed. J. L. Hollander (Lea & Febiger, Philadelphia 1960).
97. Büchner, F. und Lucadou, W.: Elektrokardiographische Veränderungen und disseminierte Nekrosen des Herzmuskels bei experimenteller Koronarinsuffizienz. Beitr. path. Anat. *93:* 169 (1934).
98. Bürger, M. und Seidel, K.: Innere Sekretion. Münch. med. Wschr. *102:* 2174 (1960).
99. Bykov, K. M.: The cerebral cortex and the internal organs; translated by W. H. Gantt (Chemical Publ., New York 1957).
100. Campanacci, M.: Osservazioni istochimiche sul neurosecreto ipotalamo-postipofisario nel ratto. Boll. Soc. ital. Biol. sper. *35:* 241 (1959).
101. Campbell, H. J.; George, R. and Harris, G. W.: The acute effects of injection of thyrotrophic hormone or of electrical stimulation of the hypothalamus on thyroid activity. J. Physiol., Lond. *152:* 527 (1960).
102. Cannon, C. and Booker, W. M.: Acute toxic effects of cortisone on the heart. Fed. Proc. *16:* 287 (1957).
103. Cannon, P. R.; Frazier, L. E. and Hughes, R. H.: Sodium as a toxic ion in potassium deficiency. Metabolism *2:* 297 (1953).
104. Cannon, W. B.: Bodily changes in pain, hunger, fear and rage (Appleton, New York 1929).
105. Cannon, W. B.: The wisdom of the body (W. W. Norton, New York 1939).
106. Carlson, A. S.; Kellner, A. and Bernheimer, A. W.: Selective inhibition by preparations of streptococcal filtrates of the oxidative metabolism of mitochondria procured from rabbit myocardium. J. exp. Med. *104:* 577 (1956).
107. Carter, A. E.: Elastase production in the canine pancreas. Science *123:* 669 (1956).
108. Casentini, S.; De Poli, A.; Hukovic, S. and Martini, L.: Studies on the control of corticotrophin release. Endocrinology *64:* 483 (1959).
109. Cavelti, P. A.: Studies on the pathogenesis of rheumatic fever. Amer. med. ass. Arch. Pathol. *44:* 1 (1947).
110. Cavelti, P. A.: Cardiac lesions produced in rats by means of autoantibodies to heart and connective tissue. Amer. med. ass. Arch. Pathol. *44:* 13 (1947).
111. Chaikoff, I. L. and Kaplan, A.: On the survival of the completely depancreatized dog. J. Nutr. *14:* 459 (1937).
112. Chance, M. R. A.: Aggregation as factor influencing toxicity of sympathomimetic amines in mice. J. Pharmacol., Baltimore *87:* 214 (1946).
113. Chance, M. R. A.: Factors influencing toxicity of sympathomimetic amines to solitary mice. J. Pharmacol., Baltimore 289 (1947).
114. Char, D. F. B. and Wagner, B. M.: The cardiac effects of group A streptococcal sonicates in rabbits. Ann. N. Y. Acad. Sci. *86:* 1009 (1960).

115. Charvat, J.; Schreiber, V. and Kmentova, V.: Effect of hypothalamic extracts on pituitary phosphatases in vitro: an increase in the activity of acid phosphatase. Rev. czechoslov. Med. *5:* 1 (1959).
116. Chauvet, J. et Achier, R.: Influence de la vasopressine sur la sécrétion de la corticotropine (ACTH). Ann. Endocrin. *20:* 111 (1959).
117. Christensen, L. K.: Pituitary regulation of thyroid activity. Acta endocrin., Kbh. *33:* 111 (1960).
118. Christian, J. J.: The roles of endocrine and behavioral factors in the growth of mammalian populations; in: Comparative endocrinology, ed. A. Gorbmann p. 71 (Wiley & Sons, New York 1959).
119. Christian, J. J.: Adrenocortical and gonadal responses of female mice to increased population density. Proc. Soc. exp. Biol., N. Y. *104:* 330 (1960).
120. Clampit, J.: Chemotherapy of allergic arteritis in the rabbit. Fed. Proc. *9:* 263 (1950).
121. Clawson, B. J. and Bell, E. T.: Incidence of fatal coronary disease in nondiabetic and in diabetic persons. Amer. med. ass. Arch. Pathol. *48:* 105 (1949).
122. Codaccioni, J. L. et Pache, R.: Les facteurs nerveux et hormonaux de la faim. Sud. med. chir., Marseille *94:* 634 (1959).
123. Cohen, H.; Megel, H. and Kleinberg, W.: Pancreatic elastase. I. Observations on cellular source and endocrine influence. Proc. Soc. exp. Biol., N. Y. *97:* 8 (1958).
124. Colby, R. W. and Frye, C. M.: Effect of feeding various levels of calcium, potassium and magnesium to rats. Amer. J. Physiol. *166:* 209 (1951).
125. Cole, R. I.: Experimental streptococcus arthritis in relation to the etiology of acute articular rheumatism. J. infect. Dis. *1:* 74 (1904).
126. Collens, M. W.; Banowitch, M. M. and Colsky, J.: Lipoprotein studies in diabetics with arteriosclerotic disease. J. amer. med. Ass. *155:* 814 (1955).
127. Comroe, J. H., Jr.: The pharmacological actions of nicotine. Ann. N. Y. Acad. Sci. *90:* 48 (1960).
128. Conway, E. J. and Hingerty, D.: The effects of cortisone, desoxycorticosterone and other steroids on the active transport of sodium and potassium ions in yeast. Biochem. J. *55:* 455 (1953).
129. Cook, E. B. and Wherry, R. J.: The urinary 17-ketosteroid output of Naval Submarine enlisted candidates during two stressful situations. Human Biol. *22:* 104 (1950).
130. Cook, L.; Davidson, A.; Davis, D. L. and Kelleher, R. T.: Epinephrine, norepinephrine and acetylcholine as conditioned stimuli for avoidance behavior. Science *131:* 990 (1960).
131. Corbin, A. and Schottelius, H. A.: Effects of posterior hypothalamic lesions on sexual maturation of immature female albino rats. Proc. Soc. exp. Biol., N.Y. *103:* 208 (1960).
132. Cordier, D. et Touze, M.: Troubles de l'absorption intestinale du glucose au cours du choc traumatique. C. R. Soc. Biol. *142:* 91 (1948).
133. Covian, M. R.; Migliorini, R. H. and Tramezzani, J. H.: Endocrine changes in hemidecorticated rats. Acta physiol. latinoamer. *9:* 24 (1959).
134. Critchlow, V.: Blockade of ovulation in the rat by mesencephalic lesions. Endocrinology *63:* 596 (1958).
135. Crossfield, H. C.; Da Vanzo, J. P. and Swingle, W. W.: Alteration of electrocardiographic pattern and cardiac rhythm by adrenal steroids in normal and adrenalectomized dogs. Circulation *18:* 710 (1958).
136. Croxatto, H. Natural and synthetic related substances having neurohypophyseal hormone-like activities. Acta endocrin., Kbh. (Suppl. 50) *34:* 33 (1960).
137. Cruz, A. R.: Sur l'existence d'un système porte dans la neuro-hypophyse des amphibiens anoures. Acta anat. *36:* 153 (1959).

138. Currie, A. R.; Adamsons, H. and Van Dyke, H. B.: Vasopressin and oxytocin in the posterior lobe of the pituitary of man. J. clin. Endocrin. *20:* 947 (1960).
139. Dale, H. H. and Laidlaw, P. P.: The significance of the suprarenal capsule in the action of certain alkaloids. J. Physiol., Lond. *45:* 1 (1912).
140. D'Angelo, S. A.: Ovarian and adrenal function in hyperthyroid hypothalamic-lesioned rats. Fed. Proc. *18:* 33 (1959).
141. D'Angelo, S. A. and Kravatz, A. S.: Gonadotrophic hormone function in persistent estrous rats with hypothalamic lesions. Proc. Soc. exp. Biol., N. Y. *104:* 130 (1960).
142. Daniel, P. M.; Prichard, M. M. L. and Smith, B.: The extent of the infarct in the anterior pituitary found soon after pituitary stalk section in the baboon and the rhesus monkey. Proc. Soc. Physiol. (1959). – J. Physiol. Lond. *146:* 2 (1959).
143. Danowski, T. S.: Diabetes mellitus. With emphasis on children and young adults (Williams & Wilkins, Baltimore 1957).
144. Dare, J. G. and Mogey, G. A.: Rabbit responses to human threshold doses of a bacterial pyrogen. J. Pharmacol., Baltimore *6:* 325 (1954).
145. Daume, E. und Hohlweg, W.: Über die Wirkung intrazerebral verabreichten Thyroxins bei Ratten. Endokrinologie *38:* 51 (1959).
146. Davidson, J. M. and Ganong, W. P.: The effect of hypothalamic lesions on the testes and prostate of male dogs. Endocrinology *66:* 480 (1960).
147. Davis, S. W. and Elmadjiann, F.: A study of combat stress: Korea 1952. Operations Research Office, Johns Hopk. Univ. (1952).
148. Dear, W. E. and Guillemin, R.: Adrenal sensitivity to ACTH as a function of time after hypothalamic lesion and after hypophysectomy. Proc. Soc. exp. Biol., N. Y. *103:* 356 (1960).
149. Dearing, W. H.; Barnes, A. R. and Essex, H. E.: Experiments with calculated therapeutic and toxic doses of digitalis. I. Effects on the myocardial cellular structure. Amer. Heart J. *25:* 648 (1943).
150. Decourt, J. et Michard, J. P.: Le retentissement endocrinien des maigreurs par oligophagie d'origine psycho-névrotique. Sem. Hôp. Paris *7:* 355 (1960).
151. Delgado, J. M. R.: Circulatory effects of cortical stimulation. Physiol. Rev. (Suppl. 4) *40:* 146 (1960).
152. Dellmann, H. D.: Beitrag zur Kenntnis des Hypothalamus-Hypophysen-Systems beim Rind. I. Anat. Anz. *106:* 202 (1959).
153. Dellmann, H. D.: Beitrag zur Kenntnis des Hypothalamus-Hypophysen-Systems beim Rind. II. Morphologische Untersuchungen am Hypothalamus-Hinterlappen-System. Anat. Anz. *107:* 230 (1959).
154. Dellmann, H. D.: Untersuchungen über Morphologie und Entstehung besonderer nervöser Strukturen in der Neurohypophyse des Rindes und ihre Bedeutung als Bildungsstätte des Neurosekrets. Dtsch. Z. Nervenheilk. *180:* 509 (1960).
155. Denamour, R. et Martinet, J.: Le rôle du système nerveux de la glande mammaire dans l'entretien de la lactation. Arch. Sci. physiol. *13:* 217 (1959).
156. Dierickx, K.; Van den Abeele, A. et Rysenaer, M.: Phénomènes d'activité cyclique dans le système hypothalamo-hypophysaire de Rana temporaria. Arch. Anat. micr. *49:* 73 (1960).
157. Dolger, H.: An assessment of oral antidiabetic therapy. J. Mt. Sinai Hosp. *27:* 33 (1960).
158. Donovan, B. T. and Werff-Bosch, J. J.: The hypothalamus and sexual maturation in the rat. J. Physiol., Lond. *147:* 78 (1959).
159. Dragstedt, L. R.: The role of the pancreas in arteriosclerosis. Biol. Symposia *11:* 118 (1945).
160. Dreyfuss, F.: Role of emotional stress preceding coronary occlusion. Amer. J. Cardiol. *3:* 590 (1959).

161. DREYFUSS, F. and CZACZKES, J. W.: Blood cholesterol and uric acid of healthy medical students under stress of an examination. Arch. intern. Med. *103:* 708 (1959).
162. DRILL, V. A. and RIEGEL, B.: Structural and hormonal activity of some new steroids. Laurentian Hormone Conf., 1957. Recent Progr. Hormone Res. *14:* 29 (1958).
163. DUCHENSE, P. Y.: Evolution de la neurosécrétion hypothalamique avec l'âge. Acta neurol. belg. *59:* 1258 (1959).
164. DUFF, G. L.; BRECHIN, D. J. H. and FINKELSTEIN, W. E.: The effect of alloxan diabetes and experimental cholesterol atherosclerosis in the rabbit. J. exp. Med. *100:* 371 (1954).
165. DUFF, G. L. and PAYNE, T. P. B.: The effect of alloxan diabetes on experimental cholesterol atherosclerosis in the rabbit. J. exp. Med. *92:* 299 (1950).
166. DULIN, W. E.; BOWMAN, B. J. and STAFFORD, R. O.: Effects of 2-methylation on glucocorticoid activity of various C-21 steroids. Proc. Soc. exp. Biol., N. Y. *94:* 303 (1957).
167. DUNCAN, C. H.; STEVENSON, I. P. and WOLFF, H. G.: Live situations, emotions, and exercise tolerance. Psychosom. Med. *13:* 36 (1951).
168. DUNCAN, G. G.: Diabetes mellitus. Disorders of metabolism, ed. G G. DUNCAN, 3rd edition (Saunders, Philadelphia 1952).
169. DZIENATKOWSKI, D. D.: Radioautographic studies of sulfate-sulfur ($S^{35}$) metabolism in articular cartilage and bone of suckling rats. J. exp. Med. *95:* 489 (1952).
170. EGDAHL, R. H.: Adrenal cortical and medullary responses to trauma in dogs with isolated pituitaries. Endocrinology *66:* 200 (1960).
171. EHRICH, W. E.; SEIFTER, J. and FERMAN, C. J.: Experimental serum disease: a pathogenetic study. J. exp. Med. *89:* 23 (1948).
172. EKMAN, B.; THARESE, S. and TRUIDSON, E.: Investigations of viscosity and hyaluronidase inhibitors in joint exudate after intra-articular cortisone injection. Scand. J. clin. Lab. Invest. *5:* 175 (1953).
173. ELLIS, J. T.: Necrosis and regeneration of skeletal muscles in cortisone-treated rabbits. Amer. J. Pathol. *32:* 993 (1956).
174. ELWERS, M. and CRITCHLOW, V.: Precocious ovarian stimulation following hypothalamic and amygdaloid lesions in rats. Amer. J. Physiol. *198:* 381 (1960).
175. EMELE, J. F. and BONNYCASTLE, D. D.: Cardiotonic activity of some adrenal steroids. Amer. J. Physiol. *185:* 103 (1956).
176. ENAMI, M.: The morphology and functional significance of the caudal neurosecretory system of fishes; in: Comparative endocrinology, ed. A. GORBMAN, p. 897 (Wiley, New York 1959).
177. ENGEL, F. L.: A consideration of the roles of the adrenal cortex and stress in the regulation of protein metabolism. Proc. Laurentian Hormone Conf., 1950. – Recent Progr. Hormone Res. *6:* 277 (1951).
178. ENGEL, F. L.: Some thoughts on the biochemistry of the steroid hormones; in: essays in biochemistry, ed. S. GRAFF, p. 85 (Wiley, New York 1955)
179. ENGEL, F. L. and FREDERICKS, J.: Contribution to understanding of mechanism of permissive action of corticoids. Proc. Soc. exp. Biol., N. Y. *94:* 593 (1957).
180. ENGLERT, E., Jr.; BROWN, H.; WALLACH, S. and SIMONS, E. L.: Metabolism of free and conjugated 17-hydroxycorticosteroids in subjects with liver disease. J. clin. Endocrin. *17:* 1395 (1957).
181. EPSTEIN, F. H. and LEVITIN, H.: Cerebral salt-wasting: an example of sustained inappropriate release of antidiuretic hormone. 51st ann. Meet. amer. Soc. clin. Invest. (Atlantic City 1959).
182. ERB, W.: Experimentelle und histologische Studien über Arterienerkrankung nach Adrenalininjektionen. Arch. exp. Path. Pharmakol. *53:* 173 (1905).
183. EULER, U. S. v.; GEMZELL, C. A.; LEVI, L. and STRÖM, G.: Cortical and medullary adrenal activity in emotional stress. Acta endocrin., Kbh. *30:* 567 (1959).

184. Everett, J. W.: Neuroendocrine mechanisms in control of the mammalian ovary; in: Comparative endocrinology, ed. A. Gorbman, p. 174 (Wiley, New York 1959).
185. Farrell, G.: Glomerulotropic activity of an acetone extract of pineal tissue. Endocrinology *65:* 239 (1959).
186. Farrell, G.: The physiological factors which influence the secretion of aldosterone. Proc. Laurentian Hormone Conf. 1958. – Recent Progr. Hormone Res. *15:* 275 (1959).
187. Farrell, G.: The control of aldosterone secretion: influence of the epiphysis cerebri. Acta endocrin., Kbh. (Suppl. 50) *34:* 57 (1960).
188. Favarger, H.: Die chronische Tabakvergiftung und ihren Einfluß auf das Herz und den Magen. Wien klin. Wschr. *11–14:* (1887), quoted by Ahn B. von: Tobacco smoking, the electrocardiogram, and angina pectoris. Ann. N. Y. Acad. Sci. *90:* 190 (1960).
189. Feldman, A.: The intradermal salt solution test in tuberculosis. Arch. intern. Med. *41:* 549 (1928).
190. Feldman, S. and Cohen, A. M.: A disorder of the central nervous system with hypogonadism and thyroid dysfunction. Acta endocrin., Kbh. *30:* 70 (1959).
191. Feldman, S.; Van der Heide, C. and Porter, R. W.: Evoked potentials in the hypothalamus. Amer. J. Physiol. *196:* 1163 (1959).
192. Fiedler, A.: Über akute interstitielle Myokarditis. Festschrift zur Feier des 50jährigen Bestehens des Stadtkrankenhauses zu Dresden-Friedrichstadt; abstract in: Zbl. inn. Med. *21:* 212 (1900).
193. Firket, H.: L'hypophyse. Structure et histophysiologie. Rev. méd., Liège *14:* 236 (1959).
194. Fischer, B.: Über Arterienerkrankungen nach Adrenalininjektionen. Münch. med. Wschr. *22:* 235 (1905).
195. Fiske, V. M. and Greep, R. G.: Neurosecretory activity in rats under conditions of continuous light or darkness. Endocrinology *64:* 175 (1959).
196. Fiske, V. M.; Bryant, G. K. and Putman, J.: Effect of light on the weight of the pineal in the rat. Endocrinology *66:* 489 (1960).
197. Flach, F.; Stokes, P. E.; Liang, E.; Diethelm, O. and Rawson, R. W.: The metabolic effects of thyroid analogues in psychiatric patients. Ann. N. Y. Acad. Sci. *86:* 582 (1960).
198. Fleckenstein, A.: Der Kalium-Natrium-Austausch als Energieprinzip im Muskel und Nerven (Springer, Berlin 1955).
199. Florsheim, W. H.: Influence of hypothalamus on pituitary-thyroid axis in the rat. Proc. Soc. exp. Biol., N. Y. *100:* 73 (1950).
200. Folkow, B.: Range of control of cardiovascular system by the central nervous system. Physiol. Rev. (Suppl. 4) *40:* 93 (1960).
201. Folkow, B.; Johansson, B. and Oberg, B.: A hypothalamic structure with a marked inhibitory effect on tonic sympathetic activity. Acta physiol. scand. *47:* 262 (1959).
202. Follis, R. H., Jr.: Myocardial necroses in rats on a potassium low diet prevented by thiamine deficiency. Bull. Johns Hopk. Hosp. *71:* 235 (1942).
203. Follis, R. H., Jr.: Effect of exercise on rats fed a diet deficient in potassium. Proc. Soc. exp. Biol., N. Y. *51:* 71 (1942).
204. Follis, R. H., Jr.: Deficiency disease. Functional and structural changes in mammalia which result from exogenous or endogenous lack of one or more essential nutritients (Thomas, Springfield 1958).
205. Follis, R. H., Jr.; Orent-Keiles, E. and McCollum, E. V.: The production of cardiac and renal lesions in rats by a diet extremely deficient in potassium. Amer. J. Pathol. *18:* 29 (1942).
206. Ford, D. H.: Factors influencing the histological visualization of the neurosecretory

system of the rat when stained by the Gomori chrome alum hematoxylin phloxin technique. Acta anat. *37:* 153 (1959).

207. Fortier, C.: Dual control of adrenocorticotrophin release. Endocrinology *49:* 782 (1951).

208. Fortier, C.: Comparative in vitro corticoidogenic effects of rat adenohypophysial extracts and U.S.P. reference standard corticotropin. Proc. Soc. exp. Biol., N. Y. *99:* 628 (1958).

209. Fortier, C.: Note on the extraction and storage of the rat pituitary prior to in vitro assay for ACTH. Canad. J. Biochem. *37:* 608 (1959).

210. Fortier, C.: Pituitary ACTH and plasma free corticosteroids following bilateral adrenalectomy in the rat. Proc. Soc. exp. Biol., N. Y. *100:* 13 (1959).

211. Fortier, C.; Groot, J. de and Hartfield, J. E.: Plasma free corticosteroid response to faradic stimulation in the rat. Acta endocrin., Kbh. *30:* 219 (1959).

212. Fortier, C. and Groot, J. de: Neuroendocrine relationships. Progr. Neurol. Psychiat., vol. XIV, p. 256, ed. E. A. Spiegel (Grune & Stratton, New York 1959).

213. Freed, S. C. and Friedman, M.: Depressor effect of potassium restriction on blood pressure of the rat. Proc. Soc. exp. Biol., N. Y. *78:* 74 (1951).

214. French, A. J. and Weller, C. V.: Interstitial myocarditis following the clinical and experimental use of sulfonamide drugs. Amer. J. Pathol. *18:* 109 (1942).

215. French, J. E.: Histologic study of heart lesions in potassium deficient rats. Arch. Path. *53:* 485 (1952).

216. Frick, E.: Tierexperimentelle Untersuchungen über eine tuberkulös-allergische Myokarditis. Z. ges. exp. Med. *117:* 393 (1951).

217. Fridberg, G. and Olsson, R.: The praeoptico-hypophysial system, nucleus tuberis lateralis and the subcommissural organ of Gastrosteus aculeatus after changes in osmotic stimuli. Z. Zellforsch. *49:* 531 (1959).

218. Friedman, M. and Rosenman, R. H.: Association of specific overt behavior pattern with blood and cardiovascular findings: Blood cholesterol level, blood clotting time, incidence of arcus senilis, and clinical coronary artery disease. J. amer. med. Ass. *169:* 1286 (1959).

219. Friedman, M.; Rosenman, R. H. and Carroll, V.: Changes in the serum cholesterol and blood clotting time in men subjected to cyclic variations of occupational stress. Circulation *17:* 852 (1958).

220. Friedman, S. M. and Friedman, C. L.: Self-sustained hypertension in the albino rat; a hypothesis to explain it. Canad. med. Ass. J. *61:* 596 (1949).

221. Fruhman, G. J.: The mobilization of neutrophils. Trans. N. Y. Acad. Sci. *23:* 30 (1960).

222. Fukuda, T. and Matsumoto, O.: Endogenous factors concerning the febrile and the leucocytic response to bacterial endotoxin in relation to the adrenal cortex. Jap. J. Physiol. *9:* 274 (1959).

223. Gabrielli, E.; Goldman, L. M. and Bernstein, A.: Effect of chemical hypothermia (hibernation) on experimental myocardial infarction in dogs. J. Newark Beth Israel Hosp. *10:* 201 (1959).

224. Gadek, A. and Paszko, Z.: Poszukiwania osrodkow podwzgorza pobudzajacych przysadke mozgowa do wydzielania hormonu adrenokortykotropowego u szczura. Endokryn. polska *9:* 125 (1958)

225. Gagnon, J. et Leblanc, R.: Sclérose cérébrale diffuse avec mélanodermie atrophique surrénale (maladie d'Addison-Scholz). Un. méd. Canada *88:* 392 (1959).

226. Gallien, L.: Endocrine basis for reproductive adaptations in amphibia; in: Comparative endocrinology, ed. A. Gorman, p. 479 (Wiley, New York 1959).

227. Ganong, W. F.: Adrenal-hypophyseal interrelations; in: Comparative endocrinology, ed. A. Gorbman, p. 187 (Wiley, New York 1959).

228. Ganong, W. F. and Forsham, P. H.: Adenohypophysis and adrenal cortex. Annu. Rev. Physiol., p. 579 (Annual Rev. Inc., Palo Alto 1960).

229. GELLERT, R. J. and GANONG, W. E.: Precocious puberty in rats with hypothalamic lesions. Acta endocrin., Kbh. *33:* 569 (1960).
230. GELLHORN, E.: Autonomic imbalance and the hypothalamus (Univ. of Minnesota Press, Minneapolis 1957).
231. GEORGE, R. and WAY, E. L.: The role of the hypothalamus in pituitary-adrenal activation and antidiuresis by morphine. J. Pharmacol., Baltimore *125:* 111 (1959).
232. GLASER, R. J.; THOMAS, W. A.; MORSE, S. I. and DARNELL, J. E., Jr.: The incidence and pathogenesis of myocarditis in rabbits after group A streptococcal pharyngeal infections. J. exp. Med. *103:* 173 (1956).
233. GOLD, M. I.; MACFARLANE, D. A. and MOORE, F. D.: Quantitative urinary 17-hydroxycorticoid patterns: effect of ACTH and 'operative stress'. J. clin. Endocrin. *16:* 282 (1956).
234. GOLDBERG, M. and FINE, J.: Traumatic shock XI. Intestinal absorption in hemorrhagic shock. J. clin. Invest. *24:* 445 (1945).
235. GOLDSCHMIDT, W.: Man's way, p. 122, 126 (Holt, New York 1959).
236. GOODOF, I. I. and MACBRYDE, C. M.: Heart failure in Addison's disease with myocardial changes of potassium deficiency. J. clin. Endocrin. *4:* 30 (1944).
237. GORBMAN, A. (ed.): Comparative endocrinology (Wiley, New York 1959).
238. GORBMAN, A. and ISHII, S.: Stimulation of neurosecretion in shark embryos by thyroid hormones. Proc. Soc. exp. Biol., N. Y. *103:* 865 (1960).
239. GORDON, A. S.; SIEGEL, C. D.; DORNFEST, B. S.; HANDLER, E. S.; LOBUE, J.; NERI, R. O. and EISLER, M.: Humoral regulation of leukocyte numbers. Trans. N. Y. Acad. Sci. *23:* 39 (1960).
240. GOVIER, W. M. and FEENSTRA, E. S.: The effect of certain hormones and miscellaneous compounds on serum disease in the rabbit. Amer. Heart J. *42:* 266 (1951).
241. GRASCHENKOV, N. I. and SEVASTYANOVA, G. A.: Endocrine disturbances in lesions of the diencephalic area (Russian text). Probl. Endocrin. *4:* 37 (1958 .– Ref.: Ex. Med. (Sect. III) *13:* 390 (1959).
242. GRAUX, P.: Le système neuro-végétatif. Données physiol. clin. Lille méd. *3:* 658 (1959).
243. GRAY, S. J. and RAMSEY, C. G.: Adrenal influences upon the stomach and the gastric responses to stress. Recent Progr. Hormone Res. Proc. Laurentian Hormone Conf. 1956 (Acad. Press, New York/London) *13:* 583 (1957).
244. GRAY, S. J.; BENSON, J. A., Jr. and REIFENSTEIN, R. W.: Effect of ACTH upon gastric secretion. Proc. Soc. exp. Biol., N. Y. *78:* 338 (1951).
245. GRAY, S. J.; BENSON, J. A., Jr. and REIFENSTEIN, R. W.: Chronic stress and peptic ulcer. I. Effect of corticotrophin (ACTH) and cortisone on gastric secretion. J. amer. med. Ass. *147:* 1529 (1951).
246. GREEN, D. E. and JÄRNEFELT, J.: Enzymes and biological organization. Perspect. Biol. Med. *2:* 163 (1959).
247. GREEN, D. M.: Hypertension. Third annu. Rep. on Stress, ed. H. SELYE and A. HORAVA, p. 277 (Acta, Montreal 1953).
248. GREEN, D. M.; SAUNDERS, F. J.; WAHLGREEN, N. and CRAIG, R. L.: Selfsustaining, post DCA hypertensive cardiovascular disease. Amer. J. Physiol. *170:* 94 (1952).
249. GREEN, J. D. and MAXWELL, D. S.: Comparative anatomy of the hypophysis and observations on the mechanism of neurosecretion; in: Comparative endocrinology, ed. A. GORBMAN, p. 368 (Wiley, New York 1959).
250. GREENBERG, D. M.; ANDERSON, C. E. and TUFTS, E. V.: Pathological changes in the tissues of rats reared on diets low in magnesium. Proc. 30th annu. Meet. amer. Soc. Biol. Chem., 1936.
251. GREER, M. A.; YAMADA, T. and IINO, S.: The participation of the nervous system in the control of thyroid function. Ann. N. Y. Acad. Sci. *86:* 667 (1960).

252. Griffiths, J. D. and Hoppe, E.: Effect of metabolic 'stress' on development of tumor following inoculation of Walker carcinosarcoma cells. Proc. Soc. exp. Biol., N. Y. *104:* 467 (1960).
253. Groot, J. de: The rat hypothalamus in stereotaxic coordinates. J. comp. Neurol. *113:* 389 (1959).
254. Grosvenor, C. E. and Turner, C. W.: Effects of oxytocin and blocking agents upon pituitary lactogen discharge in lactating rats. Proc. Soc. exp. N Y. Biol., *97:* 463 (1958).
255. Grosvenor, C. E. and Turner, C. W.: Pituitary lactogenic hormone concentration during pregnancy in the rat. Endocrinology *66:* 96 (1960).
256. Grundy, S. H. and Griffin, A. C.: Effects of periodic mental stress on serum cholesterol levels. Circulation *19:* 496 (1959).
257. Guillemin, R. and Schally, A. V.: Re-evaluation of a technique of pituitary incubation in vitro as an assay for corticotropin releasing factor. Endocrinology *65:* 555 (1959).
258. Guillemin, R.; Dear, W. E.; Nichols, B., Jr. and Lipscomb, H. S.: ACTH releasing activity in vivo of a CRF preparation and lysine vasopressin. Proc. Soc. exp. Biol., N. Y. *101:* 107 (1959).
259. Gunn, J. A. and Gurd, M. R.: Action of some amines related to adrenaline cyclohexylalkylamines. J. Physiol., Lond. *97:* 453 (1940).
260. Gutmann, E. and Jakoubek, B.: Nervous regulation of conditional hyperglycemia to nociceptive stimulation. Science *131:* 1096 (1960).
261. Halász, B. und Szentágothai, J.: Histologischer Beweis einer nervösen Signalübermittlung von der Nebennierenrinde zum Hypothalamus. Z. Zellforsch. *50:* 297 (1959).
262. Halberg, F.; Bittner, J. J. and Cole, H. L.: Activity rhythm and breast cancer in pituitary-isografted C and $D_8$ mice; effect of hypothalamus. Proc. Soc. exp. Biol., N. Y. *102:* 650 (1959).
263. Hajdu, S.: Mechanism of staircase and contracture in ventricular muscle. Amer. J. Physiol. *174:* 371 (1953).
264. Halpern, M. H.: The dual blood supply of the rat heart. Amer. J. Anat. *101:* 1 (1957).
265. Hammond, C. W.; Anderle, S. K. and Miller, C. P.: Effect of daily exposure to 15 r radiation on susceptibility of mice to experimental infection. Proc. Soc. exp. Biol., N. Y. *104:* 261 (1960).
266. Hammond, C. W.; Anderle, S. K. and Miller, C. P.: Attempts to increase resistance of mice to bacterial infection by prolonged low dose irradiation. Proc. Soc. exp. Biol., N. Y. *105:* 1 (1960).
267. Handa, Y. and Kumamoto, T.: Studies on some properties of neurosecretory substance. I. Z. Zellforsch. *47:* 647 (1958).
268. Hanig, M. and Lauter, M. A.: Ultracentrifugal studies of lipoproteins in diabetic sera. Diabetes *1:* 447 (1952).
269. Harkavy, J. and Perlman, E.: Tobacco allergy in coronary artery disease. Ann. N. Y. Acad. Sci. *90:* 327 (1960).
270. Harris, G. W.: Neural control of the pituitary gland (Arnold, London 1955).
271. Harris, G. W.: The reticular formation, stress, and endocrine activity; in: Jasper, H. H. *et al.:* Reticular formation of the brain (Little, Brown, Boston/Toronto 1958).
272. Harris, G. W.: Neuroendocrine control of TSH regulation; in: Comparative endocrinology, ed.: A. Gorbman, p. 202 (Wiley, New York 1959).
273. Harris, G. W.: Central nervous control of gonadotrophic and thyrotrophic secretion. Acta endocrin., Kbh. (Suppl. 50) *34:* 15 (1960).
274. Harrison, J.: Intradermal salt solution test in lobar pneumonia in children. J. amer. med. Ass. *84:* 1258 (1925).

275. Haynes, M. A.: The effect of prolonged local treatment with adrenalcortical and sex steroids on the intradermal spreading action of hyaluronidase. Endocrinology *52:* 646 (1954).
276. Hechter, O.: Reflections about hormone action and implications for the cancer problem. Cancer Res. *17:* 512 (1957).
277. Hechter, O. and Lester, G.: Cell permeability and hormone action. Recent Progr. Hormone Res. Proc. Laurentian Hormone Conf. 1959 (Acad. Press, New York/ London) *16:* 139 (1960).
278. Heiman, M.: Reproduction: emotions and the hypothalamic pituitary function. Fertil. Steril. *10:* 162 (1959).
279. Heimburger, R. F.: Injection into pericardial sac and ligation of coronary artery of the rat. Arch. Surg. *52:* 677 (1946).
280. Heller, H.: Die Hypophysenhinterlappen- und Nebennierenrindenhormone während der ersten Lebenszeit im Zusammenhang mit der Regulation des Wasserhaushaltes. Mschr. Kinderheilk. *106:* 81 (1958).
281. Heller, H.: Antidiuretic hormones of the neurohypophysis. Acta endocrin., Kbh. (Suppl. 50) *34:* 51 (1960).
282. Heller, H. and Lederis, K.: Maturation of the hypothalamo-neurohypophysial system. J. Physiol., Lond. *147:* 299 (1959).
283. Heller, H. and Lederis, K.: Posterior pituitary hormones of the hippopotamus. Proc. Physiol. Soc., Vet. Coll. Meet., 1960; J. Physiol., Lond. *151:* 47 (1960).
284. Hench, P. S.; Kendall, E. C.; Slocumb, C. H. and Polley, H. F.: The effect of a hormone of the adrenal cortex (17-hydroxy-11-dehydrocorticosterone; compound E) and of pituitary adrenocorticotrophic hormone on rheumatoid arthritis; preliminary report. Proc. Mayo Clin. *24:* 181 (1949).
285. Hench, P. S.; Slocmub, C. H.; Barnes, A. R.; Smith, H. L.; Polley, H. F. and Kendall, E. C.: The effects of the adrenal cortical hormone 17-hydroxy-11-dehydrocorticosterone (compound E) on the acute phase of rheumatic fever; preliminary report. Proc. Mayo Clin. *24:* 277 (1949).
286. Hench, P. S.; Slocumb, C. H.; Polley, H. F. and Kendall, E. C.: Effect of cortisone and pituitary adrenocorticotrophic hormone (ACTH) on rheumatic diseases. J. amer. med. Ass. *144:* 1327 (1950).
287. Herbertson, B. M.: Patchy myocardial necrosis in rabbits after shock doses of histamine and peptone. J. Path. Bact. *72:* 137 (1956).
288. Herr, F.; Borsi, B. und Pataky, Gy.: Wirkung der Umwelttemperatur auf die Toxizität der Analgetika. Arch. exp. Path. Pharmakol. *223:* 56 (1954).
289. Hess, E. L. and Slade, H. D.: An electrophoretic examination of cell free extracts from various serological types of group A hemolytic streptococcus. Biochim. biophys. Acta *16:* 346 (1955).
290. Hickam, J. B.; Cargill, W. H. and Golden, A.: Cardiovascular reactions to emotional stimuli: effect on cardiac output, arteriovenous oxygen difference, arterial pressure, and peripheral resistance. J. clin. Invest. *27:* 290 (1948).
291. Hicks, S. P.: Brain metabolism 'in vitro'. II. The distribution of lesions caused by azide, malonitrile, plasmocid and dinitrophenol poisoning in rats. Arch. Path. *50:* 545 (1950).
292. Hill, M.; Dvorak, M. and Pospisil, M.: Stress activation of adrenal glomerulosa. Nature, Lond. *183:* 1819 (1959).
293. Hill, S. R. and Holley, H. L.: The ameliorating effect of pregnancy and jaundice on certain rheumatic diseases; in: Arthritis and allied conditions, ed.: J. L. Hollander, p. 593 (Lea & Febiger, Philadelphia 1960).
294. Hillarp, N. A.: Catecholamines: mechanisms of storage and release. Acta endocrin., Kbh. (Suppl. 50) *34:* 181 (1960).

295. Hilton, J. G.; Scian, L. F.; Westermann, C. D. and Kruesi, O. R.: Effect of synthetic lysine vasopressin on adrenocortical secretion. Science *129:* 971 (1959).
296. Hilton, J. G.; Scian, L. F.; Westermann, C. D.; Nakano, J. and Kruesi, O. R.: Vasopressin stimulation of the isolated adrenal glands: nature and mechanism of hydrocortisone secretion. Endocrinology *67:* 298 (1960).
297. Himsworth, H. P.: The physiological activation of insulin. Clin. Sci. *1:* 1 (1933).
298. Hinton, G. G. and Stevenson, J. A. F.: The effect of hypothalamic lesions on the growth of young rats. Proc. canad. Fed. Biol. Socs. *2:* 29 (1959).
299. Hirsch, E. F.; Phibbs, B. P. and Carbonaro, L.: Parallel relation of hyperglycemia and hyperlipemia (esterified fatty acids) in diabetes. Arch. intern. Med. *91:* 106 (1953).
300. Hisaw, F. L.: Endocrine adaptations of the mammalian estrous cycle and gestation; in: Comparative endocrinology, ed.: A. Gorbman, p. 533 (Wiley, New York 1959).
301. Hodges, J. R. and Vernikos, J.: Circulating corticotrophin in normal and adrenalectomized rats after stress. Acta endocrin., Kbh. *30:* 188 (1959).
302. Hoffmann, G.: Über die Herzmuskelwirkung der Nebennierenrindenhormone. Arch. exp. Path. Pharmakol. *222:* 224 (1954).
303. Hohlweg, W. und Daume, E.: Über die Wirkung intrazerebral verabreichten Dienoestroldiacetate bei Ratten. Endokrinologie *38:* 46 (1959).
304. Hoim, R. and Lasagna, L.: Effects of aggregation and temperature on amphetamine toxicity in mice. Fed. Proc. *18:* 1588 (1959).
304a. Holesh, S.: Dissecting aneurysm of the aorta. Brit. J. Radiol. *33:* 302 (1960).
305. Holman, R. L. and Jones, C. K.: Protective influence of pregnancy on experimental collagen disease lesions. Arch. Path. *56:* 231 (1953).
306. Holmes, R. L. and Zuckerman, S.: The blood supply of the hypophysis in Macaca Mulatta. J. Anat. *93:* 1 (1959).
307. Holmes, R. L.; Hughes, E. B. and Zuckerman, S.: Section of the pituitary stalk in monkeys. J. Endocrin. *18:* 305 (1959).
308. Holub, D. A. and Kitay, J. I.: Modification of stress-induced pituitary ACTH depletion by pretreatment with saline injections. Fed. Proc. *18:* 70 (1959).
309. Holub, D. A.; Kitay, J. I. and Jailer, J. W.: Effects of exogenous adrenocorticotropic hormone (ACTH) upon pituitary ACTH concentration after prolonged cortisone treatment and stress. J. clin. Invest. *38:* 291 (1959).
310. Honigmann, J.: The world of man, p. 172 (Harper, New York 1959).
311. Horava, A.: Local and systemic factors affecting the behaviour of established neoplasias as exemplified by experiments on Walker 256 tumor. Thesis Inst. chir., Univ. Montréal 1954.
312. Hoskins, R. G.: The thyroid-pituitary apparatus as a serve (feed-back) mechanism. J. clin. Endocrin. *9:* 1429 (1949).
313. Howard, J. M.: Studies of the absorption and metabolism of glucose following injury. Ann. Surg. *141:* 321 (1955).
314. Howard, J. M.; Olney, J. M.; Frawley, J. P.; Peterson, R. E.; Smith, L. H.; Davis, J. D.; Guene, S. and Dibrell, W. H.: Studies of adrenal function in combat and wounded soldiers. Ann. Surg. *141:* 314 (1955).
315. Howe, A. and Jewell, P. A.: Effects of water deprivation upon the neurosecretory material of the desert rat (Meriones meriones) compared with the laboratory rat. J. Endocrin. *18:* 118 (1959).
316. Hökfelt, B.; Luft, R.; Ikkos, D.; Olivecrona, H. and Sekkenes, J.: The immediate effect of hypophysectomy and section of the pituitary stalk on the urinary steroid excretion in man. Acta endocrin., Kbh. *30:* 29 (1959).
317. Huant, E. et Dussert, A.: La pathologie fonctionnelle. I. Milieu et adaptation. Importance des facteurs électro-ioniques et de la régulation diencéphalique (Vigot, Paris 1959).
318. Iinos, S.: Influence of the stimulation of the cervical sympathetic nerve on the

mechanism of the hormonal secretion of the thyroid gland. Folia endocrin. jap. *34:* 978 (1959). – Ref.: Endocrin. jap. *6:* 148 (1959).
319. IMOTO, T.: Histochemical studies on the hypothalamo-hypophysial neurosecretory system. Arch. Hist. jap. *14:* 11 (1958).
320. INGLE, D. J.: Parameters of metabolic problems. Proc. Laurentian Hormone Conf. 1950; Recent Progr. *6:* 159 (1951).
321. INGLE, D. J.: The role of the adrenal cortex in the etiology of disease. 5th annu. Rep. stress, ed.: H. SELYE and G. HEUSER, p. 161 (Acta, Inc., Montréal 1955–56).
323. ITOH, S. and KIKUCHI, T.: Inactivation of antidiuretic activity of vasopressin by hypothalamic tissue in the presence of pyridoxal. Jap. J. Physiol. *9:* 401 (1959).
324. JACKSON, R. L.; HARDIN, R. C.; WALKER, G. L.; HENDRICKS, A. B. and KELLY, H. G.: Degenerative changes in young diabetics in relationship to level of control. Proc. amer. Diabetes Ass. *9:* 309 (1949).
325. JAFFE, R. and HOLZ, E.: Experimental allergic myocarditis. Exp. Med. Surg. *5–6:* 189 (1947–48).
326. JAHN, H.; STEPHAN, F.; GRUNER, J. et STAHL, J.: Etudes sur l'origine des principes antidiurétiques et diurétiques posthémorragiques. C. R. Soc. Biol. *152:* 1798 (1958).
327. JENTZER, A.: Hibernation et allergie en urologie. Helv. chir. Acta *20:* 527 (1953).
328. JOHNS, T. N. P. and OLSON, B. J.: Experimental myocardial infarction. I. A method of coronary occlusion in small animals. Ann. Surg. *140:* 875 (1954).
329. JOHNSON, D. D.: Alloxan administration in the guinea pig. A study of the regenerative phase in the islands of Langerhans. Endocrinology *47:* 393 (1950).
330. JONES, R. S. and CARTER, Y.: A study of the pathogenesis of rheumatic-like lesions in the guinea pig. Amer. med. Ass. Arch. Pathol. *58:* 613 (1954).
331. JORGENSEN, C. B. and LARSEN, L. O.: Effect of neurohypophyseal principles on adenohypophyseal activity in toads. Proc. Soc. exp. Biol., N. Y. *103:* 685 (1960).
332. JOSLIN, E. P.: Diabetes for the diabetics. 9th Banting Memorial lect. Brit. Diabetic Ass.; Diabetes *5:* 137 (1956).
333. JULESZ, M.: The role of peripheral endocrine glands in the genesis of hypothalamic-pituitary diseases. Acta med. hungar. *13:* 153 (1959).
334. KAISER, H.: Kardiologie: Cortison bei Herzinfarkt? Dtsch. med. Wschr. *102:* 931 (1960).
335. KALTER, H.: Teratogenic action of a hypocaloric diet and small doses of cortisone. Proc. Soc. exp. Biol., N. Y. *104:* 518 (1960).
336. KAPLAN, M. K.: Localization of streptococcal antigens in tissues. I. Histologic distribution and persistence of M protein, types 1, 5, 12, and 19 in the tissues of the mouse. J. exp. Med. *107:* 341 (1958).
337. KARÁDY, I.; BROWNE, J. S. L. and SELYE, H.: The effect of the alarm reaction on water excretion. Quart. J. exp. Physiol. *28:* 23 (1938).
338. KARPLUS, J. P. und KREIDL, A.: Gehirn und Sympathicus: VII. Über Beziehungen der Hypothalamuszentren zu Blutdruck und innerer Sekretion. Arch. ges. Physiol. *215:* 667 (1927)
339. KATSOYANNIS, P. G. and VIGNEAUD, V.: Arginine vasotocin. Nature, Lond. *184:* 1465 (1959).
340. KATZ, L. N. and STAMLER, J.: Experimental atherosclerosis, p. 210 (Thomas, Springfield 1953).
341. KAUFMAN, N.; GAVAN, T. L. and HILL, R. M.: Experimental myocardial infarction in the rat. Arch. Path. *67:* 482 (1959).
342. KAVETSKY, R. E. and TURKEVICH, N. M.: Some functional peculiarities of the pituitary gland and nervous system in mice of a high and low tumour strain. Vopr. onkol. *5:* 275 (1959).
343. KEIDING, N. R. and TULLER, E. F.: Protein-bound carbohydrate in serum of diabetic patients with and without vascular complications. Diabetes *4:* 37 (1955).

344. Keller, A. D.: Ulceration in the digestive tract of the dog following intracranial procedures. Arch. Path. *21:* 127 (1936).
345. Keller, A. D.: Ablation and stimulation of the hypothalamus: circulatory effects. Physiol. Rev. (Suppl. 4) *40:* 116 (1960).
346. Kellner, A.: Selective necrosis of cardiac and skeletal muscles induced by means of proteolytic enzyme solutions given intravenously. J. exp. Med. *99:* 387 (1954).
347. Kellner, A. and Robertson, R.: Myocardial necrosis produced in animals by means of crystalline streptococcal proteinase. J. exp. Med. *99:* 495 (1954).
348. Keye, J. D., Jr.: Death in potassium deficiency; report of a case including morphologic findings. Circulation *5:* 766 (1952).
349. Kien, G. A.; Lasker, N. and Sherrod, T. R.: Action of cigarette smoke on cardiovascular hemodynamics and oxygen utilization in the dog. J. Pharmacol., Baltimore *124:* 35 (1958).
350. Kinsell, L. W.: Prevention of vascular disease in diabetics. Diabetes *4:* 298 (1955).
351. Kirschner, L. and Howie, J. B.: Rheumatic-like lesions in the heart of the rabbit experimentally induced by repeated inoculation with hemolytic streptococci. J. Path. Bact. *64:* 367 (1952).
352. Kiss, F.: Neurovaskuläre Mechanismen in den endokrinen Drüsen. Pathophysiol. Diencephalica, Wien p. 41. (1958).
353. Kitay, J. I.; Holub, D. A. and Jailer, W. J.: Extra-adrenal action of exogenous ACTH: inhibition of pituitary ACTH secretion. Fed. Proc. *17:* 87 (1958).
354. Kivalo, E. and Rinne, U. K.: The relation between the hypothalamic neurosecretion and the corticotrophin release in experimental conditions. Acta endocrin., Kbh. *34:* 8 (1960).
355. Kivalo, E.; Rinne, U. K. and Marjanen, P.: Diuretic effect of chlorpromazine with special reference to the hypothalamic neurosecretory substance. Ann. Med. exp. Fenn. *36:* 185 (1958).
356. Kivalo, E.; Tyrkkö, J. and Marjanen, P.: The response to diphenylhydantoin of the neurosecretory substance in the mouse. Ann. Med. intern. Fenn. *47:* 169 (1958).
357. Klein, R.; Papadatos, C.; Fortunato, J.; Byers, C. and Pontereri, A.: Serum corticoids in liver disease. J. clin. Endocrin. *15:* 943 (1955).
358. Kletzkin, M. and Berger, F. M.: Effect of meprobamate on limbic system of the brain. Proc. Soc. exp. Biol., N. Y. *100:* 681 (1959).
359. Klinge, F.: Der Rheumatismus (Bergmann, München 1933).
360. Knigge, K. M.; Penrod, C. H. and Schindler, J. W.: In vitro and in vivo adrenal corticosteroid secretion following stress. Amer. J. Physiol. *196:* 579 (1959).
361. Knowlton, A. I.: Comparison of effect of desoxycorticosterone acetate and cortisone acetate on rat skeletal muscle electrolytes. Proc. Soc. exp. Biol., N. Y. *104:* 13 (1960).
362. Krieger, D. T.: Endocrine functions of the hypothalamus. N.Y. J. Med. *59:* 643 (1959).
363. Kobayashi, T.; Sato, H.; Maruyama, M.; Arai, K. and Takezawa, S.: Persistent estrus produced in rats by hypothalamic lesions. Endocrin. jap. *6:* 107 (1959).
364. Koelsch, F.: Kreislaufschädigungen durch gewerbliche Vergiftungen. Verh. dtsch. Ges. Kreislaufforsch, p. 97 (1936).
365. Koibuchi, E.: The effects of hypothalamic lesions on the pituitary-adrenocortical system. Endocrin. jap. *5:* 89 (1958).
366. Koibuchi, E. and Fukuda, M.: Pituitary reaction following the stalk section. Endocrin. jap. *5:* 11 (1958).
367. Kornberg, A. and Endicott, K. M.: Potassium deficiency in the rat. Amer. J. Physiol. *145:* 291 (1946).
368. Korth, C. and Spang, K.: Der Wirkung des Digitoxins auf Elektrokardiogramm und Herzmuskel der Katze. Ein Beitrag zur Klärung der Frage nach der Bedeutung der Digitalisveränderungen im Elektrokardiogramm. Arch. exp. Path. Pharmakol. *184:* 349 (1937).

369. Kovács, K.: Über die hypothalamische Regulation der Adenohypophysenfunktion. Z. ges. inn. Med. *13:* 303 (1958).
370. Kovács, S.; Lissák, K. and Endröczi, E.: Effect of the lesion of paraventricular nucleus on the function of the pituitary, thyroid, adrenal cortex and gonadal systems. Acta physiol. hungar. *15:* 137 (1959).
371. Kovács, K.; Kovács, B. M. and Petri, G.: Increased antidiuretic activity of human sera in the preoperative period. Acta med. hungar. *11:* 337 (1959).
372. Kozik, M. and Walezak, M.: Wplyw ACTH na stan neurosekrecji podwzgorza swinki morskiej. Endokryn. polska *10:* 137 (1959).
373. Kup, J.: Die Rolle des zentralen Nervensystems bei der Ausbildung klinischer Erscheinungsformen der Erkrankungen des endokrinen Systems. Frankf. Z. Path. *69:* 526 (1959).
374. Külbs, F.: Erkrankungen der Zirkulationsorgane; in: Mohr-Staehelin's Hb. d. inneren Medizin, 2. Aufl. (Springer, Berlin 1928).
375. Kyser, F. A.; Ginsberg, R. and Gilbert, N. C.: The effect of certain drugs upon the cardiotoxic lesions of digitalis in the dog. Amer. Heart J. *31:* 451 (1946).
376. Kyser, F. A.; McCarter, J. C. and Stengle, J. J.: Effect of antihistamine drugs on serum-induced myocarditis in rabbits. J. Lab. clin. Med. *32:* 379 (1947).
377. Kyser, F. A.; Teloh, H. and Sutton, G. C.: The effect of digitalis and desoxy-corticosterone acetate administration upon intra-cellular potassium ion concentration. J. Lab. clin. Med. *53:* 216 (1959).
378. Labarge, O. J. and Ogilvie, O. A.: Hypoglycemic shock followed by secondary hyperglycemia. Rockey Mt. med. J. *38:* 783 (1941).
379. Laborit, H.: Stress and cellular function (Lippincott, Philadelphia 1959).
380. Laborit, H. et Morand, P.: Sur un test de résorption utilisable dans le diagnostic du choc et dans son évolution. Nat. Acad. Chir. *72:* 65 (1946).
381. Lacroix, E. and Leusen, I.: The influence of cortisone on the oxygen consumption of myocard and diaphragm slices of the rat. Arch. int. Pharmacodyn. *114:* 103 (1958).
382. Lake, M.; Pratt, G. H. and Wright, J. S.: Arteriosclerosis and varicose veins, occupational activities and other factors: study of 536 persons divided into age groups, who had been sitting, standing, walking or climbing stairs for 10 years or more at their work. J. amer. med. Ass. *119:* 696 (1942).
383. Lansing, A. I.: Some systemic effects of elastase. J. Geront. *9:* 362 (1954).
384. Lansing, A. I.; Rosenthal, T. H. and Alex, M.: Presence of elastase in teleost islet tissue. Proc. Soc. exp. Biol., N. Y. *84:* 689 (1953).
385. Lash, A. F.: Intradermal salt solution test in normal and toxaemic pregnancies. A diagnostic and prognostic aid. Surg. Gynec. Obstet. *43:* 40 (1928).
386. Laubry, C.; Waiser, J. et Degaude, L.: Action expérimentale du tabac et de la nicotine sur le débit coronarien. Bull. Acad. Méd. Belg. *109:* 595 (1933).
387. Laude, J. S.: Myocardial necrosis and fibrosis resulting from the administration of massive doses of a cardiac glycoside. J. Pharmacol., Baltimore *76:* 1 (1942).
388. Lawrence, R. D. and Buckley, O. B.: The inhibition of insulin action by toxaemias and its explanation. I. The effect of diphtheria toxin on blood sugar and insulin action in rabbits. Brit. J. exp. Path. *8:* 58 (1927).
389. Leeman, S. E. and Voelkel, E. F.: Preparation and bioassay of a hypothalamic extract that stimulates ACTH secretion in vivo. Fed. Proc. *18:* 88 (1959).
390. Legait, H.: Contribution à l'étude morphologique et expérimentale du système hypothalamo-neurohypophysaire de la poule Rhode-Island. Thesis, Univ. of Louvain Soc. d'Impress. Typgr., Nancy 1959.
391. Lehr, D.: Causative relationships of parathyroid hormone to renogenic and reniprival cardiovascular disease. Ann. N. Y. Acad. Sci. *72:* 901 (1959).
392. Lehr, D. and Churg, J.: Human and experimental arteriosclerosis. J. Mt. Sinai Hosp. *19:* 106 (1952).

393. Leonard, A. S.; Griffen, W. O., Jr. and Wangensteen, O. H.: Experimental preparation showing effect of reserpine on tissue resistance. Proc. Soc. exp. Biol., N. Y. *103:* 190 (1960).

394. Levine, R. and Goldstein, M. S.: On the mechanism of action of insulin. Recent Progr. Hormone Res. Proc. Lauretian Hormone Conf. 1954 (Acad. Press, New York/London) *11:* 343 (1955).

395. Levy, E. Z.; North, W. C. and Welh, J. A.: Modification of traumatic shock by adrenergic blocking agents. J. Pharmacol., Baltimore *112:* 151 (1954).

396. Lewitzky, A.: Über pathologisch-histologische Veränderungen des Herzens bei Digitalisvergiftungen (Kaninchen, Hunde, Katzen). Zur Frage der experimentellen Myocarditis; Inaug.-Diss. Petersburg (1904); abstract in: Zbl. Path. *16:* 532 (1905).

397. Liebelt, R. A.: Effects of goldthioglucose-induced hypothalamic lesions on mammary tumorigenesis in mice. Proc. amer. Ass. Cancer Res. *3:* 37 (1959).

398. Linquette, M.: Les inter-relations hypothalamo-hypophyso-thyroïdiennes. Lille méd. *4:* 449 (1959).

399. Lipscomb, H. S.; Schally, A. V. and Guillemin, R.: Recent studies on CRF (corticotrophin releasing factor), a peptide of hypothalamic origin which initiates ACTH release. 57th annu. Meet. amer. Soc. Zool., Oklahoma 1960. – Anat. Rec. *137:* 376 (1960).

400. Loewe, L. and Lenke, S. E.: Cardiac lesions resembling Aschoff bodies in rabbits. J. exp. Med. *71:* 89 (1940).

401. Lorenz, E.; Jacobson, L. O.; Heston, W. E.; Shimkin, M.; Eschenbrenner, A. B.; Deringer, M. K.; Boniger, J. and Schweisthal, R.: Biological effects of external X and gamma radiation; part I, chapt. 3 (McGraw Hill, New York 1954).

402. Lovett, B. R.: The intradermal salt solution test in scarlet fever. Amer. J. med. Sci. *173:* 539 (1927).

403. Lowenhaupt, E.; Schulman, M. P. and Greenberg, D. M.: Basic histologic lesions of magnesium deficiency in the rat. Amer. med. Ass. Arch. Pathol. *49:* 427 (1950).

404. Luongo, E. P.: Health habits and heart disease—challenge in preventive medicine. J. amer. med. Ass. *162:* 1021 (1956).

405. MacGregor, A. G. and Wood, D. R.: The effect of Neoantergan and of Benadryl on serum-induced myocarditis in rabbits. Brit. J. Pharmacol. *4:* 216 (1949).

406. MacIntyre, I. and Davidsson, D.: Production of secondary potassium depletion, sodium retention, nephrocalcinosis and hypercalcaemia by magnesium deficiency. Biochem. J. *70:* 456 (1958).

406a. MacPherson, C. H.: Myocardial necrosis in the potassium depleted rat: a reassessment. Brit. J. exp. Path. *37:* 279 (1956).

407. Maekawa, M.: Allergie und Immunität. First int. Congr. for Allergy, Zürich (Karger, Basel 1951); quoted by Kaplan, M. H.: The concept of autoantibodies in rheumatic fever and in postcommissurotomy state. Ann. N. Y. Acad. Sci. *86:* 974 (1960).

407a. Maetz, J.; Morel, F. and Lahlough, B.: Natriferin: a new hormonal principle in the neurohypophysis of certain vertebrates. Nature, Lond. *184:* 1236 (1959).

408. Magoun, H. W.: The waking brain (Thomas, Springfield 1958).

409. Magrassi, F.: Experimental infectious rheumatism and streptococcal focal infection. Acta rheum. scand. *5:* 2 (1933).

410. Malek, P. and Kolc, J.: Studies on the dynamics of the circulation and action of substances in the organism in conditions of shock. Physiol. Bohemoslov. *5:* 214 (1956).

411. Mallory, G. K. and Keefer, C. S.: Tissue reactions in fatal cases of streptococcus hemolyticus infection. Amer. med. Ass. Arch. Pathol. *32:* 334 (1941).

412. Mansfield, G. und Hecht, K.: Untersuchungen über die Wirkung des Tabak-

rauchens auf das Herz-Lungenpräparat von Hunden. Arch. exp. Path. Pharmakol. *172:* 362 (1933).

413. Marchetto, G. e Brigato, G.: Meno-metrorragie puberro-giovanili e diencefalo. Attual. ostet. ginec. *5:* 347 (1959).

414. Marks, B. H.; Garber, B. G. and McCoy, F. W.: The juxtaglomerular apparatus as an extra-adrenal site of ACTH action. Proc. Soc. exp. Biol., N. Y. *105:* 593 (1960).

415. Marks, P. A. and Bishop, J. S.: Glucose metabolism in subjects with neoplastic disease. Response to insulin and glucose tolerance follow-up studies. Cancer Res. *17:* 228 (1957).

416. Marks, P. A. and Bishop, J. S.: The glucose metabolism of patients with malignant disease and of normal subjects as studied by means of an intravenous glucose tolerance test. J. clin. Invest. *36:* 254 (1957).

417. Martin, F.: Congenital hyperpituitarism of hypothalamic origin. IX. int. Congr. Paediat., Montreal 1959.

418. Martini, L.; Mire, L.; Pecile, A. and Saito, S.: Neurohypophyseal hormones and release of gonadotrophins. J. Endocrin. *18:* 245 (1959).

419. Martini, L.; Pecile, A.; Saito, S. and Tani, F.: The effect of midbrain transection on ACTH release. Endocrinology *66:* 501 (1960).

420. Mason, J. W.: Psychological influences on the pituitary-adrenal cortical system. Recent Progr. Hormone Res. Proc. Laurentian Hormone Conf. 1958 *15:* 345 (1959).

421. Masson, G.: Sensibilité à l'insuline pendant le syndrome général d'adaptation. Ann. Endocrin. *2:* 11 (1941).

422. Masson, G.: Action of nocuous agents on insulin and adrenalin sensitivity and on glucose tolerance. Endocrinology *29:* 453 (1941).

423. McAllen, P. M.: Myocardial changes occurring in potassium deficiency. Brit. Heart. J. *17:* 5 (1955).

424. McAllister, F. F.; Bertsch, R.; Jacobson, J. and D'Alessio, G.: The accelerating effect of muscular exercise on experimental atherosclerosis. Arch. Surg. *80:* 54 (1960).

425. McCann, S. M.: The ACTH-releasing activity of extracts of the posterior lobe of the pituitary in vivo. Endocrinology *60:* 664 (1957).

426. cCann, S. M. and Haberland, P.: Relative abundance of vasopressin and corticotrophin-releasing factor in neurohypophysial extracts. Proc. Soc. exp. Biol., N. Y. *102:* 319 (1959).

427. McCann, S. M. and Haberland, P.: Further studies on the regulation of pituitary ACTH in rats with hypothalmic lesions. Endocrinology *66:* 217 (1960).

428. McCann, S. M.; Fruit, A. and Fulford, B. D.: Studies on the loci of action of cortical hormones in inhibiting the release of adrenocorticotrophin. Endocrinology *63:* 29 (1958).

429. McCann, S. M.; Taleisnik, S. and Friedman, H. M.: LH-releasing activity in hypothalamic extracts. Proc. Soc. exp. Biol., N. Y. *104:* 432 (1960).

430. McClure, W. B. and Aldrich, C. A.: Time required for disappearance of intradermally injected salt solution. J. amer. med. Ass. *81:* 293 (1923).

431. McCullagh, E. P.; Reynolds, C. W. and McKenzie, J. M.: Hyperthyroidism after section of the pituitary stalk for malignant exophthalmos: report of a case. J. clin. Endocrin. *20:* 1029 (1960).

432. McManus, J. F. A.: The development of intercapillary glomerulosclerosis. Proc. amer. Diabetes Ass. *9:* 303 (1949).

433. Meites, J. and Hopkins, T. F.: Induction of lactation and mammary growth by pituitary grafts in intact and hypophysectomized rats. Proc. Soc. exp. Biol., N. Y. *104:* 263 (1960).

434. Meites, J.; Nicoll, C. S. and Talwalker, P. K.: Induction and maintenance of lactation in rats by electrical stimulation of uterine cervix. Proc. Soc. exp. Biol., N. Y. *102:* 127 (1959).

435. Meites, J.; Talwalker, P. K. and Nicoll, C. S.: Induction of mammary growth and lactation in rabbits with epinephrine, acetylcholine and serotonin. Proc. Soc. exp. Biol., N. Y. *104:* 192 (1960).
436. Meites, J.; Talwalker, P. K. and Nicoll, C. S.: Initiation of lactation in rats with hypothalamic or cerebral tissue. Proc. Soc. exp. Biol., N. Y. *103:* 298 (1960).
437. Mendell, P.: Effect of electrolytes on digitoxin intoxication in the rat (personal communication).
438. Mess, B.: Die Rolle der Nuclei habenulae bei der auf erhöhten Thyroxin-Blutspiegel eintretenden zentral-nervösen Hemmung der thyreotrophen Aktivität des Hypophysenvorderlappen. Endokrinologie *37:* 104 (1959).
439. Metuzals, J.: Hypothalamic nerve fibers in the pars tuberalis and piaarachnoid tissue of the cat and their degeneration pattern after a lesion in the hypothalamus. Experientia *15:* 36 (1959).
440. Metuzals, J.: The structure of the hypothalamic final common path to the adenohypophysis in the cat. I. The periventricular area of the nucleus arcuatus and the eminentia mediana. J. comp. Neurol. *113:* 103 (1959).
441. Meyer, J. H.; Grunert, H. R.; Zeppelin, M. T.; Grummer, R. H.; Bohstedt, G. and Phillips, P. H.: Effect of dietary levels of sodium and potassium on growth and on concentration in blood plasma and tissues of white rat. Amer. J. Physiol. *162:* 182 (1950).
442. Michon, P. et Larcan, A.: L'excitabilité neuro-musculaire en endocrinologie. Sem. Hôp. Paris *35:* 22 (1959).
443. Mietkiewski, K. and Kozik, M.: Badania histochemiczne nad jadrem nadwzrokowym i przykomorowym u kota. Endokryn. polska *10:* 1 (1959).
444. Migliorini, R. H. y Covian, M. R.: Vesiculas seminales y ovarios en ratones hemidecorticados. Rev. Soc. argent. Biol. *34:* 248 (1958).
445. Migliorini, R. H. y Penhos, J. C.: Accion del eter sobre la hipoglucemia por sulfonamidas. Rev. Soc. argent. Biol. *33:* 144 (1957).
446. Mihailovic, L. and Krzalic, L.: The effect of insulin upon the blood sugar and potassium levels in deep hypothermia. Arch. int. Physic. *66:* 526 (1958).
447. Miller, C. P.: Attempts to transmit rheumatic fever to rabbits and guinea pigs. J. exp. Med. *40:* 525 (1924).
448. Mishra, R. K.: Studies on experimental magnesium deficiency in the albino rat. Thesis, Univ. de Montréal (1959).
449. Moll, J.: Localization of hypothalamic lesions inhibiting adrenal weight maintenance in the rat. Acta endocrin., Kbh. *34:* 19 (1960).
450. Montastruc, P.: Recherches sur quelques corrélations physiologiques de l'hormone antidiurétique. Thesis, Univ. de Toulouse (Imp. Sud, Toulouse 1959).
451. Moon, R. C. and Turner, C. W.: Effect of reserpine on thyroid activity in rats. Proc. Soc. exp. Biol. *100:* 679 (1959).
452. Moon, R. C. and Turner, C. W.: A mode of action for thyroid inhibition by reserpine. Proc. Soc. exp. Biol., N. Y. *102:* 134 (1959).
453. Moore, W. W. and Selkurt, E. E.: Effect of hydrocortisone on the blockade of ovulating hormone release in the rat. Physiologist *2:* 83 (1959).
454. Mora, J. M.: The intracutaneous salt-solution test in thyrotoxicosis. Amer. J. med. Sci. *177:* 219 (1929).
455. Mora, J. M. and Jirka, F. J.: The effect of jaundice on intradermally injected salt solution. J. Lab. clin. Med. *20:* 719 (1935).
456. More, R. H.; Waugh, D. E. and Kobernick, S. A.: Cardiac lesions produced in rabbits by massive injections of bovine serum gamma globulin. J. exp. Med. *89:* 555 (1949).
457. Morgane, P. J. and Kosman, A. J.: Relationship of the middle hypothalamus to amygdalar hyperphagia. Amer. J. Physiol. *198:* 1315 (1960).

458. Morris, J. N.; Heady, J. A.; Raffle, P. A. B.; Roberts, C. G. and Parks, J. W.: Coronary heart disease and physical activity of work. Lancet, p. 1053, p. 1111 (1953).
459. Morrison, A. B.: Potassium metabolism in rats with chronic renal insufficiency. Proc. Soc. exp. Biol., N. Y. *103:* 500 (1960).
460. Moyson, F. et Toussaint, J.: Absorption intestinale des phosphates dans le shock. Acta gastro-ent. belg. *12:* 321 (1949).
461. Murdock, G. P.: How culture changes; in: Man, culture and society, ed.: H. Shapiro, p. 247 (Oxford Univ. Press, New York 1959).
462. Murphy, G. E.: Evidence that Aschoff bodies of rheumatic myocarditis develop from injured myofibers. J. exp. Med. *95:* 319 (1952).
463. Murphy, G. E. and Swift, H. F.: The induction of rheumatic-like cardiac lesions in rabbits by repeated focal infections with group A streptococci. J. exp. Med. *91:* 485 (1950).
464. Mushett, C. W.: The pancreas and cardiovascular disease. Ann. N. Y. Acad. Sci. *72:* 989 (1959).
465. Myasnikov, A. L.: Influence of some factors on development of experimental cholesterol atherosclerosis. Circulation *17:* 99 (1958).
466. Nahas, G.: Effect of hydrocortisone on acidotic failure on the isolated heart. Circulation *5:* 489 (1957).
467. Nalbandov, A. V.: Neuroendocrine reflex mechanisms: bird ovulation; in: Comparative endocrinology, ed.: A. Gorbman, p. 161 (Wiley, New York 1959).
468. Nauta, W. J. H.: Limbic system and hypothalamus: anatomical aspects. Physiol. Rev. (Suppl. 4) *40:* 102 (1960).
469. Nasmyth, P. A.: The effect of corticosteroids on the isolated mammalian heart and its response to adrenaline J. Physiol., Lond. *139:* 323 (1957).
470. Nickerson, M.: Adrenergic mediators. Canad. J. Biochem. *37:* 331 (1959).
471. Niebroj, T.: Wplyw soli kobaltu na histofizjologie jader neurosekrecyjnych podwzgora swinki morskiej. I. and II. Endokryn. polska *10:* 7, 17 (1959).
472. Nikitovitch-Winer, M. and Everett, J. W.: Functional restitution of pituitary grafts re-transplanted from kidney to median eminence. Endocrinology *63:* 916 (1958).
473. Nikitovitch-Winer, M. and Everett, J. W.: Histocytologic changes in grafts of rat pituitary on the kidney and upon retransplantation under the diencephalon. Endocrinology *65:* 357 (1959).
474. Noble, R. L.: Neurohypophyseal secretion. Canad. J. Biochem. *37:* 309 (1959).
475. Norlin, G.: Experimental heart granulomatosis in rabbits and its relation to rheumatic carditis. Acta rheum. scand. *5:* 85 (1959).
476. O'Connor, J. F.: Psychoses associated with systemic lupus erythematosus. Ann. intern. Med. *51:* 526 (1959).
477. Okinaka, S.; Ibayashi, M.; Motobashi, K.; Fujita, T.; Yoshida, S. and Ohsawa, N.: Regulation of the pituitary-adrenocortical function through the central nervous system: limbic system and reticular formation. Trans. 1st Asia and Oceania Reg. Congr. Endocrin., Kyoto 1959.
478. Okinaka, S.; Ibayashi, H.; Motohashi, K.; Fujita, T.; Yoshida, S. and Ohsawa, N.: Effect of electrical stimulation of the limbic system on pituitary-adrenocortical function: posterior orbital surface. Endocrinology *67:* 319 (1960).
479. Okinaka, S.; Ibayashi, H.; Motohashi, K.; Fujita, T.; Yoshida, S. and Ohsawa, N.: The effect of splanchnic nerve stimulation on adrenocortical secretion. Endocrin. jap. *7:* 19 (1960).
480. Oliver, M. F. and Boyd, G. S.: Some current views on the aetiology of coronary artery disease. Brit. Heart J. *19:* 582 (1957).
481. Olmsted, H. C.: Intradermal salt solution in cardiac disease in children. Arch. intern. Med. *37:* 281 (1926).

482. Olsen, J. M.; Meinecke. K. H. und Olsen, K. J.: Ursache der Wasserretention bei Adipositas unter besonderer Berücksichtigung des Nebennierenrindenhormons Aldosteron. Acta endocrin., Kbh. *31:* 384 (1959).

483. Otomo, E. and Michaelis, M.: Penetration of radioactive phosphorus into normal and shocked rat's brain. Proc. Soc. exp. Biol., N. Y. *104:* 259 (1960).

484. Packer, L.; Michaelis, M. and Martin, W. R.: Effect of shock on rat heart and brain mitochondria. Proc. Soc. exp. Biol., N. Y. *98:* 164 (1958).

485. Parker, B. M.; Thomas, W. A.; Smith, J. R. and Ahlvin, R. C.: Myocarditis and valvulitis in dogs subsequent to cardiovascular stress. Amer. med. Ass Arch. Pathol. *64:* 522 (1957).

486. Pasqualini, R. G. and Codevilla, A.: Thirst-suppressing (anti-dipsetic) effect of pitressin in diabetes insipidus. Acta endocrin., Kbh. *30:* 37 (1959).

487. Pavlov, I. P.: Lectures on conditioned reflexes; translated by W. H. Gantt (International Publ., New York 1928).

488. Pazianos, A. G.; Benua, R.; Ray, B. S. and Pearson, O. H.: Persistent thyroid function following hypophysectomy. J. clin. Endocrin. *20:* 1051 (1960).

489. Pearce, R. M.: Experimental myocarditis: a study of the histological changes following intravenous injections of adrenalin. J. exp. Med. *8:* 400 (1900).

490. Pelloja, M.: Sulla attivazione della tossina tetanica da parte del muscolo e degli estratti muscolari. Med. sper. *21:* 1 (1949).

491. Perera, G. A.; Pines, K. L.; Hamilton, H. B. and Vislocky, K.: Clinical and metabolic study of 11-dehydro-17-hydroxy-corticosterone acetate (Kendall compound E) in hypertension, Addison's disease and diabetes mellitus. Amer. J. Med. *7:* 56 (1949).

492. Perdue, H. S. and Phillips, P. H.: Effect of high fat diet on the potassium deficiency syndrome in the rat. Proc. Soc. exp. Biol., N. Y. *81:* 405 (1952).

493. Pickering, B. T. and Heller, H.: Chromatographic and biological characteristics of fish and frog neurohypophysial extracts. Nature, Lond. *184:* 1463 (1959).

494. Porter, R. W.; Movius, H. J. and French, J. D.: Hypothalamic influences on hydrochloric acid secretion of the stomach. Surgery *33:* 875 (1953).

495. Porter, R. W.; Brady, J. V.; Conrad, D.; Mason, J. W.; Galambos, R. and Rioch, D. M.: Some experimental observations on gastro-intestinal lesions in behaviorally conditioned monkeys. Psychosom. Med. *20:* 379 (1958).

496. Poutsiaks, J. W.; Thomas, B. G. and Linegar, C. R.: Effect of fluorohydrocortisone on gastrointestinal and renal excretion of cations by the dog. Proc. Soc. exp. Biol., N. Y. *96:* 712 (1957).

497. Premachandra, B. N. and Turner, C. W.: Reserpine and thyroid activity in fowls. Proc. Soc. exp. Biol., N. Y. *104:* 306 (1960).

498. Prioreschi, P.: Stress e anestesia da bromuro di sodio. Atti Soc. lomb. Sci. med. biol. *14:* 215 (1959).

499. Purves, H. D.: On the mechanism of hypothalamic control of thyrotrophin secretion. Acta endocrin., Kbh. (Suppl. 50) *34:* 21 (1960).

500. Purves, H. D. and Averill, B. L. W.: Effects of hypothalamic lesions on reproduction and lactation in rats. Trans. 1st Asia and Oceania Reg. Congr. Endocrin., Kyoto 1959.

501. Raab, W.: Hormonal and neurogenic cardiovascular disorders (Williams & Wilkins, Baltimore 1953).

502. Raab, W.: Neurohormonal atherogenesis. Amer. J. Cardiol *1:* 113 (1958).

503. Raab, W.: Int. Symp. Arteriosclerosis and Coronary Disease, Mexico, D. F. 1959.

504. Raab, W.; Stark, E. and Gigee, W. R.: The catecholamines in cardiovascular pathology. First int. Symp. Catecholamines in Cardiovascular Pathology, p. 15 (Burlington, Vermont 1959).

505. Ragan, C. E.; Howes, E. L.; Platz, C. M.; Meyer, K. and Blunt, J.: Effect of

cortisone on production of granulation in the rabbit. Proc. Soc. exp. Biol., N. Y. *72:* 718 (1949).

506. Rahman, M. H.; Frazier, L. E.; Hughes, R. H. and Cannon, P. R.: Electrolyte imbalance and intracellular potassium-sodium exchange. Amer. med. Ass. Arch. Pathol. *63:* 154 (1957).
507. Ralph, C. L. and Fraps, R. M.: Long-term effects of diencephalic lesions on the ovary of the hen. Amer. J. Physiol. *197:* 1279 (1959).
508. Ralph, C. L. and Fraps, R. M.: Effect of hypothalamic lesions on progesterone-induced ovulation in the hen. Endocrinology *65:* 819 (1959).
509. Ralph, C. L. and Fraps, R. M.: Induction of ovulation in the hen by injection of progesterone into the brain. Endocrinology *66:* 269 (1960).
510. Redgate, E. S.: Inspiratory area excitability and the hypothalamus. Amer. J. Physiol. *198:* 1299 (1960).
511. Redgate, E. S.: Hypothalamus and respiratory minute volume. Amer. J. Physiol. *198:* 1304 (1960).
512. Rees, L.: The role of stress in the aetiology of psychosomatic disorders. Proc. roy. Soc. Med. *52:* 274 (1959).
513. Reichlin, S.: Mechanism of growth failure in rats with lesions of the hypothalamus. J. Lab. clin. Med. *54:* 937 (1959).
514. Reichlin, S.: Thyroid response to partial thyroidectomy, thyroxine and 2,4-dinitrophenol in rats with hypothalamic lesions. Endocrinology *66:* 327 (1960).
515. Reichlin, S.: Thyroid function, body temperature regulation and growth in rats with hypothalamic lesions. Endocrinology *66:* 340 (1960).
516. Reilly, J.: Le rôle du système nerveux en pathologie rénale (Masson, Paris 1942).
517. Renaud, S.: Stress et toxicité des antibiotiques. Thèse, Univ. de Montréal (1960).
518. Revzin, A. M. and Costa, E.: Effects of exogenous serotonin on paleocortical excitability. Amer. J. Physiol. *198:* 959 (1960).
519. Rich, A. R. and Gregory, J. E.: Experimental evidence that lesions with basic characteristics of rheumatic carditis can result from anaphylactic hypersensitivity. Bull. Johns Hopk. Hosp. *73:* 239 (1943).
520. Ricketts, H. T.: Serum lipids and atherosclerosis. Diabetes *2:* 316 (1953).
521. Ricketts, H. T.: The problem of degenerative vascular disease in diabetes. Amer. J. Med. *19:* 933 (1955).
522. Rinne, U. K. and Kivalo, E.: Effect of dehydration and rehydration on the acid phosphatase activity of the hypothalamic magnocellular nuclei. Ann. Med. exp. Fenn. *36:* 350 (1958).
523. Rinzer, S. H.; Travell, D.; Karp, D. and Charleson, D.: Detection of coronary atherosclerosis in the living rabbit by the eryngovine cigarette test. Amer. J. Physiol. *184:* 605 (1956).
524. Roberts, R. C.; Crockett, K. A. and Laipply, T. C.: Effects of salicylates and benadryl on experimental anaphylactic hypersensitive vascular and cardiac lesions. Amer. med. Ass. Arch. intern. Med. *83:* 48 (1949).
525. Robinson, J. J.: Attempts to produce rheumatic carditis in laboratory animals by means of streptococcic injury. Amer. med. Ass. Arch. Pathol. *51:* 602 (1951).
526. Rochefort, G. J.; Rosenberger, J. and Saffran, M.: Depletion of pituitary corticotrophin by various stresses and by neurohypophysial preparations. J. Physiol., Lond. *146:* 105 (1959).
527. Rodeck, H.: Die Entwicklung der neurosekretorischen Regulation des Wasserhaushaltes beim Säugling. Mschr. Kinderheilk. *106:* 87 (1958).
528. Rodeck, H.: Neurohypophyse-Hypothalamus; in: Linneweh, F., Die physiologische Entwicklung des Kindes (Springer, Berlin 1959).
529. Rodeck, H.: Neurosecretory system and regulation of water metabolism in infancy. IX. int. Congr. Paediat. Montreal 1959.

530. Rodeck, H.: Das neurosekretorische hypothalamo-neurohypophysäre System der weißen Maus. Z. ges. exp. Med. *133:* 78 (1960).

531. Rodriguez, C. E.; Wolfe, A. L. and Bergstrom, V. W.: Hypokalemic myocarditis. Report of two cases. Amer. J. clin. Path. *20:* 1050 (1950).

532. Rodrigues, J. A.: Influencia de la corteza cerebral sobre el ciclo sexual de la rata blanca. Rev. Soc. argent. Biol. *35:* 5 (1959).

533. Rogoff, J. M. and Stewart, G. N.: Studies on adrenal insufficiency in dogs. I. Control animals not subjected to any treatment. Amer. J. Physiol. *78:* 683 (1926).

534. Rona, G.; Chappel, C. I.; Balázs, T. and Gaudry, R.: The effect of breed, age, and sex on myocardial necrosis produced by isoproterenol in the rat. J. Geront. *14:* 169 (1959).

535. Root, H. F.; Bland, E. F.; Gordon, W. K. and White, P. D.: Coronary atherosclerosis in diabetes mellitus: a post mortem study. J. amer. med. Ass. *113:* 27 (1939).

536. Root, H. E.; Pote, W. H., Jr. and Frehner, H.: Triopathy of diabetes: sequence of neuropathy, retinopathy and nephropathy in 155 patients. Arch. intern. Med. *94:* 931 (1954).

537. Rose, S.; Nelson, J. and Bradley, T. R.: Regulation of TSH release. Ann. N. Y. Acad. Sci. *86:* 647 (1960).

538. Rosenman, R. H. and Friedman, M.: The possible relationship of the emotions to clinical coronary heart disease; in: Hormones and atherosclerosis, ed.: G. Pincus, p. 283 (Academic Press, New York/London 1959).

539. Roth, M.: The phenomenology of depressive states. Canad. Psychiat. A. J. *4:* 32 (1959).

540. Royce, P. C. and Sayers, G.: Purification of hypothalamic corticotropin releasing factor. Proc. Soc. exp. Biol., N. Y. *103:* 447 (1960).

541. Rumsfeld, H. W., Jr. and Porter, J. C.: Investigation of the activation of the pituitary-adrenal axis. Fed. Proc. *18:* 132 (1950).

542. Russek, H. I. and Zohman, B. L.: Relative significance of heredity, diet and occupational stress in coronary heart disease of young adults: Based on an analysis of 100 patients between the ages of 25 and 40 years and a similar group of 100 normal control subjects. Amer. J. med. Sci. *235:* 266 (1958).

543. Saffran, M.: Activation of ACTH release by neurohypophysial peptides. Canad. J. Biochem. *37:* 319 (1959).

544. Saffran, M. and Saffran, J.: Adenohypophysis and adrenal cortex. Annu. Rev. Physiol. *21:* 403 (1959).

545. Saito, S. and Tani, F.: Biological characterization of the crude thyrotrophin releasing principle from urine. Endocrin. jap. *7:* 13 (1960).

546. Salgado, E. D.: Production d'une hypertension metacorticoïde avec des doses minimes de DCA. Rev. canad. Biol. *12:* 316 (1953).

547. Sambhi, M. P. and White, F. N.: The electrocardiogram of the normal and hypertensive rat. Circulation *8:* 129 (1960).

548. Samorajski, T. and Fitz, G. R.: Histochemical analysis of phosphomonoesterase in the hypothalamus and pituitary gland of the rat. Lab. Invest. *9:* 517 (1960).

549. Sandberg, A. A.; Eik-Nes, K.; Samules, L. T. and Tyler, F. H.: The effects of surgery on the blood levels and metabolism of 17-hydroxycorticosteroids in man. J. clin. Invest. *33:* 1509 (1954).

550. Sanders, A. E. and Rennels, E. G.: Evidence on the cellular source of luteotrophin derived from a study of rat pituitary autografts. Z. Zellforsch. *49:* 263 (1959).

551. Sano, Y. und Knoop, A.: Elektronenmikroskopische Untersuchungen am kaudalen neurosekretorischen System von Tinca vulgaris. Z. Zellforsch. *49:* 464 (1959).

552. Sayers, G.; Redgate, E. S. and Royce, P. C.: Hypothalamus, adenohypophysis and adrenal cortex. Annu. Rev. Physiol. *20:* 243 (1958).

553. Sayers, G.: Discussion. Proc. Laurentian Hormone Conf. 1958; Recent Progr. Hormone Res. *15:* 385 (1959).
554. Sayers, G.: Hypothalamus and adenohypophysis: with special reference to corticotrophin release. Acta endocrin., Kbh. (Suppl. 50) *34:* 25 (1960).
555. Sawyer, W. H.: Activation and blockade of the release of pituitary gonadotropin as influenced by the reticular formation; in: Jasper, H. R. *et al.,* Reticular formation of the brain (Little, Brown, Boston/Toronto 1958).
556. Sawyer, W. H.: Increased water permeability of the bullfrog (Rana catesbiana) bladder in vitro in response to synthetic oxytocin and arginine vasotocin and to neurohypophysial extracts from nonmammalian vertebrates. Endocrinology *66:* 112 (1960).
557. Sawyer, W. H.; Munsick, R. A. and Van Dyke, H. B.: Pharmacological evidence for the presence of arginine vasotocin and oxytocin in neurohypophysial extracts from coldblooded vertebrates. Nature, Lond. *184:* 1464 (1959).
557a. Schacher, J.; Browne, J. S. L. and Selye, H.: Effect of various sterols on thymus in the adrenalectomized rat. Proc. Soc. exp. Biol., N. Y. *36:* 488 (1937).
558. Schallek, W. and Kuehn, A.: Effects of psychotropic drugs on limbic system of cat. Proc. Soc. exp. Biol., N. Y. *105:* 115 (1960).
559. Schally, A. V. and Guillemin, R.: Concentration of corticotropin releasing factor by chromatography on carboxylmethylcellulose. Proc. Soc. exp. Biol., N. Y. *100:* 138 (1959).
560. Schally, A. V.; Saffran, M. and Zimmermann, B.: A corticotrophin-releasing factor: partial purification and amino acid composition. Biochem. J. *70:* 97 (1958).
561. Scharrer, B.: General and phylogenetic interpretations of neuro-endocrine interrelations; in: Comparative endocrinology, ed.: A. Gorbman, p. 233 (Wiley, New York 1959).
562. Scharrer, B.: The role of neurosecretion in neuroendocrine integration; in: Comparative endocrinology, ed.: A. Gorbman, p. 134 (Wiley, New York 1959).
563. Schapiro, S. and Katz, J.: Preferential concentration of $C^{14}$ in posterior pituitary following hydrocortisone $C^{14}$ injection. Proc. Soc. exp. Biol., N. Y. *102:* 609 (1959).
564. Schapiro, S. and Marmorston, J.: Response to stress: differing responses of atherosclerotic and normal dog to electric shock or cold. Proc. Soc. exp. Biol., N. Y. *103:* 520 (1960).
565. Schmitthenner, J. E.; Reigel, C. and Hafkenshiel, J. H.: Effects of increased cardiac work on coronary blood flow and left ventricular metabolism: effect of nicotine. Fed. Proc. *15:* 164 (1958).
566. Schrader, G. A.; Prickett, C. O. and Sakmon, W. D.: Symptomatology and pathology of potassium and magnesium deficiencies in the rat. J. Nutrit. *14:* 35 (1937).
567. Schreiber, V. und Kmentova, V.: Die Zusammenhänge zwischen der Aktivität der sauren Phosphatasen in der Hypophyse und der Produktion des thyreotropen Hormons. Endokrinologie *38:* 69 (1959).
568. Schreiber, V. and Kmentova, V.: The effect of thyroidectomy on acid phosphatases in the pituitary and on the hypothalamic factor activating acid phosphatases in the pituitary in vitro. Physiol. bohemoslov. *8:* 506 (1959).
569. Schreiber, V.; Charvat, J. and Kmentova, V.: Fractionation of brain extracts for acid phosphatase-elevating activity. Nature, Lond. *183:* 473 (1959).
570. Schon, M. and Sutherland, A. M.: The role of hormones in human behavior. III. Changes in female sexuality after hypophysectomy. J. clin. Endocrinol. *20:* 833 (1960).
571. Schottstaedt, W. W.; Pinsky, R. H.; Mackler, D. and Wolf, S.: Sociologic, psychologic and metabolic observations on patients in the community of a metabolic ward. Amer. J. Med. *25:* 243 (1958).

572. SCHÖNBAUM, E.: Adrenocortical function in rats exposed to low environmental temperatures. Fed. Proc. (Suppl. 5) *19:* 85 (1960).
573. SCHWARTZ, L.; FONG, C. T. G.; POPENOE, E. A.; SILVER, L. and SCHOESSLER, M. A.: Evidence for a covalent attachment of the antidiuretic hormone to its receptor site in the kidney. 51st annu. Meet. amer. Soc. clin. Invest., Atlantic City 1959.
574. SCHWEINBURG, F. B. and FINE, J.: Host resistance to bacteria in hemorrhagic shock. II. Effect of transient vascular collapse on sensitivity to endotoxin. Proc. Soc. exp. Biol., N. Y. *88:* 589 (1955).
575. SEHRA, K. B.: Carbohydrate metabolism in injury. Indian J. med. Sci. *12:* 313 (1958).
576. SEIFERT, J. and BAEDER, D. H.: Hormonal control of permeability and mobilization of fat depots. Ann. N. Y. Acad. Sci. *72:* 1031 (1959).
577. SEIP, M. F.: Congenital hyperpituitarism of hypothalamic origin. IX. int. Congr. Paediat., Montreal 1959.
578. SELYE, H.: Morphologische Studie über die Veränderungen nach Verfütterung von bestrahltem Ergosterin (Vigantol) bei der weißen Ratte. Krankheitsforsch. *7:* 290 (1929).
579. SELYE, H.: Knochenveränderungen bei den jungen Vigantol-behandelten Tieren. Verein. dtsch. Ärzte, Prag 1928. – Med. Klin. *25:* 167 (1929).
580. SELYE, H.: A syndrome produced by diverse nocuous agents. Nature, Lond. *138:*32 (1936).
581. SELYE, H.: Thymus and adrenals in the response of the organism to injuries and intoxications. Brit. J. exp. Path. *17:* 234 (1936).
582. SELYE, H.: The alarm reaction. Canad. med. Ass. J. *34:* 706 (1936).
583. SELYE, H.: The significance of the adrenals for adaptation. Science *85:* 247 (1937).
584. SELYE, H.: Experimental production and prevention of appendicitis with histamine. Canad. med. Ass. J. *36:* 462 (1937).
585. SELYE, H.: Studies on adaptation. Endocrinology *21:* 169 (1937).
586. SELYE, H.: The significance of the adrenal glands for adaptation. Arch. int. Pharmacodyn. *55:* 431 (1937).
587. SELYE, H.: The prevention of adrenalin lung oedema by the alarm reaction. Amer. J. Physiol. *122:* 347 (1937).
588. SELYE, H.: Über den Einfluß der Alarmreaktion und der Histaminbehandlung auf den Wasserstoffwechsel bei Nierenschädigung. Klin. Wschr. *17:* 666 (1938).
589. SELYE, H.: The effect of the alarm reaction on the absorption of toxic substances from the gastro-intestinal tract. J. Pharmacol., Baltimore *64:* 138 (1938).
590. SELYE, H.: Experimental evidence supporting the conception of 'adaptation energy'. Amer. J. Physiol. *123:* 758 (1938).
591. SELYE, H.: Interactions between various steroid hormones. Canad. med. Ass. J. *42:* 113 (1940).
592. SELYE, H.: On the production of malignant hypertension by chronic exposure to various damaging agents. Rev. canad. Biol. *2:* 501 (1943).
593. SELYE, H.: The general adaptation syndrome and the disease of adaptation J. clin. Endocrin. *6:* 117 (1946).
594. SELYE, H.: Effect of ACTH and cortisone upon an 'anaphylactoid reaction'. Canad. med. Ass. J. *61:* 553 (1949).
595. SELYE, H.: Further studies concerning the participation of the adrenal cortex in the pathogenesis of arthritis. Brit. med. J., p. 1129 (1949).
596. SELYE, H.: Interactions between gluco-corticoid and mineralocorticoid hormones. J. clin. Invest. *29:* 845 (1950).
597. SELYE, H.: Stress. The physiology and pathology of exposure to stress (Acta Inc., Montreal 1950).
598. SELYE, H.: Effect of desoxycorticosterone upon the toxic actions of somatotrophic hormone. Proc. Soc. exp. Biol., N. Y. *76:* 510 (1951).

599. Selye, H.: The influence of STH, ACTH and cortisone upon resistance to infection. Canad. med. Ass. J. *64:* 489 (1951).
600. Selye, H.: Role of the adrenals in the production of renal and cardiovascular damage by anterior pituitary preparations. Lancet, p. 483 (1951).
601. Selye, H.: The story of the adaptation syndrome (Acta Inc., Montreal 1952).
602. Selye, H.: Induction of local 'crossed resistance' to various necrotizing agents. J. exp. Med. *11:* 81 (1953).
603. Selye, H.: Induction of topical resistance to acute tissue injury. An experimental study with the 'granuloma pouch technique'. Surg. Clin. N. Amer. *33:* 1417 (1953).
604. Selye, H.: The part of inflammation in the local adaptation syndrome. Rev. canad. Biol. *12:* 155 (1953).
605. Selye, H.: 'Conditioning' versus 'permissive' actions of hormones. J. clin. Endocrin. *14:* 122 (1954).
606. Selye, H.: An experimental model illustrating the pathogenesis of the diseases of adaptation. J. clin. Endocrin. *14:* 997 (1954).
607. Selye, H.: Sensitization of individual vascular territories to the antiphlogistic effect of hydrocortisone. An example of 'selective conditioning'. Circulation *2:* 53 (1954).
608. Selye, H.: Effect of somatotropic hormone (STH) upon inflammation; in: The hypophyseal growth hormone, nature and actions, ed.: R. W. Smith, C. H. Gaebler and , H. C. Long (Blakiston Div., McGraw-Hill, New York 1955).
609. Selye, H.: The stress of life (McGraw-Hill, New York 1956).
610. Selye, H.: Protection by pregnancy against the development of experimental arteriosclerosis and metastatic calcification. Amer. J. Obstet. Gynec. *74:* 289 (1957).
611. Selye, H.: Lathyrism. Rev. canad. Biol. *16:* 1 (1957).
612. Selye, H.: Skeletal lesions produced by chronic treatment with somatotrophic hormone (STH) and aminoacetonitrile (AAN). J. Geront. *12:* 270 (1957).
613. Selye, H.: The chemical prevention of cardiac necroses (Ronald Press, New York 1958).
614. Selye, H.: Prophylactic treatment of an experimental arteriosclerosis with magnesium and potassium salts. Amer. Heart J. *55:* 805 (1958).
615. Selye, H.: Humoral 'conditioning' for the production of a suppurative, acute myocarditis by the oral administration of sodium phosphate. Amer. Heart J. *55:* 1 (1958).
616. Selye, H.: Conditioning by cortisol for the production of acute massive myocardial necroses during neuromuscular exertion. Circulation *6:* 168 (1958).
617. Selye, H.: The humoral production of cardiac infarcts. Brit. med. J., *1:* 599 (1958).
618. Selye, H.: Synergism between mineralo and glucocorticoids in the production of the 'phosphate-steroid-cardiopathy'. Acta endocrin., Kbh. *28:* 279 (1958).
619. Selye, H.: Cardiopatia infartoide. Folia clin. internac. *8:* 97 (1958).
620. Selye, H.: Protection by pregnancy against the development of 'phosphate-steroid-cardiopathy' and nephrocalcinosis. J. Obstet. Gynaec. brit. Emp. *65:* 588 (1958).
621. Selye, H.: Production with sodium sulphates of an 'electrolyte-steroid-cardiopathy' characterized by necroses (ESCN), and its prevention by $MgCl_2$ and KCl. Canad. J. Biochem. *36:* 717 (1958).
622. Selye, H.: Production of 'electrolyte-steroid-cardiopathy' with $NaClO_4$, and its prevention by $MgCl_2$ and KCl. Angiology *9:* 262 (1958).
623. Selye, H.: Prevention by $MgCl_2$ and KCl of the vascular hypersensitivity induced by pretreatment with dihydrotachysterol (DHT). Int. Arch. Allergy *12:* 145 (1958).
624. Selye, H.: Infarctoid cardiopathy elicited by temporary obstruction of the pylorus in humorally conditioned animals. Tohoku J. exp. Med. *67:* 335 (1958).
625. Selye, H.: Perspectives in stress research. Perspect. Biol. Med. *2:* 403 (1959).
626. Selye, H.: Wechselwirkungen zwischen Streß, Elektrolyten und Steroiden beim Entstehen verschiedener Kardiopathien und Myopathien. Endokrinologie *38:* 195 (1959).

627. SELYE, H.: Protection by a steroid-spirolactone against certain types of cardiac necroses. Proc. Soc. exp. Biol., N. Y. *104:* 212 (1960).
628. SELYE, H.: The pluricausal cardiopathies: Beaumont lecture for 1961 (Thomas, Springfield 1961).
629. SELYE, H.: Nonspecific resistance. Ergebn. allg. Path. path. Anat. *41:* 208 (1961).
630. SELYE, H. und BAJUSZ, E.: Beiträge der Streßforschung zur Kardiologie. Herznekrosen und ihre Verhütung. Schweiz. med. Wschr. *88:* 1147 (1958).
631. SELYE, H. und BAJUSZ, E.: Experimentelle Beiträge zur Frage der relativen Beteiligung von Streß und Anoxämie bei der Pathogenese gewisser Herznekrosen. Beitr. path. Anat. *119:* 333 (1958).
632. SELYE, H. and BAJUSZ, E.: Provocation and prevention of potassium deficiency by various ions. Proc. Soc. Biol., N. Y. *98:* 580 (1958).
633. SELYE, H. and BAJUSZ, E.: Prevention by $MgCl_2$ and KCl of the myocardial necroses normally produced by papain. Cardiologia *33:* 305 (1958).
634. SELYE, H. and BAJUSZ, E.: Effect of denervation on experimentally induced changes in the growth of bone and muscle. Amer. J. Physiol. *192:* 297 (1958).
635. SELYE, H. and BAJUSZ, E.: Stress and the electrolyte-steroid-cardiopathy. Acta physiol. latinoamer. *8:* 147 (1958).
636. SELYE, H. and BAJUSZ, E.: Zatez a srdecni infarkty. Vesmir, Prague *37:* 271 (1958).
637. SELYE, H. and BAJUSZ, E.: Effect of various stressors on muscular contraction induced by $NaH_2PO_4$. Amer. J. Physiol. *196:* 681 (1959).
638. SELYE, H. and BAJUSZ, E.: Role of sodium in production of myocardial necroses by stress. Proc. Soc. exp. Biol., N. Y. *100:* 11 (1959).
639. SELYE, H. and BAJUSZ, E.: Sensitization by potassium-deficiency for the production of myocardial necroses by stress. Amer. J. Path. *35:* 525 (1959).
640. SELYE, H. und BAJUSZ, E.: Die Bedeutung von Elektrolyten bei der Prophylaxe experimenteller Herznekrosen. Arzneimittelforsch. *9:* 281 (1959).
641. SELYE, H. and BAJUSZ, E.: Influence of blood pressure upon the production of myocardial necroses by various agents. Arch. int. Physiol. *67:* 78 (1959).
642. SELYE, H. and BAJUSZ, E.: Sensitization by potassium deficiency for the production of myocardial necrosis by stress. Amer. J. Path. *35:* 525 (1959).
643. SELYE, H. and BAJUSZ, E.: Sensitization by dihydrotachysterol (DHT) for induction of cardiac lesions by various agents. Amer. J. Cardiol. *4:* 102 (1959).
644. SELYE, H. and BAJUSZ, E.: Stress and cardiac infarcts: effect of sodium deficiency upon necrotizing cardiopathies produced by various agents. Angiology *10:* 412 (1959).
645. SELYE, H. and BAJUSZ, E.: Sensitization by K- or Mg-deficiency for the production of myocardial necroses by papain. Z. Vitamin-, Hormon-, Fermentforsch. *10:* 39 (1959).
646. SELYE, H. and BAJUSZ, E.: Conditioning by corticoids for the production of cardiac lesions with noradrenaline. Acta endocrin., Kbh. *30:* 183 (1959).
647. SELYE, H. and BAJUSZ, E.: Effect of various electrolytes upon cardiac and skeletal musculature. Brit. J. Pharmacol. *14:* 83 (1959).
648. SELYE, H. and BAJUSZ, E.: Interactions between electrolytes, corticoids and dihydrotachysterol (DHT) in the production of cardiovascular disease and nephrocalcinosis. Lab. Invest. *8:* 1499 (1959).
649. SELYE, H. und BAJUSZ, E.: Erzeugung und Verhütung von Herznekrosen bei der dehydrotachysterin sensibilisierten Ratte. Arch. Path. *332:* 140 (1959).
650. SELYE, H. and BAJUSZ, E.: The age factor in the production of various experimental cardiopathies. J. Geront. *14:* 164 (1959).
651. SELYE, H. and BAJUSZ, E.: Sensitization by dihydrotachysterol (DHT) for the induction of cardiac lesions by various agents. Amer. J. Cardiol. *4:* 102 (1959).

652. Selye, H. and Bajusz, E.: A stress-kutatas újabb eredményei és a stress-elmélet szerepe a modern kórtani kutatómunkában. I. Mi a stress? Orv. Hetil. *101:* 1 (1960).
653. Selye, H. and Bajusz, E.: A stress-kutatás újabb eredményei és a stress-elmélet szerepe a modern kórtani kutatómunkában. II. Kondicionálo tényezök az infarktoid kardiopathiák patomechanizmusában. Orv. Hetil. *101:* 145 (1960).
654. Selye, H. and Bajusz, E.: The stress concept as applied to traumatology (Part I). Acta chir. hungar. *1:* 305 (1960).
655. Selye, H. and Bajusz, E.: The stress concept as applied to traumatology (Part II). Acta chir. hungar. *1:* 347 (1960).
656. Selye, H. and Bajusz, E.: Stress and rheumatic diseases; in: Arthritis and allied conditions, 6th ed., p. 607, ed.: J. L. Hollander (Lea & Febiger, Philadelphia 1960).
657. Selye, H. and Bajusz, E.: The prevention of experimental myopathies by various chlorides. J. Nutrit. *72:* 37 (1960).
658. Selye, H. and Bajusz, E.: Adrenal cortex in essential hypertension. Prague Conf. int. Symp. Pathogenesis of Essential Hypertension, Prague 1960.
659. Selye, H. and Bajusz, E.: Protection afforded by stress against humorally induced cardiac necroses. Dr. Sodi Pallares' Memorial vol. (Mexico, D. F., p. 359, 1961).
660. Selye, H. and Bajusz, E.: Unpublished; quoted by Selye, H. The pluricausal cardiopathies (Thomas, Springfield 1961).
661. Selye, H.; Bajusz, E. and Cantin, M.: Pathogenic actions of hormones. Z. Vitamin-, Hormon-, Fermentforsch. *12:* 262 (1962).
662. Selye, H.; Bajusz, E.; Grasso, S. and Mendell, P.: Simple techniques for the surgical occlusion of coronary vessels in the rat. Angiology *11:* 398 (1960).
663. Selye, H.; Bajusz, E. and Renaud, S.: Effect of pregnancy upon myocardial lesions produced by various agents. Monit. ostet.-ginec. *30:* 7 (1959).
664. Selye, H.; Bajusz, E. und Renaud, S.: Über die Mitwirkung verschiedener Elektrolyte bei der Erzeugung von Herzläsionen durch Dihydrotachysterin (DHT). Z. Kreislaufforsch. *48:* 237 (1959).
665. Selye, H.; Bajusz, E.; Renaud, S. and Lemire, Y.: Sensitization by dihydrotachysterol (DHT) and calcium acetate for the induction of cardiac lesions by various agents. Amer. Hearth J. *57:* 88 (1959).
666. Selye, H.; Bajusz, E.; Renaud, S. et Nádasdi, M.: Progrès récents dans l'étude de la pathogénie et de la prophylaxie des nécroses cardiaques. Ars med. *15:* 831 (1960).
667. Selye, H.; Bajusz, E. and Strebel, R.: Cross-resistance to cardiotoxic agents. Canad. J. Biochem. *39:* 519 (1961).
668. Selye, H.; Bajusz, E. and Veilleux, R.: Production of dissecting aneurysm by chronic isoproterenol treatment. Cor & Vasa *2:* 273 (1960).
669. Selye, H. and Bois, P.: Effect of STH on experimental lathyrism. Proc. Soc. exp. Biol., N. Y. *94:* 133 (1957).
670. Selye, H. and Bois, P.: Effect of corticoids upon experimental lathyrism. Endocrinology *60:* 507 (1957).
671. Selye, H. and Collip, J. B.: Fundamental factors in the interpretation of stimuli influencing endocrine glands. Endocrinology *20:* 667 (1936).
672. Selye, H. and Dosue, C.: Influence of traumatic shock on blood sugar of adrenalectomized rats treated with adrenal cortical extracts. Proc. Soc. exp. Biol., N. Y. *48:* 532 (1941).
673. Selye, H.; Hall, C. R. and Rowley, E. M.: Malignant hypertension produced by treatment with desoxycorticosterone acetate and sodium chloride. Canad. med. Ass. J. *49:* 88 (1943).
674. Selye, H. and Hall, C. E.: Pathologic changes induced in various species by overdosage with desoxycorticosterone. Arch. Path. *36:* 19 (1943).
675. Selye, H. and Hall, C. E.: The pathology of desoxycorticosterone overdosage in various species. Fed. Proc. *2:* 44 (1943).

676. Selye, H. and Heuser, G.: Experimental studies concerning the role of hormonal, vascular and nervous factors in the regulation of the 'anaphylactoid reaction' of the rat. Int. Arch. Allergy *5:* 52 (1954).
677. Selye, H.; Horava, A. and Heuser, G.: 1st–5th Ann. Rev. on stress (Acta Inc., Montreal 1951–55/56).
678. Selye, H. and Jasmin, G.: Screening of possible therapeutic agents by means of replicas of connective-tissue diseases. Ann. N. Y. Acad. Sci. *64:* 481 (1956).
679. Selye, H.; Jasmin, G.; Bois, P. and Richer, C. L.: Role of corticoids in the production of an experimental polyarthritis in the rat. J. clin. Endocrin. *16:* 918 (1956).
680. Selye, H.; Jean, P. et Bajusz, E.: Résistance croisée et prévention des cardiopathies expérimentales produites par un dérivé de la vitamine D. Sem. Hôp. Paris *9:* 331 (1961).
681. Selye, H.; Jean, P. and Cantin, M.: Prevention by stress and cortisol of gastric ulcers normally produced by 48/80. Proc. Soc. exp. Biol., N. Y. *105:* 444 (1960).
682. Selye, H.; Jean, P. and Veilleux, R.: Sensitization by thallium to dihydrotachysterol overdosage. Proc. Soc. exp. Biol., N.Y. *106:* 408 (1961).
683. Selye, H.; Mintzberg, J. and Rowley, E. M.: Effect of various electrolytes upon the toxicity of desoxycorticosterone acetate. J. Pharmacol., Baltimore *85:* 42 (1945).
684. Selye, H. and Mishra, R. K.: Prevention of the 'phosphate-steroid-cardiopathy' by various electrolytes. Amer. Heart J. *55:* 163 (1958).
685. Selye, H. and Pentz, E. I.: Pathogenetical correlations between periarteritis nodosa, renal hypertension and rheumatic lesions. Canad. med. Ass. J. *49:* 264 (1943).
686. Selye, H.; Prioreschi, P. and Jean, P.: Production of cardiac necroses and nephrocalcinosis by stress in adrenalectomized rats. Proc. Soc. exp. Biol., N. Y. *104:* 68 (1960).
687. Selye, H. and Renaud, S.: Humoral conditioning for the production of acute, massive myocardial necroses by neuromuscular exertion. Proc. Soc. exp. Biol., N. Y. *96:* 512 (1957).
688. Selye, H. et Renaud, S.: Prévention, par le chlorure de potassium, d'une myocardite expérimentale. Presse méd. *66:* 99 (1958).
689. Selye, H.; Renaud, S. and Nádasdi, M.: Nonspecificity of the mechanism that elicits myocardial necroses in humorally conditioned rats. Endocrinology *62:* 541 (1958).
690. Selye, H.; Renaud, S. and Nádasdi, M.: Ability of various steroids to produce 'infarctoid cardiopathy' in rats conditioned by $NaH_2PO_4$. J. Pharmacol., Baltimore *122:* 504 (1958).
691. Selye, H. and Salcedo, I. de: 'Infarctoid cardiopathy' produced by combined treatment with hydrocortisone and monobasic sodium phosphate. Arch. intern. Med. *102:* 551 (1958).
692. Selye, H.; Stone, H. and Timiras, P. S.: Influence of sodium chloride upon the actions of desoxycorticosterone acetate. Amer. Heart J. *37:* 1009 (1949).
693. Selye, H.; Sylvester, O.; Hall, C. E. and Leblond, C. P.: Hormonal production of arthritis. J. amer. med. Ass. *124:* 201 (1944).
694. Selye, H.; Veilleux, R. and Grasso, S.: Protection, by coronary ligature, against isoproterenol-induced myocardial necroses. Proc. Soc. exp. Biol., N. Y. *104:* 343 (1960).
695. Selye, H. and Ventura, J.: Effect of hypophysectomy and substitution therapy with STH upon experimental bone lathyrism. Amer. J. Pathol. *33:* 919 (1957).
696. Shelton, M.; Becker, W. M.; Adeyemo, A. and Allen, G.: Effects of cortisone on the perfused rabbit heart. Fed. Proc. *15:* 482 (1956).
697. Shibusawa, K.; Nishi, K. and Abe, C.: Further observations of the hypothalamic control of the thyroid gland. Endocrin. jap. *6:* 31 (1959).

698. Shibusawa, K.; Yamamoto, T.; Nishi, K.; Abe, C. and Tomie, S.: Studies on the tissue concentrations of TRF in the normal dog. Endocrin. jap. *6:* 137 (1959).

699. Shibusawa, K.; Yamamoto, T.; Nishi, K.; Abe, C. and Tomie, S.: Urinary excretion of TRF in various functional states of the thyroid. Endocrin. jap. *6:* 131 (1959).

700. Shimizu, T.: The hypothalamic neurosecretory phenomena and the activity of thyroid gland in partially thyroidectomized rats. Endocrin. jap. *6:* 75 (1959).

701. Shoji, H.: Studies on the effective fractions isolated from myocardium; cephalin as a determinant group of an antigen in heart allergy. Jap. Circulat. J. *19:* 327 (1955).

702. Sideman, M. and Sobel, H.: ACTH releasing factor active in the guinea pig. Proc. Soc. exp. Biol., N. Y. *103:* 274 (1960).

703. Simpson, G. G.: The major features of evolutions, p. 100, 166 (Columbia Univ. Press, New York 1953).

704. Simpson, G. G.; Pittendrigh, C. and Tiffany, L.: Life, p. 434 (Harcourt Brace, New York 1957).

705. Slusher, M. A.: Dissociation of adrenal ascorbic acid and corticosterone responses to stress in rats with hypothalamic lesions. Endocrinology *63:* 412 (1958).

706. Slusher, M. A.: Effect of brainstem lesions on stress-induced corticosteroid release in female rats. Endocrinology *67:* 347 (1960)

707. Smelik, P. G.: Autonomic nervous involvement in stress-induced ACTH secretion. Thesis, Univ. of Groningen (N. V. Druk. V. H. H. Born, Assen 1959).

708. Smelik, P. G.: The role of the posterior lobe of the pituitary gland in the corticotrophic response to acute stress. Proc. Netherl. Soc. Endocr., Amsterdam 1959. – Acta physiol. pharmacol. néerl. *9:* 125 (1960).

709. Smelik, P. G.: Mechanism of hypophysial response to psychic stress. Acta endocrin., Kbh. *33:* 437 (1960).

710. Smith, C. A., Jr.; Jabbur, S. J.; Rushmer, R. G. and Lasher, E. P.: Role of hypothalamic structures in cardiac control. Physiol. Rev. (Suppl. 4) *40:* 136 (1960).

711. Smith, S. G.: Magnesium-potassium antagonism. Arch. Biochem. *20:* 473 (1949).

711a. Smith, S. G.: Respiration and paralysis as they relate to magnesium-potassium antagonism. Amer. J. Physiol. *164:* 702 (1951).

712. Snyder, D. D. and Campbell, G. S.: Effect of aortic constriction on experimental atherosclerosis in rabbits. Proc. Soc. exp. Biol., N. Y. *99:* 563 (1958).

713. Solomon, J. and Greep, R. O.: The effect of alterations in thyroid function on the pituitary growth hormone content and acidophil cytology. Endocrinology *65:* 158 (1959).

714. Solomon, N.; Travis, R. H. and Sayers, G.: Corticosteroids and the functional capacity of the rat heart-lung preparation. Endocrinology *64:* 535 (1959).

715. Solomon, R. L. and Wynne, L. C.: Avoidance conditioning in normal dogs and in dogs deprived of normal autonomic functioning. Amer. Psychologist *5:* 264 (1950).

716. Sommerville, W.: The effect of cortisone on the cardiogram in chronic adrenal insufficiency. Brit. med. J. *2:* 860 (1950).

717. Soskin, S. and Levine, R.: Carbohydrate metabolism (Univ. of Chicago Press, Chicago 1940).

718. Soulairac, A. et Soulairac, M. L.: Actions de la gonadotrophine chronique et de la testostérone sur le comportement sexuel et le tractus génital du rat mâle porteur de lésions hypothalamiques postérieures. Ann. Endocrin. *20:* 137 (1959).

719. Speransky, A. D.: A basis for the theory of medicine (International Publ., New York 1943).

720. Spire, H. M.; Reifenstein, R. W. and Gray, S. J.: The effect of adrenocorticotropic hormone upon uropepsin excretion. J. Lab. clin. Med. *35:* 899 (1950).

721. Stamler, J.; Boleme, C.; Harris, R. and Katz, L. N.: Effect of choline and inositol on plasma and tissue lipids and atherosclerosis in the cholesterol-fed chick. Circulation *2:* 714 (1950).

722. STAMMLER, J. and KATZ, L. N.: The effect of pancreatectomy on lipemia, tissue lipoidosis and atherogenesis in chicks. Circulation *4:* 255 (1951).

723. STEENBURG, R. W. and GANONG, W. F.: Observations on the influence of extra-adrenal factors on circulating 17-hydroxycorticoids in the surgically stressed, adrenalectomized animal. Surgery *38:* 92 (1955).

724. STEFFEN, A.: Zur akuten Myocarditis. Ann. paediat., Basel *27:* 223 (1388).

725. STETSON, C.: Occurrence of leukocyte-platelet thrombosis in rheumatic carditis. J. exp. Med. *94:* 493 (1957).

726. STETTEN, W. DE, Jr. and TOPPER, Y. J.: The metabolism of carbohydrates. Amer. J. Med. *19:* 96 (1955).

727. STEVENSON, I. P.; DUNCAN, C. R. and WOLFF, H. G.: Circulatory dynamics before and after exercises in subjects with and without structural heart disease during anxiety and relaxation. J. clin. Invest. *28:* 1534 (1949).

728. STEVENSON, I. P.; DUNCAN, C. H. and RIPLEY, H. S.: Variations in electrocardiogram changes in emotional state. J. amer. Ass. Geriatr. *6:* 164 (1951).

729. STEWARD, J.: Theory of culture change, p. 39 (Univ. of Illinois, Urabana 1955).

730. STIGLIANI, R.: Sulle sostanze MacManus- e Gomori-positive nello stroma dei plessi corioidei dell'umo. Arch. «de Vecchi» anat. pat. *29:* 331 (1959).

731. STOLKOWSKI, J. et REINBERG, A.: Recherches sur le mécanisme de l'action de quelques hormones corticostéroïdes sur le potassium cellulaire. I. Influence du glucose et de l'acide adenosine-triphosphorique (A.T.P.) sur les mouvements du K cellulaire. Ann. Endocrin. *17:* 137 (1959).

732. STURTEVANT, F. M.: The biology of metacorticoid hypertension. Ann intern. Med. *49:* 1281 (1958).

733. SUPEK, Z.; KECKES, S. and VOJVODIC, S.: The influence of chlorpromazine on the antidiuretic and chloruretic effects of nicotine and posterior pituitary extracts. Arch. int. Pharmacodyn. *123:* 260 (1960).

734. SUPEK, Z.; KECKES, S. and VOJVODIC, S.: The action of chlorpromazine on water and chloride excretion in rats. Arch. int. Pharmacodyn. *123:* 253 (1960).

735. SUZUKI, T.; ROMANOFF, E. B.; KOELLA, W. P. and LEVY, C. K.: Effect of diencephalic stimuli on 17-hydroxycorticosteroid secretion in unanesthetized dogs. Amer. J. Physiol. *198:* 1312 (1960).

736. SWIFT, H. F.: The nature of rheumatic fever. J. Lab. clin. Med. *21:* 551 (1936).

737. SWINGLE, W. W.; DAVANZO, J. P.; GLENISTER, D.; WAGLE, G.; OSBORNE, M. and ROWEN, R.: Effect of mineralo- and glucocorticoids on fasted adrenalectomized dogs subjected to electroshock. Proc. Soc. exp. Biol., N. Y. *104:* 184 (1960).

738. SZENTGYÖRGYI, A.: Chemistry of muscular contraction, 2nd ed. (Academic Press, New York 1951).

739. SZENTGYÖRGYI, A.: Chemical physiology of contraction in body and heart muscle (Academic Press, New York 1953).

740. SZENTGYÖRGYI, A.: Bioenergetics (Academic Press, New York 1957)

741. TALEISNIK, S. and MCCANN, S. M.: Alterations in behavior and endocrine function in rats with hypothalamic constant estrus. Physiologist *3:* 161 (1960).

742. TANZ, R. D.: Studies on the action of cortisone acetate on isolated cardiac tissue. J. Pharmacol., Baltimore *128:* 168 (1960).

743. TANZ, R. D.; WHITEHEAD, R. W. and WOIR, G. J., Jr.: Cardiotonic activity of 9-alpha fluorohydrocortisone. Proc. Soc. exp. Biol., N. Y. *94:* 258 (1957).

744. TENNENT, D. M.; ZANETTI, M. E.; OTT, W. H.; KURON, G. W. and SPIEGEL, H.: Influence of crystalline elastase on experimental atherosclerosis in the chicken. Science *124:* 588 (1956).

745. THACKER, E. J.: The mineral composition of the albino rat as affected by chloride deficiency. J. Nutr. *26:* 431 (1943).

746. THOMAS, C. B. and MURPHY, E. A.: Further studies on cholesterol levels in the

Johns Hopkins medical students: Effect of stress at examinations. J. chron. Dis. *8:* 661 (1958).
747. Thomas, C. B. and Murphy, E. A.: Circulatory responses to smoking in healthy young men. Ann. N. Y. Acad. Sci. *90:* 266 (1960).
748. Thomas, L. and Gamble, C. N.: Morphologic changes in rabbits following the intravenous administration of meningococcal toxin. II. Two appropriately spaced injections; the role of fibrinoid in the generalized Shwartzman reaction. Amer. J. Pathol. *31:* 655 (1955).
749. Thomas, R. M.; Mylon, E. and Winternitz, M. C.: Myocardial lesions resulting from dietary deficiency. Yale J. Biol. Med. *12:* 345 (1940).
750. Thomas, L.; Denny, F. W. and Floyd, J.: Studies on the generalized Shwarztman reactions. III. Lesions of the myocardium and coronary arteries accompanying the reaction in rabbits prepared by infection with group A streptococci. J. exp. Med. *97:* 751 (1955).
751. Thorp, R. H.: The effect of exercise upon the response of rabbits to insulin. Quart. J. exp. Pharmacol. *17:* 75 (1949).
752. Tuchmann-Duplessis, H.: Thyroïde et corrélations hypophysothyroïdiennes chez l'anencéphale humain. Ann. Endocrin. *20:* 569 (1959).
753. Tufts, E. V. and Greenberg, D. M.: The biochemistry of magnesium deficiency. II. The minimum magnesium requirement for growth, gestation, and lactation, and the effect of the dietary calcium level thereon. J. biol. Chem. *122:* 715 (1938).
754. Turevich, N. M.: Effect of experimental neurosis on the gonadotropic function of the hypophysis an precancerous changes in the mammary glands in mice of the $C_3HA$ strain. Fiziol. zhur. *5:* 58 (1959).
755. Uhley, H.; Friedman, M. and Ayello, C.: Atherosclerotic response of 'aggressive' and 'passive' groups of chickens to a cholesterol enriched diet. Proc. Soc. exp. Biol., N. Y. *96:* 244 (1957).
756. Urasov, I. G.: Besonderheiten des Baues der Neurologia der Hypophyse bei Säugetieren. Z. mikr.-anat. Forsch. *65:* 98 (1959).
757. Van Liere, E. J.; David, N. A. and Lough, D. H.: Absorption of water from small intestine at various degrees of anoxemia. Amer. J. Physiol. *115:* 239 (1936).
758. Van Liere, E. J. and Sleeth, C. K.: Absorption of sodium chloride from small intestine at various degrees of anoxemia. Amer. J. Physiol. *117:* 309 (1936).
759. Van Liere, E. J.; Northup, D. W. and Sleeth, C. K.: The effect of acute hemorrhage on absorption from the small intestine. Amer. J. Physiol. *124:* 102 (1938).
760. Van Slyke, C. B. and Larson, P. S.: Observations on the role of the adrenal medulla in the blood pressure response to nicotine. J. Pharmacol., Baltimore *98:* 400 (1950).
761. Van Wyk, J. J.; Dugger, G. S.; Newsome, J. F. and Thomas, P. Z.: The effect of pituitary stalk section on the adrenal function of women with cancer of the breast. J. clin. Endocrin. *20:* 157 (1960).
762. Vignolbe, J.; Berthaux, P.; Gouygou, Ch.; Colas-Belcour, J. F.; Lemarchal, A. and Hammel, A.: Hypogonadisme hypogonadotrophique associé à une maladie de Friedreich. Ann. Endocrin. *20:* 172 (1959).
763. Volpé, R.; Vale, J. and Johnston, M. W.: The effect of certain physical and emotional tensions and strains on fluctuations in the level of serum protein-bound iodine. J. clin. Endocrin. *20:* 415 (1960).
764. Voris, L. and Thacker, E. J.: The effects of substitution of bicarbonate for chloride in the diet of rats on growth, energy and protein metabolism. J. Nutrit. *23:* 365 (1942).
765. Wachstein, M. and Meisel, E.: Succinic dehydrogenase activity in myocardial infarction and in induced myocardial necrosis. Amer. J. Pathol. *31:* 353 (1955).
766. Waidl, E. und Semm, K.: Der Beginn der hypothalamischen Neurosekretion in der Fetalzeit. Arch. Gynäk. *192:* 269 (1960).

767. Wagener, H. P.; Dry, T. J. S. and Wilder, R. M.: Retinitis in diabetes. New Engl. J. Med. *211:* 1131 (1934).
768. Wagner, B. M.: Relationship of the Aschoff body to experimental carditis. Fed. Proc. *16:* 376 (1957).
769. Wagner, B. M.; Vanace, P. and McGrath, J.: Hypersensitivity myocarditis in rabbits and swine. Fed. Proc. *17:* 462 (1958).
770. Warren, S. and LeCompte, P. M.: The pathology of diabetes mellitus, 3rd ed. (Lea & Febiger, Philadelphia 1952).
771. Weiss, B. and Laties, V. G.: Amphetamine toxicity in rats subjected to aversive stimulation. Fed. Proc. *18:* 457 (1959).
772. Weiss, E.; Dolin, B.; Rollin, H. R.; Fischer, H. K. and Bepler, C. R.: Emotional factors in coronary occlusion. I. Introduction and general summary. Arch. intern. Med. *99:* 628 (1957).
773. Weitze, M.: Factors influencing the sensitivity of mice to insulin. Rep. Sten. Hosp. Nordisk Insulin Lab. *7:* 186 (1958).
774. Wells, L. J.: Functioning of the anterior hypophysis in the fetal rat; in: Comparative endocrinology, ed.: A. Gorbman, p. 444 (Wiley, New York 1959).
775. Welsh, J. H.: Neuroendocrine substance; in: Comparative endocrinology, ed.: A. Gorbman, p. 121 (Wiley, New York 1959).
776. Welt, L. G.; Hollander, W., Jr.; Blythe, W. B. and Hill, C.: The consequences of potassium depletion. J. chron. Dis. *11:* 213 (1960).
777. Westlake, P. T.; Wilcox, A. A.; Haley, M. I. and Peterson, J. E. Relationship of mental and emotional stress to serum cholesterol levels. Proc. Soc. exp. Biol., N. Y. *97:* 163 (1958).
778. White, P. and Waskow, E.: Clinical pathology of diabetes in young patients. Sth. Med. J. *41:* 561 (1948).
779. Wied, D. de and Mirsky, I. A.: The effect of $\triangle^1$-hydrocortisone on the antidiuretic and adrenocorticotropic responses to noxious stimuli. Endocrinology *64:* 955 (1959).
780. Wilgram, G. F.: Cardiovascular changes induced in choline-deficient rats by growth hormone. Ann. N. Y. Acad. Sci. *72:* 863 (1959).
781. Wingstrand, K. G.: Attempts at a comparison between the neurohypophysial region in fishes and tetrapods, with particular regard to amphibians; in Comparative endocrinology, ed.: A. Gorbman, p. 393 (Wiley, New York 1959).
782. Winkler, G.; Biebel, R. und Tonutti, E.: 17-Corticoidausscheidung bei Meerschweinchen mit Läsionen im mittleren Hypothalamus. Acta neuroveg. *20:* 230 (1959).
783. Winternitz, W. W.; Dintzis, R. and Long, C. N.: Further studies on the adrenal cortex and carbohydrate metabolism. Endocrinology *61:* 724 (1957).
784. Wissler, R. W.; Smull, K. and Lesh, J.: The effects of various horse serum fractions producing cardiovascular and renal lesions in rabbits. J. exp. Med. *90:* 577 (1949).
785. Wolf, G. A., Jr. and Wolff, H. G.: Studies on the nature of certain symptoms associated with cardiovascular disorders. Psychosom. Med. *8:* 293 (1946).
786. Wolf, S.: Stress and heart disease. Mod. Conc. cardiovasc. Dis. *29:* 599 (1960).
787. Wolf, S.; Cardon, P. V., Jr.; Shepard, E. M. and Wolff, H. G.: Life stress and essential hypertension: Study of circulatory adjustments in man (Williams & Wilkins, Baltimore 1955).
788. Woodbury, D. M. and Koch, A.: Effects of aldosterone and desoxycorticosterone on tissue electrolytes. Proc. Soc. exp. Biol., N. Y. *94:* 720 (1957).
789. Worthington, W. C., Jr.: Vascular responses in the pituitary stalk. Endocrinology *66:* 19 (1960).
790. Wright, I. S.: Coronary artery disease: progress and problems. J. amer. Geriatr. Soc. *8:* 237 (1960).

791. Wynn, V.: Electrolyte disturbances associated with failure to metabolise glucose during hypothermia. Lancet *2:* 575 (1954).
792. Wyrwicka, W. and Dobrzecka, C.: Relationship between feeding and satiation centers of the hypothalamus. Science *132:* 805 (1960).
793. Yamada, T.: Studies on the mechanism of hypothalamic control of thyrotropin secretion: effect of intrahypothalamic thyroxine injection on thyroid hypertrophy induced by propylthiouracil in the rat. Endocrinology *65:* 216 (1959).
794. Yamada, T. and Greer, M. A.: Studies on the mechanism of hypothalamic control of thyrotropin secretion: effect of thyroxine injection into the hypothalamus or the pituitary on thyroid hormone release. Endocrinology *65:* 559 (1959).
795. Yamada, T. and Greer, M. A.: The effect of bilateral ablation of the amygdala on endocrine function in the rat. Endocrinology *66:* 565 (1960).
796. Yokoyama, A. and Ota, K.: The effect of hypothalamic lesions on litter growth in rats. Endocrin. jap. *6:* 14 (1959).
797. Yokoyama, A. and Ota, K.: Studies on the mammary glands of lactating rats bearing hypothalamic lesions. Endocrin. jap. *7:* 1 (1960).
798. Ziegler, K.: Über die Wirkung intravenöser Adrenalininjektion auf das Gefäßsystem und ihre Beziehung zur Arteriosklerose. Beitr. path. Anat. *38:* 229 (1905).
799. Zsotér, T.; Pintér, I. and Nádasdi, M.: Electrocardiographic studies on experimental cardiac necrosis of rats. Cardiologia *34:* 218 (1959).
800. Zweifach, B. W.; Hershey, S. G.; Rovewstine, E. A.; Lee, R. E. and Chambers, R.: Anesthetic agents as factors in circulatory reactions induced by hemorrhage. Surgery *18:* 48 (1945).
801. Zweifach, B. W. and Thomas, L.: The relationship between vascular manifestations of shock produced by endotoxin, trauma and hemorrhage. I.: Certain similarities between the reactions in normal and endotoxin-tolerant rats. J. exp. Med. *106:* 385 (1957).
802. Bajusz, E.: The role of some essential nutrients in the pathogenesis of cardiac necroses. Studies on K-, Mg-, Na- and Cl-deficiencies. Rev. canad. Biol. *20:* 713 (1961).
803. Bajusz, E.: Nutritional factors in the pathogenesis of cardiac necroses. Z. Ernährungswissenschaft *2:* 229 and *3:* 1 (1962).
804. Bajusz, E.: The relationship of general adaptive reactions to cardiovascular pathology. Amer. Coll. Chest Phys. Meet., Chicago 1962.
805. Bajusz, E.: Neuroendocrine relationships, part 3; in: Progress in Neurology and psychiatry, ed. E. A. Spiegel, vol. XVII, p. 222 (Grune & Stratton, New York 1962).
806. Bajusz, E.: Neuroendocrine relationships (part 4); in: Progress in neurology and psychiatry, ed.: E. A. Spiegel, vol. XVIII (Grune & Stratton, New York 1963) (in press).
807. Bajusz, E.: Nutritional factors in the pathogenesis of necrotizing cardiopathies. Seventh int. Congr. 'Diseases of the Chest', New Delhi 1963.
808. Bajusz, E.: The participation of the vegetative nervous system in the neuroendocrine regulation of adaptive reactions; in: Das vegetative Nervensystem, ed.: K. H. von Monakow (Karger, Basel 1963) (in press).
809. Bajusz, E. and Jasmin, G.: Protective action of serotonin against certain chemically and surgically induced cardiac necroses. Rev. canad. Biol. *21:* 51 (1962).
810. Bajusz, E. and Jasmin, G.: Effect of aldactone, an antimineralocorticoid steroid spirolactone, on inflammation. Rev. canad. Biol. *20:* 829 (1961).
811. Bajusz, E. and Jasmin, G.: Morphologic and histochemical observations on chemically induced cardiac necroses as compared with occlusive infarcts. IV. int. Congr. int. Acad. Pathol., Zürich 1962. – Proc. of the Congr., p. 9 (1962).
812. Bajusz, E. and Jasmin, G.: On the mechanism of the anti-inflammatory effect of

aldactone, an antimineralocorticoid steroid spirolactone. Fourth Acta Endocrin. Congr., Geneva 1962. – Acta endocrin., Kbh. Suppl. 67, 104 (1962).

813. BAJUSZ, E. and JASMIN, G.: Effect of the monoamine oxidase inhibitor, nialamide, upon certain chemically and surgically induced cardiac necroses. IV. World Congr. Cardiology, Mexico, D. F. 1962. – Proc. IV. World Congr. of Cardiology, p. 15 (1962).
814. BAJUSZ, E. and JASMIN, G.: Effect of serotonin on experimental cardiac necroses. Int. Acad. Pathol. Meeting, Montreal 1962. – Lab. Invest. *11:* 673 (1962).
815. BAJUSZ, E. and JASMIN, G.: Studies on the activity and distribution of oxidative and hydrolytic enzymes in the skeletal and cardiac muscle of dystrophic mice kept on various diets. Rev. canad. Biol. *21:* 409 (1962).
816. BAJUSZ, E. and JASMIN, G.: Studies on factors that selectively influence calcification of the myocardium. Cardiologia 1963 (in press).
817. BAJUSZ, E.; JASMIN, G. and MONGEAU, A.: Influence of the thyroparathyroid system upon the myocardial calcification due to coronary vein obstruction. Amer. Physiol. Soc. Fall Meeting, Buffalo, N. Y. 1962. – Physiologist *5:* 102 (1962).
818. BAJUSZ, E.; JASMIN, G. and MONGEAU, A.: Mechanisms through which the thyroparathyroid system governs myocardial calcification. 30th annu. Congr. Ass. canad. franç. pour l'avancement des sciences, Montreal 1962.
819. BAJUSZ, E.; SELYE, H. and STREBEL, R.: Neuroleptic phenothiazine derivatives and stress-induced cardiac necroses. Proc. 3rd World Congr. Psychiatr., vol. II, p. 924 (McGill Univ. Press, Montreal 1961).
820. JASMIN, G. and BAJUSZ, E.: Myocardial lesions in strain 129 dystrophic mice. Nature, Lond. *193:* 181 (1962).
821. JASMIN, G. et BAJUSZ, E.: Action de la sérotonine, du 48/80 et de la réserpine sur des lésions de calcinose provoquées par divers agents chez le rat. Rev. canad. Biol. *21:* 135 (1962).
822. JASMIN, G. et BAJUSZ, E.: Etude histochimique des lésions du myocarde induites par divers agents. 30th annu. Congr. Ass. canad.-franç. pour l'avancement des sciences, Montreal 1962.
823. SELYE, H. and BAJUSZ, E.: Prevention of cross-resistance to cardiotoxic agents by low chloride intake. Amer. J. Path. *38:* 481 (1961).
824. SELYE, H. and BAJUSZ, E.: A szervezet nem-fajlagos rezisztenciájának néhány alapvetö kérdéséröl. Orvosi Hetilap *103:* 385, 529 (1962).
825. SELYE, H.; CANTIN, M.; JEAN, P. and BAJUSZ, E.: Protection by systemic stress against the induction of various organ lesions. Annu. Meet. Royal Soc. canad., Montreal 1961. – Proc. roy. Soc. Canada, p. 46 (1961).
826. STREBEL, R.; BAJUSZ, E. and SELYE, H.: Fasting as a protective stressor against the potential cardiotoxic action of various agents. Cardiologia *41:* 179 (1962).
827. ZSOTÉR, T. and BAJUSZ, E.: Electrocardiograms in surgically induced cardiopathies in the rat. Cardiologia *40:* 290 (1962).
828. BAJUSZ, E. and JASMIN, G.: Studies on the activity and distribution of oxidative and hydrolytic enzymes in the skeletal and cardiac muscle of dystrophic mice kept on various diets. Rev. canad. Biol. *21:* 409 (1962).
829. BAJUSZ, E.; JASMIN, G. and MONGEAU, A.: Thyroid-parathyroid interrelationships in processes governing myocardial calcification. Endocrinology 1963 (in press).
830. BAJUSZ, E. and JASMIN, G.: Action of parathyroidectomy and dihydrotachysterol on myocardial calcification due to coronary vein obstruction. Proc. Soc. exp. Biol., N.Y. 1963 (in press).
831. BAJUSZ, E.: Role of dietary chloride intake in age-dependent disease susceptibility of myocardium. 6th int. Congr. of Gerontology, Copenhagen 1963.
832. BAJUSZ, E. and JASMIN, G.: Enzyme histochemistry of various necrotizing cardiopathies. 47th Annual Meet. of Fed. Amer. Socs. Exp. Biol., Atlantic City 1963.